Trauma, Resilience, an
in LGBT Patients

MW00838249

Kristen L. Eckstrand • Jennifer Potter

Editors

Trauma, Resilience, and Health Promotion in LGBT Patients

What Every Healthcare Provider Should Know

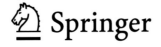 Springer

Editors
Kristen L. Eckstrand, MD, PhD
Western Psychiatric Institute and Clinic,
    Department of Psychiatry
University of Pittsburgh Medical Center
Pittsburgh, PA, USA

Jennifer Potter, MD
Associate Professor of Medicine and Advisory Dean
    and Director, William B. Castle Society
    Harvard Medical School

Director, Women's Health Center
Beth Israel Deaconess Medical Center

Director, Women's Health Program
Fenway Health Center

Director, Women's Health Research
The Fenway Institute
Boston, MA, USA

Illustrations
Katja Tetzlaff, MS
University of Illinois at Chicago
Medical Illustrator, ktetzlaff.com
Chicago, IL USA

ISBN 978-3-319-54507-3   ISBN 978-3-319-54509-7   (eBook)
DOI 10.1007/978-3-319-54509-7

Library of Congress Control Number: 2017942792

© Springer International Publishing AG 2017
This work is subject to copyright. All rights are reserved by the Publisher, whether the whole or part of the material is
concerned, specifically the rights of translation, reprinting, reuse of illustrations, recitation, broadcasting, reproduction
on microfilms or in any other physical way, and transmission or information storage and retrieval, electronic
adaptation, computer software, or by similar or dissimilar methodology now known or hereafter developed.
The use of general descriptive names, registered names, trademarks, service marks, etc. in this publication does not
imply, even in the absence of a specific statement, that such names are exempt from the relevant protective laws and
regulations and therefore free for general use.
The publisher, the authors and the editors are safe to assume that the advice and information in this book are believed
to be true and accurate at the date of publication. Neither the publisher nor the authors or the editors give a warranty,
express or implied, with respect to the material contained herein or for any errors or omissions that may have been
made. The publisher remains neutral with regard to jurisdictional claims in published maps and institutional
affiliations.

Printed on acid-free paper

This Springer imprint is published by Springer Nature
The registered company is Springer International Publishing AG
The registered company address is: Gewerbestrasse 11, 6330 Cham, Switzerland

Preface

Prior to the preliminary definition of trauma in the *Diagnostic and Statistical Manual of Mental Disorders (DSM-III)* in 1980 as a catastrophic stressor outside the range of typical human experience, it was well understood that certain adverse experiences can cause acute clinical manifestations. The long-term sequelae of trauma, however, were frequently misdiagnosed as primary psychiatric disorders or unexplained physical syndromes. Trauma research and informed care have progressed significantly since that time. For example, it is now known that exposure to a traumatic experience can have epigenetic, neuropsychiatric, and transgenerational effects that can persist over the course of a person's – or their offspring's – lifetime. Further, what constitutes a traumatic experience is no longer narrowly defined (e.g., war, rape, natural disaster). Trauma is both context and person dependent, in that one individual may experience traumatic sequelae from a specific event while another might not. Finally, trauma may have myriad mental, physical, and behavioral effects that are not always easily classified.

As the conceptualization of trauma diversifies, so too does the understanding of how being identified as a member of a minority group can expose individuals to a unique set of experiences that can be traumatic. Individuals with diverse sexual orientations, gender identities, and expressions are more likely to experience bias, harassment, discrimination, and violence compared to heterosexual, cisgender populations. They may also face unique internal challenges associated with the coming out process. As suggested by the minority stress model, the combination of these internal and external stressors can place lesbian, gay, bisexual, and transgender (LGBT) individuals at higher risk for mental and physical health concerns. This vulnerability may be compounded for individuals with multiple stigmatized intersectional identities and expressions.

Fortunately, traumatic experiences are frequently paralleled by the development of coping strategies that permit affected individuals to recover and even thrive. The ability to adapt positively or cope with adversity – otherwise known as resilience – is difficult to measure construct that nonetheless portends improved psychosocial function and higher quality of life. Understanding the specific adversities experienced by different communities is a crucial first step in the development of a resilience promotion approach. This book educates healthcare professionals on the impact of traumas experienced by LGBT populations and outlines strategies that can be used in the clinical encounter to facilitate recovery and resilience.

One important theme that emerges is the use of terminology. While numerous acronyms exist to describe LGBT populations including sexual and gender minority (SGM) or sexual and gender diverse (SGD), "LGBT" will be used throughout this text to describe individuals with diverse sexual orientations and gender identities as this acronym is currently the most widely used. However, at a clinical level, terminology is personal and healthcare professionals should be well-equipped to communicate with their patients regarding sexual orientation and gender identity using a variety of terms.

The first section of the text provides an overview of trauma in LGBT populations, followed by a review of how resilience changes across the life span. Characteristics of resilience development are then examined in particularly vulnerable LGBT communities, including transgender and gender nonconforming individuals, people of color, sexual minority women, migrant communities, and incarcerated individuals. Finally, experts in the field present strategies clinicians can use when working with LGBT individuals to facilitate adaptation and healthy coping.

A critical theme throughout this text is that *all* clinicians play a critical role in making healthcare and the healthcare environment trauma informed. While certain specialties may play a more specific role in treating the psychological sequelae of trauma, the myriad manifestations of chronic stigma and trauma necessitate interdisciplinary and wide-reaching individual, organizational, and systems changes. These changes are not arduous or cumbersome; rather, they simply require an ongoing investment by all healthcare professionals in to understanding, recognizing, contextualizing, and managing trauma. By addressing trauma in LGBT communities using the strategies described in this text, we hope that not only will the health disparities faced by LGBT communities be reduced, but that clinicians themselves can serve as role models for the larger societal changes necessary to eliminate the stigma, violence, and discrimination faced by LGBT individuals.

Pittsburgh, PA, USA   Kristen L. Eckstrand, MD, PhD
Boston, MA, USA   Jennifer Potter, MD

Contents

Part IV   Resilience Promotion in Clinical Practice

Contributors

Edward J. Alessi, PhD, LCSW School of Social Work, Rutgers, The State University of New Jersey, Newark, NJ, USA

Ashley Austin, PhD, LCSW School of Social Work, Barry University, Miami Shores, FL, USA

Nathan Brewer, MSW, LICSW Simmons College, Boston, MA, USA

Lauren Brinkley-Rubinstein, PhD Department of Social Medicine, University of North Carolina-Chapel Hill, Chapel Hill, NC, USA

Center for Health Equity Research, University of North Carolina-Chapel Hill, Chapel Hill, NC, USA

Kerith J. Conron, ScD, MPH Blachford-Cooper Research Director and Distinguished Scholar, The Williams Institute, UCLA School of Law and Affiliated Investigator, The Fenway Institute, Fenway Health, Boston, MA, USA

Shelley L. Craig, PhD, RSW, LCSW Factor-Inwentash Faculty of Social Work, University of Toronto, Toronto, ON, Canada

E. Kale Edmiston, PhD Vanderbilt University Medical Center, Program for LGBTI Health, Nashville, TN, USA

Mickey Eliason, PhD Faculty Development and Scholarship, College of Health and Social Sciences, San Francisco, CA, USA

Laura Erickson-Schroth, MD, MA Mount Sinai Beth Israel, Hetrick Martin Institute, New York, NY, USA

Elizabeth Glaeser, BS The Department of Child and Adolescent Psychiatry, NYU Langone Medical Center, New York, NY, USA

Rebecca Hopkinson, MD Department of Psychiatry and Behavioral Medicine, University of Washington, Seattle, WA, USA

Charles P. Hoy-Ellis, MSW, PhD, LICSW College of Social Work, University of Utah, Salt Lake City, UT, USA

Brian Hurley, MD, MBA, DFASAM Los Angeles County Department of Mental Health, Robert Wood Johnson Foundation Clinical Scholar, David Geffen School of Medicine of the University of California, Los Angeles, CA, USA

Katie Imborek, MD Department of Family Medicine, University of Iowa Hospitals and Clinics, Iowa City, IA, USA

Laura A. Jacobs, LCSW-R New York, NY, USA

Suni Niranjan Jani, MD, MPH Massachusetts General Hospital/McLean Hospital, Harvard Medical School, Child and Adolescent Psychiatry Department, Yawkey Center for Outpatient Care 6A, Boston, MA, USA

Blake E. Johnson, ScM UNC School of Medicine, The University of North Carolina at Chapel Hill, Chapel Hill, NC, USA

Philip Jai Johnson, PhD Program for the Study of LGBT Health, Division of Gender, Sexuality, and Health, Columbia University, New York, NY, USA

Robert-Paul Juster, PhD Program for the Study of LGBT Health, Division of Gender, Sexuality, and Health, Columbia University, New York, NY, USA

Kevin Kapila, MD Fenway Health, Fenway South End, Boston, MA, USA

Eva S. Keatley, MA Department of Psychology, University of Windsor, Windsor, ON, Canada

Kenny Lin, MD Massachusetts General Hospital, Child and Adolescent Psychiatry Department, Boston, MA, USA

James I. Martin, PhD, MSW Silver School of Social Work, New York University, New York, NY, USA

Erin McCauley, MEd Department of Policy Analysis and Management, College of Human Ecology, Cornell University, Ithaca, NY, USA

Heather L. McCauley, ScD, MS Human Development and Family Studies, Michigan State University, Pittsburgh, PA, USA

Matthew J. Mimiaga, ScD, MPH Epidemiology and Behavioral & Social Health Sciences, Institute for Community Health Promotion, Brown University, Providence, RI, USA

Sarah M. Peitzmeier, MSPH, PhD Johns Hopkins Bloomberg School of Public Health, Department of Population, Family and Reproductive Health, Baltimore, MD, USA
The Fenway Institute, Boston, MA, USA

Shannon Phillips, PA-C Denver Health, Denver, CO, USA

Tonia C. Poteat, PhD, MPH, PA-C Johns Hopkins School of Public Health, Baltimore, MD, USA

Jennifer Potter, MD William B. Castle Society, Harvard Medical School, Boston, MA, USA
Women's Health Center, Beth Israel Deaconess Medical Center, Boston, MA, USA
Women's Health Program, Fenway Health Center, Boston, MA, USA
Women's Health Research, The Fenway Institute, Boston, MA, USA

Tia Powell, MD Montefiore Einstein Center for Bioethics, Bronx, NY, USA

Asa E. Radix, MD, MPH Director of Research and Education at Callen-Lorde Community Health Center, Assistant Clinical Professor of Medicine at New York University, New York, NY, USA

R.J. Robles, MDiv Vanderbilt University Medical Center, Program for LGBTI Health, Nashville, TN, USA

Andrés Felipe Sciolla, MD University of California, Davis, Department of Psychiatry & Behavioral Sciences, Sacramento, CA, USA

Sophia Shapiro, MD Emergency Medicine Department, NYUMC/Bellevue Hospital Center, New York, NY, USA

Anneliese A. Singh, PhD Department of Counseling and Human Development Services, The University of Georgia, Athens, GA, USA
Avondale Estates, GA, USA

Nathan Grant Smith, PhD Department of Psychological, Health, and Learning Sciences, University of Houston, Houston, TX, USA

Carl G. Streed Jr., MD General Internal Medicine & Primary Care, Brigham & Women's Hospital, Boston, MA, USA

Dana van der Heide, MD, MPH Carver College of Medicine, University of Iowa, Iowa City, IA, USA

Jennifer A. Vencill, PhD Program in Human Sexuality, Department of Family Medicine & Community Health, University of Minnesota Medical School, Minneapolis, MN, USA

Part I

Overview of Trauma in LGBT Populations

Intersection of Trauma and Identity

Edward J. Alessi and James I. Martin

In the last four decades, lesbian, gay, bisexual, and transgender (LGBT) people have made significant progress in gaining social acceptance and securing legal rights in many parts of the world. Same-sex sexual and gender-nonconforming behavior used to be considered morally, pathologically, and legally aberrant throughout the world, but LGBT identities are now increasingly affirmed and celebrated in many countries. However, the trauma that LGBT people have experienced throughout history remains part of their shared identity. Moreover, even in relatively accepting parts of the world (e.g., North America, Western Europe), LGBT people continue to encounter verbal abuse, physical and sexual victimization, and structural oppression [1]. The increased risk of experiencing such events results in a "fundamental ecological threat," forcing sexual and gender minorities to choose between expressing their authentic selves or the identities validated by society [2, p246]. Constant exposure to marginalization and the frequent fear of victimization contribute to unrelenting vigilance that may ultimately become integrally linked to identity.

The primary aim of this chapter is to describe the intersection of trauma and identity among LGBT people. First, we will review diagnostic criteria for posttraumatic stress disorder (PTSD) and then discuss how current conceptualizations of trauma overlook associations between non-traumatic events and PTSD-like disorder. Next, we will discuss minority stress among sexual and gender minorities and draw upon microsociological theories to understand the impact of the social environment on the mental health of LGBT people. We will follow this discussion with the developmental impact of homophobia and transphobia and then focus on the connection between PTSD and traumatic and non-traumatic events. Finally, we will conclude with a clinical case to illustrate the concepts discussed in this chapter.

Any discussion about LGBT people must acknowledge their extraordinary diversity. Although LGBT people are often discussed as if they comprise a single population, we understand that the experiences and identities of lesbians may be quite different from those of gay men; those of bisexual and transgender people are likely to differ from lesbians and gay men even more [3]. Additionally, there are LGBT people in every part of the world [4], and they have a broad spectrum of life experiences influenced not only by their sexual orientation and gender identity but also by other intersecting identities, including race, ethnicity, social class, culture, religion, age, and ability status [5–10]. The intersection of these sociocultural characteristics results in highly diverse identities [11], life course trajectories [12], and experiences of privilege or marginalization and discrimination [4, 13]. Furthermore, all of these identities must be taken into consideration when attempting to understand how trauma impacts the mental health of LGBT individuals.

Traumatic Versus Non-traumatic Events

The term trauma is widely used in vernacular language and commonly refers to an experience "that is emotionally painful, distressful, or shocking" [14]. Traumatic experiences can precipitate a myriad of psychiatric disorders including depressive and anxiety disorders, and, of course, PTSD. PTSD is a commonly occurring disorder that can seriously impair an individual's psychosocial functioning, resulting in mood vacillations, disorganized thinking, dissociation, impaired judgment, hyperarousal, and the use of maladaptive coping

E.J. Alessi (✉)
School of Social Work, Rutgers, The State University of New Jersey, 360 Martin Luther King Jr. Blvd, Hill Hall, Room 401, Newark, NJ 07102, USA
e-mail: ealessi@ssw.rutgers.edu

J.I. Martin
Silver School of Social Work, New York University, 1 Washington Square North, New York, NY 10003-6654, USA
e-mail: james.martin@nyu.edu

© Springer International Publishing AG 2017
K.L. Eckstrand, J. Potter (eds.), *Trauma, Resilience, and Health Promotion in LGBT Patients*,
DOI 10.1007/978-3-319-54509-7_1

strategies [14]. In the United States, the lifetime prevalence of PTSD ranges from about 6% to 9% [15–19]. Although initially categorized as an anxiety disorder, PTSD was removed from the chapter on anxiety disorders and included in a new chapter on Trauma- and Stressor-Related disorders in the 5th edition of the *Diagnostic and Statistical Manual of Mental Disorders* (*DSM-5*; [20]). All of the disorders in the Trauma- and Stressor-Related disorders chapter account for the various clinical presentations that can emerge following exposure to a traumatic or stressful event [21]. See Table 1.1 for a list of Trauma- and Stressor-Related disorders in *DSM-5*.

According to *DSM-5*, traumatic events involve "exposure to actual or threatened death, serious injury, or sexual violence" [20, p271]. Exposure to traumatic events can occur in one or more of the following ways: (a) directly experiencing the event, (b) witnessing the event as it happened to others, (c) learning that the event occurred to a loved one, or (d) experiencing repeated or extreme exposure to aversive details of the event [20]. To be diagnosed with PTSD, individuals are required to have at least one intrusion symptom (spontaneous memories, nightmares, flashbacks), one avoidance symptom (avoidance of distressing memories or external reminders of the event), two symptoms of negative alteration in cognition and mood (estrangement from others, distorted sense of blame, diminished interest in activities), and two symptoms of marked alterations in arousal and activity (difficultly sleeping or concentrating, hypervigilance, self-destructive behavior). These symptoms must be present for a least 1 month following the traumatic event and cause significant impairment in social and/or occupational functioning (Fig. 1.1).

Studying the mental health consequences of life-threatening events and sexual violence has obvious value and importance; however, focusing solely on such events tends to ignore the psychological impact of so-called "non-traumatic" events [22]. The use of the term non-traumatic is not intended to minimize the psychological impact of these events, but to clearly demonstrate how they differ from events considered traumatic by the *DSM*. Non-traumatic events include major life events such as ending a marriage/relationship, psychological or emotional abuse, employment issues, homelessness, financial concerns, nonlife-threatening medical problems, and the expected death of a loved one. Ignoring the connection between non-traumatic events and symptoms that look very much like PTSD may overlook the suffering of many individuals and result in the use of inappropriate or ineffective treatment interventions [23].

The debate over whether events must involve threat to life or physical integrity to qualify as traumatic has existed since PTSD was first introduced as a psychiatric disorder in 1980 [24]. In our study of PTSD [23], we joined that debate by investigating the stressor criterion, which sets the threshold for the types of events qualifying as traumatic [25]. Referred to as Criterion A1 in *DSM-IV*, the stressor criterion defined traumatic events as those that involve "actual or threatened death or serious injury, or a threat to the physical integrity of oneself or others" [25, p427]. Although the stressor criterion originated from the concept of PTSD as an expectable response following exposure to extraordinary events [26], it is still unclear why events that do not pose threat to life or physical integrity are excluded from the stressor criterion [27]. Excluding these events is contradictory to what is already well established in the trauma literature—that reactions to stressful events are inherently subjective. Moreover, studies consistently show that non-traumatic events can be associated with symptoms suggestive of PTSD

Table 1.1 Trauma-spectrum disorders in *DSM-5*

Trauma and stressor-related disorders in *DSM-5* include disorders in which exposure to a traumatic or stressful event is necessary to make a diagnosis
Reactive attachment disorder
Disinhibited social engagement disorder
Posttraumatic stress disorder
Specifiers:
With dissociative systems (depersonalization or derealization)
With delayed expression (full diagnostic criteria are not met until at least 6 months after the event)
Acute stress disorder
Adjustment disorders
With depressed mood
With anxiety
With mixed anxiety and depressed mood
With disturbance of conduct
With mixed disturbance of emotions and conduct
Unspecified
Other specified trauma and stressor-related disorder
Unspecified trauma and stressor-related disorder

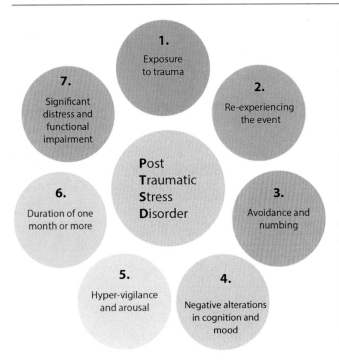

Fig. 1.1 Abbreviated *DSM-5* diagnostic criteria for posttraumatic stress disorder

traumatic events also emerge following non-traumatic events [23]. Ultimately, the adjustment disorder specifier *with PTSD-like symptoms* was not included, although the *DSM-5* does indicate that an adjustment disorder is "diagnosed when the symptom pattern of PTSD occurs in response to a stressor that does not meet PTSD Criterion A (e.g., spouse leaving, being fired)" [20, p279]. While the adjustment disorder specifiers account for symptoms of anxiety and depression, they do not the capture the core symptoms of PTSD (re-experiencing, avoidance, and hyperarousal; for a comparison of diagnostic criteria between PTSD and adjustment disorder see Table 1.2). Furthermore, adjustment disorders must be diagnosed within 3 months of the onset of the stressor, and symptoms cannot persist longer than 6 months following termination of the stressor [20]. In contrast, symptoms do not have to emerge within a specific time frame to diagnose PTSD, although a delayed expression subtype is used when individuals do not manifest the full set of PTSD symptoms until 6 months after the trauma [20]. Therefore, clinicians may overlook the symptoms suggestive of PTSD following exposure to a non-traumatic event, particularly if those symptoms emerge more than 3 months following exposure to the stressor.

[23, 28–31]. Specifically, in these studies individuals presented with the requisite number of symptoms from each *DSM-IV* cluster (re-experiencing, avoidance, and hyperarousal) to meet criteria for PTSD, although they were exposed to a non-traumatic event.

Given the potential pitfalls of using the stressor criterion, some suggested removing it from PTSD diagnostic criteria in *DSM-5* [32]. Doing so would have allowed clinicians and researchers to focus on the symptoms following a stressful event rather than whether the event met Criterion A1. However, others were concerned that removing the stressor criterion would increase PTSD prevalence and diffuse the suffering of those exposed to catastrophic events such as war, natural disasters, concentration camp imprisonment, and extreme violence [33]. Arguing in favor of retaining the stressor criterion, Friedman [24] explained that traumatic events are distinct from non-traumatic events because exposure to a traumatic stressor results in discontinuity between the way individuals view themselves before and after the event. However, exposure to non-traumatic events may also result in a similar process [34].

To address the validity issues related to Criterion A1, the *DSM-5* work group initially proposed adding a new adjustment disorder specifier that could be used when PTSD symptoms were present following exposure to non-traumatic events [23]. However, adding this specifier would not have resolved the ongoing conceptual problems because it still does not explain why symptoms considered unique to

Minority Stress

The marginalized status of sexual and gender minorities increases their vulnerability to traumatic and non-traumatic stressors; therefore, understanding the effects of PTSD and trauma-related disorders among LGBT people is critical for providing culturally sensitive health and mental health care. Prejudice related to homophobia and transphobia characterize the social environment for LGBT people and precipitate stressful events, commonly referred to as minority stress. Meyer [35] proposed a model of minority stress in which sexual minorities encounter stress "along a continuum from distal stressors, which are typically defined as objective events and conditions, to proximal personal processes, which are by definition subjective because they rely on individual perceptions and appraisals" (p676). Four specific minority stress processes provide the framework for Meyer's [35] minority stress model: (a) external, objective stressful events, (b) the expectation of minority stress and the vigilance this expectation requires (stigma), (c) the internalization of negative societal attitudes (internalized homophobia), and (d) sexual orientation concealment. Scholars initially used minority stress-based hypotheses to explain the higher prevalence of mental health problems among sexual minorities as compared to heterosexuals; in recent years, however, minority stress theory has also been used to explain negative mental health outcomes among gender minorities [36, 37].

Table 1.2 Comparision of trauma- and stressor-related disorders in *DSM-5*

Criteria for trauma and stress-related disorders in *DSM-5*[a]	Posttraumatic stress disorder (PTSD)[b]	Acute stress disorder	Adjustment disorders
Time frame			
Duration of disturbance is more than 1 month	✓		
Symptom duration of 3 days to 1 month after traumatic event		✓	
Symptoms develop within 3 months of onset of stressor(s); when stressor and consequences cease, symptoms do not persist for more than an additional 6 months			✓
Symptoms			
Exposure to actual or threatened death, serious injury, or sexual violence (i.e., traumatic event)	✓	✓	
Development of emotional or behavioral symptoms (e.g., anxiety, depression) in response to stressor of any severity			✓
Intrusion symptoms associated with traumatic event	✓	✓	
Persistent avoidance of stimuli associated with traumatic event	✓	✓	
Negative alterations in cognitions and mood associated with traumatic event	✓	✓	
Alterations in arousal and reactivity associated with traumatic event (i.e., angry outbursts, reckless behavior, sleep disturbance)	✓	✓	
Symptoms persist more than 1 month after traumatic event	✓		
Significant distress or impairment in major areas of functioning	✓	✓	✓
Disturbance is not due to medication, substance use, developmental disability, or other disorder	✓	✓	✓

[a]All criteria are further specified in *DSM-5*; this figure is not all-inclusive, but highlights important features of each disorder
[b]Separate diagnostic criteria for children and adolescents and for children age 6 or younger

To explain how particular minority stress processes influence the well-being of LGBT identities, we draw from microsociological theorists such as Charles Horton Cooley and Erving Goffman. Their theories were critical to the development of Meyer's minority stress model [35]. Cooley's [38] concept of the looking-glass self suggests that the way in which individuals see themselves is determined by how others view them. Cooley questioned the concept of the self, since one's feelings are always connected to the ways in which others think about him or her. According to Cooley, the self is really a social self consisting of three principal components: how we imagine our appearance to another person, the way we imagine another person judges our appearance, and the specific self-feeling that results from this judgment such as pride or mortification (Fig. 1.2). Thus, the formulation of our self-concept is dependent on the ways in which others perceive us. Since LGBT people are likely to face discrimination based on their sexual orientation and/or gender identity, Cooley's theory may help to explain why these experiences contribute to hypervigilance, insecurity, shame, avoidance, and self-loathing. For instance, homophobic and transphobic attitudes are constantly being communicated to sexual and gender minority individuals. These negative societal attitudes are then reflected onto sexual and gender minority people, which in turn influence how they feel about themselves.

Goffman's work also increases our understanding of how stigma affects the lives of LGBT people. According to

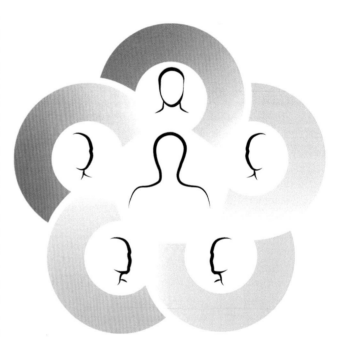

Fig. 1.2 Visual representation of Cooley's looking-glass self which proposes that an individual's sense of self develops from interpersonal actions with and perceptions of others

Goffman [39], stigmatized individuals are likely to interpret their interactions as being undermined by the dominant group, as they may justifiably anticipate rejection based on their marginalized status. Consequently, they must continually discern what others think about them [22]. Those who do not adhere to heterosexual and cisgender norms are therefore ascribed deviant status. The deviant is "cleanly stripped of many of his [sic] accustomed affirmations, satisfactions, and defenses, and is subjected to a rather full set of mortifying experiences" [39, p365]. For LGBT people, mortifying experiences can include harassment and hate crimes, alienation from family and friends, termination from certain types of employment, and exposure to propaganda portraying LGBT persons as sick or mentally ill [22]. As a result of these mortifying experiences, LGBT people may have difficulty sustaining any of their previously assumed roles, such as student, worker, friend, spouse, or partner. The only role society acknowledges is the deviant one [40]. Essentially, mortifying experiences result in a withdrawal of environmental support for LGBT people, and to cope, they may use avoidance, isolation, and/or conceal their identities, to protect themselves from further experiences of prejudice. Although these strategies serve an adaptive function by fostering a greater sense of control, their use may also result in feelings of disconnection, or lead LGBT people to overestimate danger in contexts in which they are free to express their authentic selves [41, 42].

Empirical research has demonstrated the relationship between social stigma and negative health and mental health outcomes among sexual minorities [43–45] as well as gender minorities [36, 46]. Because sexual and gender minority people grow up in homophobic and transphobic environments, they inevitably internalize these negative attitudes or direct them inward. When applied to lesbian, gay, and bisexual (LGB) people, these internalizations have commonly been called internalized homophobia [47]; other terms include internalized heterosexism and internalized sexual stigma (see [48]). Internalized homophobia has been connected to psychological distress in this population and has been shown to predict PTSD symptom severity in lesbian and gay survivors of child abuse [49] as well as sexual assault [50, 51]. More research is needed to understand the influence of internalized transphobia among transgender populations [37], though emerging evidence suggests that internalized stigma mediates the relationship between gender identity and a host of negative health outcomes as well as depression among transgender older adults [52].

Even sexual minority individuals who "pass" as heterosexual must contend with the consequences of concealing their stigmatized status [22]. Pachankis [53] contends that those who conceal their stigmatized identity must cope with the constant threat of being discovered, which leads to four psychological responses: cognitive (vigilance, suspiciousness, preoccupation), affective (shame, guilt, anxiety, depression), behavioral (social avoidance, the need for feedback, impaired relationships), and self-evaluation (identity ambivalence, negative view of self, diminished self-efficacy). Interestingly, these psychological consequences

also are associated with PTSD, indicating that concealing a stigmatized identity may in and of itself be traumatic [22]. Researchers have begun to use population-based studies to investigate the effects of concealing a stigmatized identity, with one study revealing that women who were recently out were less likely to be depressed than closeted women, although this was not the case for men who were out when compared to closeted men [54]. Men who were recently out were more likely to have major depressive disorder or generalized anxiety than men who were closeted, suggesting that because of strict gender norms, men who are out may experience greater minority stress than women who are out, which in turn negatively impacts their mental health [54]. There is limited research on the effects of concealing a stigma among transgender individuals, though one study of transgender adults aged 50 and older showed that identity concealment explained the effect of gender identity on perceived stress, with concealment being related to higher levels of stress [52].

Developmental Impact of Homophobia and Transphobia

To gain a comprehensive understanding of trauma among LGBT people we must consider the impact of minority stress on childhood and adolescent development. Growing up in an environment where one's experiences of gender and sexuality do not conform to societal standards contributes to conditions in which there is a high potential for trauma and identity to intersect. Studies demonstrate that sexual and gender minority youth experience high numbers of victimization events and that these events are associated with negative mental health outcomes such as depression [55, 56] and PTSD [57, 58]. Given the increased levels of stress encountered by sexual and gender minority youth, it is not surprising that they have a higher prevalence of mood and anxiety disorders [59] – as well as depressive symptoms and suicidality [60, 61] – than heterosexual youth. Even sexual and gender minority children and adolescents who grow up in supportive environments must deal with structural forces that marginalize those who do not conform to heterosexual or cisgender identities. Therefore, they too may be at greater risk for negative mental and physical health outcomes. In fact, evidence suggests that age may be an important modifier of physical health disparities among sexual minority individuals. A study using a general population sample in Sweden revealed that LGB individuals had more physical health symptoms and conditions as compared to heterosexual individuals and that these disparities differed by age, with adolescents and young adults reporting worse self-rated health than older individuals, indicating that minority stress may be exacerbated for youth [62].

Institutional heterosexism and binary gender bias can be especially traumatic for LGBT children and youth who are in the beginning stages of formulating their sexual and gender identities. Evidence suggests that children who experience traumatic events are predisposed to depressive and anxiety disorders and that they are at risk for developing PTSD in adulthood [63, 64]. Parsing out the impact of abuse and other traumatic events on sexual and gender minority children and adolescents is essential for understanding how these events may contribute to adult functioning in LGBT individuals. Roberts and colleagues [65] found that increased prevalence of PTSD among sexual minority individuals was related to greater exposure to child abuse and interpersonal violence. Previous studies that investigated the victimization experiences of sexual minority individuals have reported similar findings. For example, Balsam, Rothblum, and Beauchaine [66] compared 557 lesbian/gay and 163 bisexual individuals with 525 of their heterosexual siblings and found that sexual orientation predicted victimization throughout the lifespan. Sexual minority individuals reported more experiences of child psychological and physical abuse by parents and child sexual abuse, as well as more adult experiences of intimate partner violence (IPV) and sexual assault. Additionally, heterosexual and nonheterosexual men who displayed gender-nonconforming behavior in childhood were more likely to report child sexual abuse than their gender conforming counterparts [67].

Prolonged exposure to trauma, particularly during childhood, suggests that some LGBT people may be at higher risk for developing complex PTSD. Complex PTSD refers to a distinct trauma syndrome that can emerge due to repeated instances or multiple forms of trauma [68, p615]. Herman [69], one of the first scholars to discuss complex trauma syndromes, proposed that diagnostic criteria for PTSD did not fully capture the symptoms exhibited by victims of prolonged interpersonal trauma, such as intimate partner violence and child abuse. Individuals with complex PTSD typically manifest symptoms of PTSD *in addition to* severe dissociation, difficulty relating with others, somatization, and alteration in affect and impulses, in self-perception and perception of the perpetrator, and in systems of meaning [70, 71]. The *DSM-5* has expanded PTSD criteria to include some symptoms of complex PTSD, including negative changes in cognition and mood (Criterion D), and aggressive, irritable, self-destructive, and suicidal behavior (Criterion E). It also added a new dissociative subtype [24]. However, complex PTSD was not included in the *DSM-5* because field trials showed that mostly everyone who met criteria for complex PTSD also met criteria for PTSD [24]. Therefore, the *DSM-5* considers complex PTSD to be a severe form of PTSD.

Research on complex PTSD among LGBT populations is limited, although emerging evidence suggests that LGBT individuals who have fled persecution based on sexual orientation or gender identity may be at a greater risk for developing this disorder [72, 73]. LGBT refugees and asylees report a history of multiple traumatic events, including physical and emotional abuse, assault, shunning, blackmail, forced heterosexual marriage, corrective rape, and pressure to participate in conversion therapy [73]. A retrospective study of LGBT refugees and asylees revealed that they encountered severe child and adolescent abuse (e.g., harassment, public humiliation, and physical and sexual abuse) at home, in school, and in the community [72]. Furthermore, they had little protection from family members or authority figures, and in many cases an adult perpetrated the abuse.

PTSD Among LGBT Individuals

Because sexual minorities are exposed to more acute stressors, including prejudice-related events [74], they may be at higher risk for PTSD. Additionally, LGBT individuals contend with many of the risk factors associated with PTSD, such as prior trauma exposure [75, 76], preexisting anxiety and affective disorders [77, 78], and life stress [79–81]. Although findings are mixed [23, 82], research tends to show that sexual minorities are more likely to have PTSD than heterosexuals [65, 83]. The increased risk for PTSD may be even higher for gender minorities who are at especially high risk for violence throughout their lives, including sexual assault [84]. One study showed that 91% of transgender participants ($N = 97$) had encountered multiple traumatic events and 17.8% manifested clinically significant symptoms of PTSD [85]. Potentially traumatic events include experiencing, witnessing, or being confronted with life-threatening events such as hate crimes.

The Federal Bureau of Investigation defines a hate crime as a "criminal offense against a person or property motivated in whole or in part by an offender's bias against a race, religion, disability, ethnic origin or sexual orientation" [86]. Using a probability-based sample ($N = 662$), Herek [87] found 13.1% of sexual minority adults living in the United States experienced at least one hate crime, or incident of violence due to sexual orientation bias, in their adult life. Approximately 14.9% of the sample experienced property crimes, while 20% experienced both a property crime and an incident of physical violence [87]. In 2013, approximately 20.8% of the 5922 single-bias hate crimes reported to the Federal Bureau of Investigation (FBI) involved sexual orientation bias, with antigay male bias accounting for the majority of cases [86].

Although only 0.5% ($n = 31$) of the single-bias hate crimes reported to the FBI in 2013 were due to transgender or gender-nonconforming bias [86], this may be due to the underreporting of such crimes. According to the National Coalition of Anti-Violence Programs [88], which collected data across 14 US states from 16 of its member programs, transgender women were 1.6 times more likely to experience physical and sexual violence compared to lesbian, gay, and bisexual (LGB) and HIV-affected people. Transgender individuals were also 5.8 times more likely to experience police violence than LGB and HIV-affected people. Additionally, although transgender people are only about 8% of the LGBT population, more than half (55%) of the 20 documented homicides in the report were transgender women, with 50% being transgender women of color [88]. Of course, LGBT people may also be victimized because of their race, religion, or gender, and they can experience multiple-bias hate crimes as well [89, 90]. The least affluent LGBT people of all – those who are homeless – experience particularly high prevalence of victimization [91].

In addition to experiencing assaultive violence related to sexual orientation and gender identity, LGBT people may encounter violence within their intimate relationships. Although relatively understudied in comparison to heterosexual partner violence, increased societal acceptance of LGBT people has resulted in greater awareness of this serious problem [92–94]. A systematic review of research on domestic violence indicated that the prevalence of domestic violence among sexual minorities and heterosexuals was similar (i.e., between 25% and 75% [95]). Because domestic violence tends to be underreported among sexual minorities, prevalence might even be higher in this population. Fear of discrimination, inequality in legal protection, and feelings of shame may contribute to apprehension about reporting or seeking services [95], suggesting a critical need for health and mental health providers to conduct assessments that specifically ask LGBT people questions about intimate partner violence (IPV). IPV tends to be higher among gay men, LGBT people of color, bisexual women, LGBT youth, and transgender individuals [95]. In fact, one study showed that transgender individuals were two times more likely to face threats/intimidation, and 1.8 times more likely to experience harassment, than LGB and HIV-affected people, with transgender women and people of color being at particular risk for IPV [96].

Non-traumatic Events and PTSD-Like Disorder

PTSD-like disorders may also be present after experiencing non-traumatic events, especially those involving prejudice. LGB individuals [87, 97, 98], as well as trans individuals [46, 52, 99, 100], experience a high prevalence of nonviolent forms of victimization, such as verbal assault, harassment, and employment and housing discrimination. Experiencing these types of events has the potential to precipitate PTSD-like disorders among LGBT people.

Current knowledge about the relationship between non-traumatic events and PTSD is informed by attempts to understand the psychological effects of prejudice events among people of color [34, 101–103] and women [104]. For example, events motivated by racial prejudice—regardless of whether these events involve actual or threatened death—can be considered cognitive and affective assaults on one's identity, and therefore they "strike the core of one's selfhood" [34, p480]. Thus, scholars have proposed that exposure to nonlife-threatening racism-related events can also contribute to posttrauma symptoms, such as avoidance and numbing, self-blame, feelings of shame, and hypervigilance [34, p480].

Initial studies of trauma, beginning in the early twentieth century, focused primarily on white men who had served in combat [104]. Although these studies played a major role in how scholars currently conceptualize traumatic stress, they failed to consider how differences in socialization between white men and other marginalized groups could impact their responses to stressful events [104]. Despite these differences, these early formulations continued to inform how trauma was understood over time, especially when renewed interest in understanding trauma emerged during the 1960s and 1970s due to the Vietnam War, women's movement, and struggle for civil rights [104]. Consequently, the original conceptualization of trauma was inappropriately generalized to women, and minority groups such as people of color and LGBT individuals. Doing so failed to take into account that the way in which marginalized groups experience and respond to stress may be influenced by a number of social and cultural factors.

The way in which traumatic stress was initially conceptualized led to a narrow definition of trauma that mainly focused on direct traumas such as war experiences, natural disasters, childhood sexual abuse and stranger rape, and life-threatening illnesses [104]. When individuals are exposed to an isolated direct trauma (i.e., an event considered traumatic by the *DSM*) it is easier for researchers and clinicians to connect individuals' symptoms to the traumatic event. However, this is not the case when it comes to those who have been exposed to insidious trauma, which is "associated with the social status of an individual being devalued because a characteristic intrinsic to their identity is different from what is valued by those in power, for example, gender, color, sexual orientation, physical ability" [104, p240]. Repeated exposure to prejudice-related events contributes to feelings of insecurity, which in turn may lead to the feeling that one needs to remain alert to physical harm or to experiences of enacted homophobia and transphobia [104].

The effects of nonlife-threatening sexual prejudice have been discussed by Brown [105], who argued that coming out can be traumatic for sexual minority individuals when the experience involves the loss of support of one's family or religious community. Drawing from the work of Janoff-Bulman [106], Brown proposed that this loss might be traumatic because it shatters an LGB person's three basic assumptions about the world—benevolence of the world, meaningfulness of the world, and sense of self-worth. Because prejudice-related events have the potential to occur unexpectedly, sexual and gender minority individuals must constantly readjust to living in a hostile social environment. According to Brooks [107], "'readjustment' becomes, in a sense, adaptation to a perpetual state of stress" (p78). When adaptation fails, a pathological stress response such may result [22]. The consequences of trauma involving homophobia and transphobia can be enduring, and sexual and gender minorities often have little awareness of how exposure to this type of trauma may influence their current thoughts, feelings, and behavior [108].

Empirical studies do indicate that sexual minorities manifest PTSD-like disorder in response to non-traumatic events such as verbal harassment [57] and heterosexist discrimination (e.g., being treated unfairly by a friend or boss or being rejected by a family member or friends) [109]. In our study [110] that examined associations between PTSD and prejudice-related events motivated by race, sexual orientation, physical appearance, or social class, we found that sexual minority individuals were more likely than heterosexual individuals to experience a prejudice-related event. Furthermore, of the 19 LGB participants who experienced a prejudice-related event, 8 participants developed a disorder suggestive of PTSD following exposure to a nonlife-threatening prejudice event, including physical assault, child abuse, harassment, and termination from employment [110]. Given the high exposure of transgender individuals to stigma and discrimination, it is likely that they too would be at risk for developing trauma-related syndromes after exposure to nonlife-threating prejudice events.

Conclusion

Despite the major advances toward equality for sexual and gender minorities over the last 40 years, LGBT people continue to face marginalization and encounter victimization at alarming rates, even in relatively accepting parts of the world [1]. Growing up in a society that privileges heterosexual and cisgender norms contributes to a social environment in which there is high potential for trauma and identity to intersect. LGBT individuals are exposed to minority stress from an early age, and minority stress-based hypotheses are now used to explain, in part, the higher prevalence of anxiety, depression, and PTSD among in

LGBT populations. Conceptualizing trauma in ways that move beyond existing psychiatric nomenclature can help healthcare professionals to identify LGBT people who develop symptoms suggestive of PTSD following non-traumatic events. Given their culturally specific experiences of stress, and the subsequent development of trauma-related disorders, promoting culturally relevant resilience practices for LGBT populations is critical. One way for healthcare professionals to bolster resilience in LGBT people is to acknowledge the struggle of living in an environment that privileges heterosexual and cisgender norms. Healthcare providers should address the trauma precipitated by oppressive social conditions with the same care and concern offered to survivors of other traumatic experiences [34]. Doing so has the potential to not only help LGBT people recover from trauma but also to thrive in social environments that continue to marginalize their identities.

Case

Renaldo is a 33-year-old Hispanic male who was referred to you for outpatient psychotherapy by his primary care physician, who is concerned that the antidepressant medication she prescribed 6 weeks ago has not helped to improve his mood. He continues to report insomnia, irritability, anxiety, and ruminative thoughts, which began after he ended a 3-month intimate relationship with Paul, a heterosexually identified married man whom he met at church (Fig. 1.3).

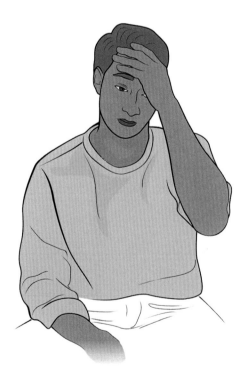

Fig. 1.3 Renaldo is a 33-year-old Hispanic male who was referred to you for outpatient psychotherapy by his primary care physician

Renaldo began attending church 6 months ago at the suggestion of his mother and sister, who believed that it could help him to live a heterosexual lifestyle. However, he doesn't think he will be able to resist his same-sex desires, even by attending church. Renaldo has felt different than others since he was young, and his family has always had trouble accepting him. While growing up, they were concerned about him being too effeminate and about his voice being too soft. And when he came out in his early 20s, they refused to speak with him for a few months. Being with Paul was the first time in his life that Renaldo felt really connected to anyone. He is devastated over the recent break-up and wants to reach out to Paul to talk. At the same time, Renaldo feels this is a bad idea because Paul is still married. He is very confused about his situation and hopes you can tell him what to do.

Discussion Questions

1. How is the loss of family support potentially traumatic for Renaldo?
2. How do structural sources of oppression (e.g., religious ideology) and intersectional factors (e.g., race/ethnicity) influence Renaldo's mental health?
3. Explain how a therapist can help Renaldo connect his current symptomatology to previous trauma related to his sexual orientation.
4. Describe the ways in which Renaldo manifests resilience. How can a therapist draw Renaldo's attention to these strengths throughout treatment?
5. What community resources are available for Renaldo?

Summary Practice Points

- Sexual and gender minorities encounter traumatic events throughout the life span in the form of verbal, physical, and sexual victimization, and these events are associated with physical problems, depression, anxiety, and traumatic stress.
- Emerging evidence suggests that structural forms of oppression, as well as non-traumatic events involving discrimination, have the potential to precipitate a traumatic stress response among LGBT individuals.
- LGBT individuals may not be able to connect their traumatic experiences, especially those of a nonlife-threatening nature, to their current emotional state. Mental health practitioners should help them to make this link.
- Healthcare professionals should account for within-group differences among LGBT populations (age, race/

ethnicity, gender, socioeconomic status), as well as their impact on mental health.
- Acknowledging the role of culture (e.g., religious and familial influences) among LGBT populations may help to facilitate treatment engagement and to bolster resilience.

Resources

1. Alessi, E. J. (2014). A framework for incorporating minority stress theory into treatment with sexual minority clients. *Journal of Gay & Lesbian Mental Health, 18,* 47–66.
2. APA Task Force on Appropriate Therapeutic Responses to Sexual Orientation. (2009). *Report of the Task Force on Appropriate Therapeutic Responses to Sexual Orientation.* Washington, DC: American Psychological Association.
3. O'Donnell, S., Meyer, I.H., & Schwartz. (2011). Increased risk of suicide attempts among Black and Latino lesbians, gay men, and bisexuals. *American Journal of Public Health, 101,* 1055–1059.
4. Severson N., Muñoz-Laboy, M., & Kaufman R. (2014). At times, I feel like I'm sinning': The paradoxical role of non-lesbian, gay, bisexual and transgender-affirming religion in the lives of behaviourally-bisexual Latino men. *Culture, Health, & Sexuality, 16,* 136–148.

References

1. Carroll A, Itaborahy LP. State-sponsored homophobia: a world survey of laws: criminalisation, protection and recognition of same-sex love. 10th ed. Geneva: ILGA; 2015.
2. Cole SW. Social threat, personal identity, and physical health in closeted gay men. In: Omoto AM, Kurtzman HM, editors. Sexual orientation and mental health: examining identity and development in gay, lesbian, and bisexual people. Washington, DC: American Psychological Association; 1996. p. 245–67.
3. Balsam KF, Mohr JJ. Adaptation to sexual orientation stigma: a comparison of bisexual and lesbian/gay adults. J Couns Psychol. 2007;54(3):306–19.
4. United Nations High Commissioner for Human Rights. Discriminatory laws and practices and acts of violence against individuals based on their sexual orientation and gender identity. 2011. [cited 2016 Jan 13]. Report No.: A/HRD/19/41.
5. Barrett DC, Pollack LM. Whose gay community? Social class, sexual self-expression, and gay community involvement. Sociol Q. 2005;46(3):437–56.
6. Dudley Jr RG. Being black and lesbian, gay, bisexual or transgender. J Gay Lesbian Ment Health. 2013;17(2):183–95.
7. Follins LD, Walker JJ, Lewis MK. Resilience in black lesbian, gay, bisexual, and transgender individuals: a critical

review of the literature. J Gay Lesbian Ment Health. 2014;18 (2):190–212.

8. Fredriksen-Goldsen KI, Kim HJ, Barkan SE. Disability among lesbian, gay, and bisexual adults: disparities in prevalence and risk. Am J Public Health. 2012;102(1):e16–21.

9. Martin JI, D'Augelli AR. Timed lives: cohort and period effects in research on sexual orientation and gender identity. In: Meezan W, Martin JI, editors. Handbook of research with lesbian, gay, bisexual, and transgender populations. New York: Routledge; 2009. p. 190–207.

10. Meyer IH. Identity, stress, and resilience in lesbians, gay men, and bisexuals of color. Couns Psychol. 2010;38(3):442–54.

11. Thing J. Gay, Mexican and immigrant: intersecting identities among gay men in Los Angeles. Social Identities. 2010;16 (6):809–31.

12. Dubé EM, Savin-Williams RC, Diamond LM. Intimacy development, gender, and ethnicity among sexual-minority youths. In: D'Augelli AR, editor. Lesbian, gay, and bisexual identities and youth. Oxford/New York: Oxford University Press; 2001. p. 129–52.

13. Reisner SL, Bailey Z, Sevelius J. Racial/ethnic disparities in history of incarceration, experiences of victimization, and associated health indicators among transgender women in the US. Women Health. 2014;54(8):750–67.

14. Straussner SLA, Calnan AJ. Trauma through the life cycle: a review of current literature. Clin Soc Work J. 2014;42(4):323–35.

15. Breslau N. The epidemiology of trauma, PTSD, and other posttrauma disorders. Trauma Violence Abuse. 2009;10 (3):198–210.

16. Breslau N, Davis GC, Andreski P, Peterson E. Traumatic events and posttraumatic stress disorder in an urban population of young adults. Arch Gen Psychiatry. 1991;48(3):216–22.

17. Kessler RC, Sonnega A, Bromet E, Hughes M, Nelson CB. Posttraumatic stress disorder in the national comorbidity survey. Arch Gen Psychiatry. 1995;52(12):1048–60.

18. Kessler RC, Berglund P, Demler O, Jin R, Merikangas KR, Walters EE. Lifetime prevalence and age-of-onset distributions of DSM-IV disorders in the National Comorbidity Survey Replication. Arch Gen Psychiatry. 2005;62(6):593–602.

19. Pietrzak RH, Goldstein RB, Southwick SM, Grant BF. Prevalence and Axis 1 comorbidity of full and partial posttraumatic stress disorder in the United States: results from wave 2 of the national epidemiologic survey on alcohol and related conditions. J Anxiety Disord. 2011;25(3):456–65.

20. American Psychiatric Association. Diagnostic and statistical manual of mental disorders. 5th ed. Washington, DC: American Psychiatric Association; 2013.

21. US Department of Veteran Affairs. Title. Washington, DC; 2015. [cited 2016 Jan 13]. Available from http://www.ptsd.va.gov/pro fessional/PTSD-overview/diagnostic_criteria_dsm-5.asp.

22. Alessi EJ. Posttraumatic stress disorder and sexual orientation: an examination of life-threatening and non-life-threatening events. Dissertation, New York University; 2010.

23. Alessi EJ, Meyer IH, Martin JI. PTSD and sexual orientation: an examination of criterion A1 and non-criterion A1 events. Psychol Trauma. 2013;5(2):149–57.

24. Friedman MJ. Finalizing PTSD in DSM-5: getting here from there and where to go next. J Trauma Stress. 2013;26(5):548–56.

25. American Psychiatric Association. Diagnostic and statistical manual of mental disorders: DSM-IV. Washington, DC: American Psychiatric Association; 1994.

26. Spitzer RL, First MB, Wakefield JC. Saving PTSD from itself in DSM-V. J Anxiety Disord. 2007;21(2):223–41.

27. Carlson EB, Dalenberg C. A conceptual framework for the impact of traumatic experiences. Trauma Violence Abuse. 2000;1 (1):4–28.

28. Gold SD, Marx BP, Soler-Baillo JM, Sloan DM. Is life stress more traumatic than traumatic stress? J Anxiety Disord. 2005;19 (6):687–98.

29. Long ME, Elhai JD, Schweinle A, Gray MJ, Grubaugh AL, Frueh BC. Differences in posttraumatic stress disorder diagnostic rates and symptom severity between criterion A1 and non-criterion A1 stressors. J Anxiety Disord. 2008;22(7):1255–63.

30. Roberts AL, Dohrenwend BP, Aiello AE, Wright RJ, Maercker A, Galea S, Koenen KC. The stressor criterion for posttraumatic stress disorder: does it matter? J Clin Psychiatry. 2012;73(2): e264–70.

31. Van Hooff M, McFarlane AC, Baur J, Abraham M, Barnes DJ. The stressor criterion-A1 and PTSD: a matter of opinion? J Anxiety Disord. 2009;23(1):77–86.

32. Brewin CR, Lanius RA, Novac A, Schnyder U, Galea S. Reformulating PTSD for DSM-V: life after criterion a. J Trauma Stress. 2009;22(5):366–73.

33. McNally RJ. Progress and controversy in the study of posttraumatic stress disorder. Annu Rev Psychol. 2003;54:229–52.

34. Bryant-Davis T, Ocampo C. Racist incident-based trauma. Counsel Psychologist. 2005;33(4):479–500.

35. Meyer IH. Prejudice, social stress, and mental health in lesbian, gay, and bisexual populations: conceptual issues and research evidence. Psychol Bull. 2003;129(5):674–97.

36. Bockting WO, Miner MH, Swinburne Romine RE, Hamilton A, Coleman E. Stigma, mental health, and resilience in an online sample of the US transgender population. Am J Public Health Res. 2013;103(5):943–51.

37. Hendricks ML, Testa RJ. A conceptual framework for clinical work with transgender and gender nonconforming clients: an adaptation of the minority stress model. Prof Psychol Res Pr. 2012;43(5):460–7.

38. Cooley CH. Human nature and the social order. New York: Schocken Books; 1964.

39. Goffman E. Stigma: notes on the management of spoiled identity. New York: Simon & Schuster; 1963.

40. Martin AD, Hetrick ES. The stigmatization of the gay and lesbian adolescent. J Homosex. 1988;15(1–2):163–83.

41. Alessi EJ. A framework for incorporating minority stress theory into treatment with sexual minority clients. J Gay Lesbian Ment Health. 2014;18(1):47–66.

42. Davies D. Towards a model of gay affirmative therapy. In: Davies D, Neal C, editors. Pink therapy: a guide for counsellors and therapists working with lesbian, gay and bisexual clients. Buckingham: Open University Press; 1996. p. 24–40.

43. Huebner DM, Davis MC. Perceived antigay discrimination and physical health outcomes. Health Psychol. 2007;26(5):627–34.

44. Lewis RJ, Derlega VJ, Clarke EG, Kuang JC. Stigma consciousness, social constraints, and lesbian well-being. J Couns Psychol. 2006;53(1):48–56.

45. Meyer IH. Minority stress and mental health in gay men. J Health Soc Behav. 1995;36(1):38–56.

46. Gamarel KE, Reisner SL, Laurenceau JP, Nemoto T, Operario D. Gender minority stress, mental health, and relationship quality: a dyadic investigation of transgender women and their cisgender male partners. J Fam Psychol. 2014;28(4):437–47.

47. Herek GM. Beyond "homophobia": thinking about sexual prejudice and stigma in the twenty-first century. Sex Res Social Policy. 2004;1(2):6–24.

48. Frost DM, Meyer IH. Internalized homophobia and relationship quality among lesbians, gay men, and bisexuals. J Couns Psychol. 2009;56(1):97–109.

49. Gold SD, Feinstein BA, Skidmore WC, Marx BP. Childhood physical abuse, internalized homophobia, and experiential avoidance among lesbians and gay men. Psychol Trauma. 2011;3 (1):50–60.

50. Gold SD. Dickstein, Marx BP, Lexington JM. Psychological outcomes among lesbian sexual assault survivors: an examination of the roles of internalized homophobia and experiential avoidance. Psychol Women Q. 2009;33(1):54–66.

51. Gold SD, Marx BP, Lexington JM. Gay male sexual assault survivors: the relations among internalized homophobia, experiential avoidance, and psychological symptom severity. Behav Res Ther. 2007;45(3):549–62.

52. Fredriksen-Goldsen KI, Cook-Daniels L, Kim HJ, Erosheva EA, Emlet CA, Hoy-Ellis CP, Goldsen J, Muraco A. Physical and mental health of transgender older adults: an at-risk and underserved population. Gerontologist. 2014;54(3):488–500.

53. Pachankis JE. The psychological implications of concealing a stigma: a cognitive-affective-behavioral model. Psychol Bull. 2007;133(2):328–45.

54. Pachankis JE, Cochran SD, Mays VM. The mental health of sexual minority adults in and out of the closet: a population-based study. J Consult Clin Psychol. 2015;83(5):890–901.

55. Almeida J, Johnson RM, Corliss HL, Molnar BE, Azrael D. Emotional distress among LGBT youth: the influence of perceived discrimination based on sexual orientation. J Youth Adolesc. 2009;38(7):1001–14.

56. Toomey RB, Ryan C, Diaz RM, Card NA, Russell ST. Gender-nonconforming lesbian, gay, bisexual, and transgender youth: school victimization and young adult psychosocial adjustment. Dev Psychol. 2010;46(6):1580–9.

57. D'Augelli AR, Grossman AH, Starks MT. Childhood gender atypicality, victimization, and PTSD among lesbian, gay, and bisexual youth. J Interpers Violence. 2006;21(11):1462–82.

58. Dragowski EA, Halkitis PN, Grossman AH, D'Augelli AR. Sexual orientation victimization and posttraumatic stress symptoms among lesbian, gay, and bisexual youth. J Gay Lesbian Soc Serv. 2011;23(2):226–49.

59. Bostwick WB, Boyd CJ, Hughes TL, West BT, McCabe SE. Discrimination and mental health among lesbian, gay, and bisexual adults in the United States. Am J Orthopsychiatry. 2014;84(1):35–45.

60. Marshal MP, Dietz LJ, Friedman MS, Stall R, Smith HA, McGinley J, Thoma BC, Murray PJ, D'Augelli AR, Brent DA. Suicidality and depression disparities between sexual minority and heterosexual youth: a meta-analytic review. J Adolesc Health. 2011;49(2):115–23.

61. Marshal MP, Dermody SS, Cheong J, Burton CM, Friedman MS, Aranda F, Hughes TL. Trajectories of depressive symptoms and suicidality among heterosexual and sexual minority youth. J Youth Adolesc. 2013;42(8):1243–56.

62. Bränström R, Hatzenbuehler ML, Pachankis JE. Sexual orientation disparities in physical health: age and gender effects in a population-based study. Soc Psychiatry Psychiatr Epidemiol. 2016;51(2):289–301. Epub 2015 Aug 23. PubMed.

63. Sherin JE, Nemeroff CB. Post-traumatic stress disorder: the neurobiological impact of psychological trauma. Dialogues Clin Neurosci. 2011;13(3):263–78.

64. Nemeroff CB. Neurobiological consequences of childhood trauma. J Clin Psychiatry. 2004;65(Suppl 1):118–28.

65. Roberts AL, Austin SB, Corliss HL, Vandermorris AK, Koenen KC. Pervasive trauma exposure among US sexual orientation minority adults and risk of posttraumatic stress disorder. Am J Public Health. 2010;100(12):2433–41.

66. Balsam KF, Rothblum ED, Beauchaine TP. Victimization over the life span: a comparison of lesbian, gay, bisexual, and heterosexual siblings. J Consult Clin Psychol. 2005;73(3):477–87.

67. Xu Y, Zheng Y. Does sexual orientation precede childhood sexual abuse? Childhood gender nonconformity as a risk factor and instrumental variable analysis. Sex Abuse. Epub 2015 Nov 29. pii: 1079063215618378. PubMed.

68. Cloitre M, Courtois CA, Charuvastra A, Carapezza R, Stolbach BC, Green BL. Treatment of complex PTSD: results of the ISTSS expert clinician survey on best practices. J Trauma Stress. 2011;24 (6):615–27.

69. Herman JL. Complex PTSD: a syndrome in survivors of prolonged and repeated trauma. J Trauma Stress. 1992;5 (3):377–91.

70. Pelcovitz D, van der Kolk B, Roth S, Mandel F, Kaplan S, Resick P. Development of a criteria set and a structured interview of disorders of extreme stress. J Trauma Stress. 1997;10(1):3–16.

71. Roth S, Newman E, Pelcovitz D, van der Kolk B, Mandel FS. Complex PTSD in victims exposed to sexual and physical abuse: results from the DSM-IV field trial for posttraumatic stress disorder. J Trauma Stress. 1997;10(4):539–55.

72. Alessi EJ, Kahn S, Chatterji S. 'The darkest times of my life': recollections of child abuse among forced migrants persecuted because of their sexual orientation and gender identity. Child Abuse Negl. 2016;51(1):93–105.

73. Shidlo A, Ahola J. Mental health challenges of LGBT forced migrants. Forced Migr Rev. 2013;42:9–11.

74. Meyer IH, Schwartz S, Frost DM. Social patterning of stress and coping: does disadvantaged social statuses confer more stress and fewer coping resources? Soc Sci Med. 2008;67(3):368–79.

75. Breslau N, Chilcoat HD, Kessler RC, Davis GC. Previous exposure to trauma and PTSD effects of subsequent trauma: results from the Detroit area survey of trauma. Am J Psychiatry. 1999;156 (6):902–7.

76. Breslau N, Peterson EL, Schultz LR. A second look at prior trauma and the posttraumatic stress disorder effects of subsequent trauma. Arch Gen Psychiatry. 2008;65(4):431–7.

77. Breslau N, Davis GC. Posttraumatic stress disorder in an urban population of young adults: risk factors for chronicity. Am J Psychiatry. 1992;149(5):671–5.

78. Bromet E, Sonnega A, Kessler RC. Risk factors for DSM-III-R posttraumatic stress disorder: findings from the National Comorbidity Survey. Am J Epidemiol. 1998;147(4):353–61.

79. Brewin CR, Andrews B, Valentine JD. Meta-analysis of risk factors for posttraumatic stress disorder in trauma-exposed adults. J Consult Clin Psychol. 2000;68(5):748–66.

80. Galea S, Ahern J, Tracy M, Hubbard A, Cerda M, Goldmann E, et al. Longitudinal determinants of posttraumatic stress disorder in a population-based cohort study. Epidemiology. 2008;19 (1):47–54.

81. Yehuda R, McFarlane AC. Conflict between current knowledge about posttraumatic stress disorder and its original conceptual basis. Am J Psychiatry. 1995;152(12):1705–13.

82. Gilman SE, Cochran SD, Mays VM, Hughes M, Ostrow D, Kessler RC. Risk of psychiatric disorders among individuals reporting same-sex sexual partners in the national comorbidity survey. Am J Public Health. 2001;91(6):933–9.

83. Lehavot K, Simpson TL. Trauma, posttraumatic stress disorder, and depression among sexual minority and heterosexual women veterans. J Couns Psychol. 2014;61(3):392–403.

84. Stotzer RL. Violence against transgender people: a review of United States data. Aggress Violent Behav. 2009;14(3):170–9.

85. Shipherd JC, Maguen S, Skidmore WC, Abramovtiz SM. Potentially traumatic events in a transgender sample: frequency and associated symptoms. Traumatol. 2011;17(2):56–67.

86. U.S. Department of Justice- Federal Bureau of Investigation. Hate crime statistics, 2014. Washington, DC; 2015 Nov 16. [cited 2015 Dec 11]. Available from https://www.fbi.gov/about-us/cjis/ucr/hate-crime/2014/resource-pages/hate-crime-2014-_summary.

87. Herek GM. Hate crimes and stigma-related experiences among sexual minority adults in the United States: prevalence estimates from a national probability sample. J Interpers Violence. 2009;24 (1):54–74.

88. National Coalition of Anti-Violence Programs. Lesbian, gay, bisexual, transgender, queer, and HIV-affected hate violence in 2014. New York: New York City Gay and Lesbian Anti-Violence Project, Inc.; 2015.

89. Martin JI, Alessi EJ. Stressful events, avoidance coping, and unprotected anal sex among gay and bisexual men. Am J Orthopsychiatry. 2010;80(3):293–301.

90. Meyer D. An intersectional analysis of lesbian, gay, bisexual, and transgender (LGBT) people's evaluations of anti-queer violence. Gend Soc. 2012;26(6):849–73.

91. Collaborative WWR. A fabulous attitude: low income lgbtgnc people surviving & thriving on love, shelter & knowledge. New York: Queers for Economic Justice; 2010. 76 p.

92. Balsam KF, Szymanski DM. Relationship quality and domestic violence in women's same-sex relationships: the role of minority stress. Psychol Women Q. 2005;29(3):258–69.

93. Burke LK, Follingstad DR. Violence in lesbian and gay relationships: theory, prevalence, and correlational factors. Clin Psychol Rev. 1999;19(5):487–512.

94. Goldberg NG, Meyer IH. Sexual orientation disparities in history of intimate partner violence results from the California health interview survey. J Interpers Violence. 2013;28 (5):1109–18.

95. Stiles-Shields C, Carroll RA. Same-sex domestic violence: prevalence, unique aspects, and clinical implications. J Sex Marital Ther. 2015;41(6):636–48.

96. National Coalition of Anti-Violence Programs. Lesbian, gay, bisexual, transgender, queer, and HIV-affected intimate partner violence in 2011. New York: New York City Gay and Lesbian Anti-Violence Project, Inc.; 2012.

97. Martin JI, Alessi EJ. Victimization in a nationwide sample of gay and bisexual men. J Gay Lesbian Soc Serv. 2012;24(3):260–73.

98. Otis MD, Skinner WF. The prevalence of victimization and its effect on mental well-being among lesbian and gay people. J Homosex. 1996;30(3):93–121.

99. Bradford J, Reisner SL, Honnold JA, Xavier J. Experiences of transgender-related discrimination and implications for health: results from the Virginia transgender health initiative study. Am J Public Health. 2013;103(10):1820–9.

100. Grant JM, Mottet LA, Tanis J, Harrison J, Herman JL, Keisling M. Injustice at every turn: a report of the National Transgender Discrimination Survey. Washington, DC: National Center for Transgender Equality and National Gay and Lesbian Task Force; 2011. p. 1–222.

101. Helms JE, Nicolas G, Green CE. Racism and ethnoviolence as trauma: enhancing professional training. Traumatol. 2010;16 (4):53–62.

102. Loo CM, Fairbank JA, Scurfield RM, Ruch LO, King DW, Adams LJ, Chemtob CM. Measuring exposure to racism: development and validation of a race-related stressor scale (RRSS) for Asian American Vietnam veterans. Psychol Assess. 2001;13(4):503–20.

103. Waller RJ. Application of the kindling hypothesis to the long-term effects of racism. Soc Work Ment Health. 2003;1(3):81–9.

104. Root MP. Reconstructing the impact of trauma on personality development: a feminist perspective. In: Brown LS, Ballou MB, editors. Personality and psychopathology: feminist reappraisals. New York: Guilford; 1992. p. 229–66.

105. Brown LS. Sexuality, lies, and loss: lesbian, gay, and bisexual perspectives on trauma. J Trauma Pract. 2003;2(2):55–68.

106. Janoff-Bulman R. Shattered assumptions. New York: Free Press; 1992.

107. Brooks VR. Minority stress and lesbian women. Lexington: Lexington Books; 1981.

108. Mascher J. Surviving trauma and anxiety as a result of events of discrimination. In: Whitman JS, Boyd CJ, editors. The therapist's notebook for lesbian, gay, and bisexual clients: homework, handouts, and activities for use in psychotherapy. New York: Haworth Clinical Practice Press; 2003. p. 60–8.

109. Szymanski DM, Balsam KF. Insidious trauma: examining the relationship between heterosexism and lesbians' PTSD symptoms. Traumatol. 2011;17(2):4–13.

110. Alessi EJ, Martin JI, Gyamerah A, Meyer IH. Prejudice events and traumatic stress among heterosexuals and lesbians, gay men, and bisexuals. J Aggress Maltreat Trauma. 2013;22(5):510–26.

Medical Intervention and LGBT People: A Brief History

Sophia Shapiro and Tia Powell

Introduction

This chapter provides a brief history of the lesbian, gay, bisexual, and transgender (LGBT) community and its relationship with medicine. While a full review of LGBT history cannot be covered in a single chapter, there are crucial historical developments and concepts that health-care providers should grasp in order to put their patient care in context (Fig. 2.1).

We will focus on medical interventions for LGBT individuals, and also explore some concurring social developments and artistic representations of those developments during several time periods. Throughout, we will try to shed light on issues that are useful for health-care providers. For instance, how have LGBT people and physicians in different eras understood the concept of sexual orientation – i.e., which sorts of partners a person is attracted to? How have LGBT people and medicine understood gender identity (the gender one perceives as correct for one's self) and gender expression – the choices one makes to demonstrate gender identity? This entanglement between sexual orientation, sexual behavior, sex, gender, and gender expression is what makes LGBT history so difficult to translate to the modern era. To understand LGBT patients today, clinicians should grasp what these terms mean today, and also understand how their meanings have changed over time.

S. Shapiro, MD
Emergency Medicine Department, NYUMC/Bellevue Hospital Center, New York, NY, USA

T. Powell, MD (✉)
Montefiore Einstein Center for Bioethics, 111 E 210 St, Bronx, NY 10467, USA
e-mail: Tpowell@montefiore.org

Nineteenth and Early Twentieth Century

Before the turn of the last century, the concept of a person identifying as gay, i.e., someone whose primary sexual attractions are to same-sex partners, did not exist. Sexual acts between persons of the same sex have been described since pre-history, but using sexual orientation as a way of organizing or labeling people did not begin until the 1890s. In American culture prior to this, sex outside of marriage was forbidden, but masculinity was not dependent upon heterosexuality. A man might still be "normal" and retain the stature associated with his masculinity even if he participated in sex acts outside of marriage, whether they were with men or women [2]. Essentially, same-sex sexual practices were viewed as sinful acts that any type of person could commit – that is, as behaviors in which any person might engage – rather than the actions of a specific type of stigmatized person.

In the late nineteenth and early twentieth century, physicians and others began to incorporate sexuality into the increasingly detailed taxonomy of medical and mental illness. These nineteenth-century doctors, psychologists, and scientists attempted to find a cohesive theory that would explain why some people desired members of the same sex, while others did not. One early theory was that of Richard von Krafft-Ebing, a late-nineteenth-century German psychiatrist, who argued that homosexuality resulted from an in-utero sexual "inversion," causing men and women to invert their normal sexual desire and pursue sexual interactions more typical of the other sex [3]. British psychiatrist Havelock Ellis built upon the work of Krafft-Ebing to draft his massive six-volume *Studies in the Psychology of Sex* and used the term "invert" to classify transsexuals and transvestites [4]. This work formed the basis of the early twentieth-century conception of sexual orientation as inextricably linked to gender presentation. To be attracted to women is inextricably masculine, and to be attracted to men, inextricably feminine. To invert one is

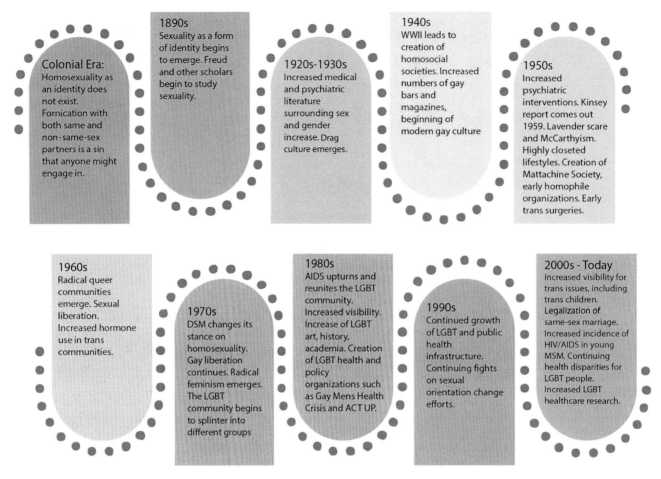

Fig. 2.1 Outline of US LGBT history

to invert the other. For instance, a man who was attracted to men was seen as more womanly, and a woman attracted to women more manly; there was simply no space for a masculine man who desired other men, or a feminine woman who similarly desired other women.

An intriguing literary example of Ellis' theory emerges from *The Well of Loneliness*, a 1929 novel by Radclyffe Hall [5]. The main character, a masculine woman whose father named her Stephen because he wished for a son, typifies the author's and society's attempt to explain same-sex desire as a simple inversion of gender. Stephen (and by extension Radclyffe Hall herself) desires women because her internal life is that of a male. When Stephen falls in love with a more feminine woman later in the novel, Hall depicts the woman's attraction to Stephen as temporary since she is also attracted to men, but also as resting upon Stephen's masculinity. The book offers no concept of a feminine woman who is attracted to women because of their femininity.

Krafft-Ebing, Ellis, and others offer a view of homosexuality as an illness rather than a moral failing. Some might see this shift from crime to illness as an improvement over earlier concepts of same-sex behavior as criminal, which commonly resulted in corporal punishment for homosexual behavior. However, the notion of illness as a kinder and gentler theory of homosexuality is a rebuttable hypothesis. For one, the aggressive medical interventions assigned to attack same-sex behavior were at times of such a damaging nature that a prison sentence would have been more humane. For another, same-sex behaviors remained criminalized in many jurisdictions, even while the concept of illness was added. This resulted in medical treatments mandated by law, as a form of punishment, without appropriate consideration of either efficacy or side effects, as we shall review below.

Freud himself accepted the work of Krafft-Ebing, and referred to homosexuals as inverts. He further delved into the theory of why homosexuality exists, suggesting that it represented a failure to fully sexually mature. However, he also cautioned that homosexuals should not be blamed for their nature. He felt that conversion to heterosexuality was unlikely in all but very unusual circumstances, and discouraged attempts to use psychoanalysis to change sexual orientation. His views were famously summarized in this letter to the mother of a gay son:

"Homosexuality is assuredly no advantage, but it is nothing to be ashamed of, no vice, no degradation; it cannot be classified as an illness; we consider it to be a variation of the sexual function, produced by a certain arrest of sexual development" [6].

This medicalization of homosexuality as an accidental deviation from normal development, rather than a moral failing, led to further study of the growing homosexual social group by scientists and doctors. However, the idea of removing blame from the development of same-sex orientation may also have had a profound impact on the emerging subculture in some major cities. This culture included those who based their lives around homosexuality, but also others who engaged in same-sex sexual acts without identifying as part of a homosexual community. At the same time, communities based around gender presentation, flamboyance, and performance flourished in the 1920s, an era that challenged long-standing restrictions on gender presentation and behavior norms, including dress and sexual behavior. During this time of Prohibition, the police ignored many acts that were officially illegal, from drinking alcohol to cross-dressing, at least within specific times and places, a lenience often supported by bribes. While same-sex attraction largely went unnoticed except during specific noteworthy events, cross-gender performance was hugely popular. There were wildly successful male impersonators during the vaudeville era, and some drew huge crowds, such as Vesta Tilley and Hetty King [7]. Various drag balls were held in major cities on Halloween and New Year's Eve, and boasted attendance by prominent members of society, as well as cross-dressing performers who made the balls so successful [2]. These cultures, one based on gender, one on sexuality, one publicly performed, and one hidden, were seen as related because frequently the participants were the same and because the social theories of the day assumed "inversion" was the only plausible cause of same-sex attraction. George Chauncey has argued that it is the urge of middle-class, masculine men to create an identity distinct from both cross-dressers and "normal" men that creates the concept of homosexuality and creates a private community distinct from both the dominant heterosexual society and the public cross-dressing, gender-inverted community [2].

Just as same-sex sexual behavior was present long before homosexual communities emerged, cross-dressing, passing as another gender, and non-binary gender identification existed long before the popularization of drag balls and cross-gender culture entered the public consciousness. Instances in which women passed as men date back centuries, as women sought to gain access to jobs, join the military, and travel without harm. However, those who passed in these situations may have done so out of external motivations, and did not create a community of like-minded individuals in the way that the drag ball culture and male and female impersonators of the late nineteenth and early twentieth century did. The birth of a subculture of nonnormative gender presentation and same-sex attraction in major cities

allowed scientists to create taxonomies describing individuals within this subculture. The application of this reductive framework shaped medical views of the culture even as it formed, sorting people into binary categories, and aligning sexuality with gender. This scientific emphasis on drawing distinctions and sorting into categories persists in modern terminology (e.g., the moniker LGBT), despite the nuanced differences in identity and lived experiences espoused by members of these communities. As we will discuss later, physicians today still face this burdensome tendency to pigeonhole patients, and instead should seek to understand patients' own self-understanding of sexual orientation and gender identity.

WWII and Beyond: The Era of Medical Intervention

The 1950s represented an era of bold moves in medicine and science. Not coincidentally, this was also a time of few ethical protections for patients and human research subjects, leading to some disastrous consequences. Post-WWII confidence levels were high, and included overwhelmingly positive views on the merits of science and medicine. Esteem for science emerged from successes like the discovery of penicillin, which provided enormous gains in the ability to treat infectious diseases. Throughout medicine, physicians took up the "battle" against other diseases in a manner that paid scant attention to the command, "first, do no harm." For example, radical mastectomies removed not only the breast from cancer patients, but sometimes substantial parts of the chest wall, the arm, and even the torso [8]. As the saying of the day went, "lesser surgery was for lesser surgeons." Similarly, early efforts in transplant medicine and cancer chemotherapy brought both medical progress as well as significant failures, at times with a frightening cost in human lives [9, 10].

Psychiatry, too, developed aggressive treatments to attack disease. Lobotomy gained traction as treatment for a wide range of mental illnesses, earning the Nobel Prize in 1949 for Egas Moniz, one of its main proponents. Lobotomy resembles other invasive psychiatric treatments of that era, in that claims of major therapeutic advances rested on a slim to absent evidentiary basis. Over the next two decades, therapeutic claims were not only discredited, but deleterious side effects emerged as far more common than previously documented [11]. Thus, this was an era in which physicians plunged ahead, hoping for scientific progress but with seemingly little concern for untoward consequences among their patients. Science meant progress, and related scandals (thalidomide, Tuskegee) had not yet emerged to tarnish its reputation and to encourage greater caution. While psychiatric treatment with electroconvulsive therapy, insulin coma, and cold packs burgeoned, rights for patients with mental illness remained severely curtailed. Physicians, with the permission of a family member or judge, could commit a patient to a psychiatric facility and administer treatments without the patient's consent. In some cases, patients were held in psychiatric facilities for years without noticeable treatment. Only in the 1970s did the US Supreme Court forbid the practice of confinement without treatment [12]. Thus, a significant and unfortunate effect of the medicalization of same-sex attraction was that it solidified in this era of bold interventions without recognition for patient rights and safety.

While all persons viewed as mentally ill were subject to the treatments prevalent at the time, LGBT people faced additional interventions purported to change sexual orientation and/or atypical gender presentation. Common methods used in the attempt to control sexuality included electroconvulsive therapy, psychosurgery, and psychoanalysis. Chemical castration was often used for gay men caught engaging in sex acts with other men. Victims of this practice included Alan Turing, the British mathematician and engineer credited with inventing the first computer during WWII. After being arrested for sexual behavior with men, he was sentenced to chemical castration. After several years he committed suicide, leaving behind an apple poisoned with cyanide, a possible allusion to his identity as a "wicked queen" like that in Snow White [13].

Turing may have been among the more famous people to suffer from legal sentences and medical treatments on the basis of sexual orientation and/or behavior, but he was hardly alone. Many narratives document the damaging legal and medical practices common through the 1960s. One young man's family, disturbed by suggestive postcards and other indications of his same-sex orientation, had him forcibly admitted to psychiatric facilities on several occasions during the 1960s, where he received extensive electroconvulsive therapy. Though these interventions had no impact on his sexual orientation, he suffered substantial memory loss and trauma for years after treatment, as noted in this interview:

> For the first eight years after shock treatment, I never knew if I would be able to connect my thoughts. I'd be walking down the street in New York and would have these flashes – and there would be nothing. I'd suddenly not know where I was. I'd think, "My God, I have to find out where I am. Why doesn't anything look familiar?" I would be typing at work and suddenly not be able to remember what city I was in…A lot of times I'd forget my name and address. That might last an hour and a half. But that's a long time when your mind is really going. The feeling was panic…The fear of loss of memory is one of the worst experiences I had after shock treatment, the fear that I might at any point experience this amnesia. That amnesia happened maybe a thousand times. [14]

In the 1950s and 1960s, doctors and social scientists produced a substantial volume of work investigating the nature and frequency of same-sex attractions and nonnormative gender identities. Much of this "scientific" work, selectively edited, reinforced existing prejudice and provided a powerful set of arguments to support social and legal harassment of LGBT people, creating a terrible era for LGBT human rights [15]. Repressive social and political culture confronted anyone who failed to fit strict codes of social conduct. Anti-communist sentiment often coincided with anti-gay fears during the McCarthy era, thus blending both the red scare and the "lavender scare." As David K. Johnson outlines in *The Lavender Scare: Cold War Persecution of Gays and Lesbians in the Federal Government*, gay men and women were thought of during the McCarthy era as "fellow travelers" to communists [16]. Anti-gay activists conjured up the circular argument that gay men and women were susceptible to blackmail by spies because of their hidden identities, ignoring the fact that this persecution is what made gay men and women susceptible to blackmail in the first place. Because of this supposed susceptibility to blackmail and theories that same-sex behavior indicated moral laxness, McCarthy succeeded in banning gay men and lesbians from many government positions. Many were fired from the Departments of State and other federal agencies, or were discharged dishonorably from the military. Job loss under this circumstance was highly damaging and could easily preclude successful employment in the private sector as well [17].

Gay men and lesbians were forced even deeper into the closet, and many sought treatment for their sexuality from medical professionals with the hope they might be able to return to prestigious jobs if "cured" of their sexuality. Others were forced into medical treatment by a legal system that understood their sex acts as a medical condition or perversion, an illness that was also a crime. Same-sex sexual interaction between males was illegal, and arrests were frequent. Police raided gay bars often, and used entrapment methods to arrest gay men in public places known as meeting locations. Patrons faced weeks of jail time for minor infractions including cross-dressing, generally defined as wearing more than three items of clothing associated with the opposite sex [18]. Beatings and sexual assault were common in jails, for both gay men and lesbians [19]. Any arrest could take people away from work with no acceptable explanation, and permanent records of the incident might make them unemployable. Instead of jail time, those convicted of "sexual perversion" might opt for medical intervention, or were ordered to undergo a medical intervention as part of their sentencing. These interventions aimed to curb sexual attraction, especially in gay men. The state claimed a vested interest in controlling the sex lives of its citizens, based on the idea of what created a moral society.

Psychiatric theory and practice of that time generally aided repressive legal actions by insisting, despite Freud's advice to the contrary, that homosexuality was an illness and that invasive treatments could "cure" it. However, some researchers began to explore sexuality in a less pejorative fashion. Notably, Kinsey's detailed reports surprised many both by their relatively neutral stance and their data documenting that same-sex behavior and attraction were far more common than previously believed [20].

Similarly, hopeful legal developments also emerged during the 1950s, either despite or because of increasing repression. Indeed, the 1950s became a tipping point, leading to the formation of the country's earliest LGBT human rights activism. These early "homophile" organizations arose from the freedom of movement and homosocial gatherings made permissible by WWII [21]. Early organizations such as the Mattachine Society and the Daughters of Bilitis protested the exclusion of gay men and women from government jobs and other prohibitions on their participation in public life.

During the post-war era, a more nuanced understanding of the difference between sexuality and gender presentation began to emerge, perhaps because of the growth of the trans identity during this era. Without the means to transition medically, it was difficult for society to understand an individual's decision to live as another gender, as distinct from choosing to present one's birth gender in a nonnormative way, or even to engage in sex acts not normally associated with that gender. Importantly, we also see the first introduction of medical treatments intended to support, rather than suppress, the needs of those outside the heterosexual mainstream. With the development of synthetic estrogen, testosterone, and early sex-reassignment surgeries, we start to hear of people who we can recognize as transgender in the modern sense. These pioneers, such as the GI-turned starlet Christine Jorgensen, showed that transsexuality was a distinct identity, rather than a continuation of the sexual desires of "inverts" [22]. Jorgensen introduced to a wider public the idea that a desire for same-sex partners was separate from an identity with a gender other than that given at birth. She was so clearly different from a gay man that people began to perceive a real difference between sexual orientation and gender identity. Thus, these two concepts begin to diverge, though they remain confusingly intertwined in much current public discourse even today.

1960s–1990s: Civil Rights in a Changing Political Era

We will highlight only the most important developments in the evolving relationship between the LGBT and medical communities between 1959 and today. The past four decades have seen drastic changes in how LGBT individuals are viewed by society and by doctors. In addition, historical moments rooted in the LGBT community have shaped the medical community, our nation, and the world at large. In this section we will cover the emergence of the gay civil rights movement in the late 1960s, the removal of homosexuality as a psychiatric illness from the DSM, the grappling of the medical and psychiatric community with transgender issues, and the AIDS crisis, which shaped gay identity and medical practice the world over.

While there were LGBT activists working for legal reform in the 1950s, the 1960s and 1970s saw a shift in the radical nature of the LGBT civil rights movement, as with other civil rights movements, and a huge boom in the number of "out" LGBT individuals. For many, the Stonewall riots of 1968 represented the first pivotal event in the LGBT rights movement. Though accounts vary, the consensus is that patrons of the Stonewall Inn, most likely a group of young, black, and Latino drag queens, butch lesbians, and transgender people, decided to resist arrest after police invaded the bar during one of their frequent roundups in the neighborhood. Instead, these young, marginalized patrons fought back, trapping the police in the bar and starting riots that lasted for several days, as more and more people from the community joined the fray to protest police abuses [18]. Other events around the country soon followed. Similar riots broke out in the Compton Cafeteria in LA, a gathering place for similarly marginalized, black and Latino gay and trans youth, when police attempted a raid. The next year, the first gay pride march commemorated the Stonewall riots. Over time, more radical protests emerged against discrimination, and called for more gay people to live their lives out of the closet. This shift in tone marked a difference from the philosophy of homophile organizations such as the Mattachine Society, which sought to project an image of respectability. These pioneering activists secured important legal victories, resulting in decreased raids on gay bars and the repeal of various anti-sodomy laws. However, some jurisdictions retained stigmatizing laws for far longer. Sodomy was still illegal in several states until the Lawrence V. Texas decision in 2003. Other states today still have limited legal protections for LGB employees, and many states have laws discriminating against trans individuals.

Large shifts also occurred in the 1960s and 1970s with regard to transgender history. Hormones became more accessible, both via doctors and black market channels. Gender affirmation surgeries improved and slowly became more accessible in the USA. At the same time, however, the LGBT community began to fragment as it grew, and many of its members tried to prioritize the voices and desires of their particular subgroup over others. Gay men began to focus more on sexual liberation, while lesbians took up radical feminism, and transgender rights were often overlooked. Some lesbians rejected members of the trans community, by describing trans women (male to female) as false women who did not belong to their community, and trans men (female to male) as self-hating misogynists. While lesbian and gay rights expanded greatly during this era, the trans community remained marginalized, both by society at large and by the LGB community.

The revision of the Diagnostic and Statistical Manual (DSM) to delete homosexuality as a psychiatric diagnosis was a critically important development in LGB history. This history is well chronicled in Ronald Bayer's excellent work, *Homosexuality and American Psychiatry: The Politics of Diagnosis* [23]. Briefly, psychiatry's annual meeting became the scene of increasingly visible protest for several years in a row. At one point a disguised psychiatrist addressed a large group, discussing his experience as a closeted gay man and physician. Initially, homosexuality as a diagnosis was removed in 1973 but replaced with the category *Sexual Orientation Disturbance* in DSM II, which still was grounded in the idea that same-sex attraction and behavior was abnormal. Activists protested the medicalization of same-sex attraction and garnered support from key American Psychiatric Association (APA) leaders, including Robert Spitzer, who had a pivotal role in drafting relevant versions of the DSM. A protracted, controversial, yet ultimately successful effort led to the elimination of homosexuality as a diagnosis in 1987.

Acquired Immune Deficiency Syndrome, or AIDS, propelled same-sex behavior and LGBT politics into the national spotlight in the 1980s. AIDS caused the deaths of hundreds of thousands of people in the USA alone [24], including many gay leaders in the fields of politics, the arts, and academia. The horror of the disease stirred widespread anti-gay sentiment, with many denouncing the LGBT community, refusing housing, medical and other services, and damning the "sinful" behavior that put people at risk for the illness. Indeed, one early medical acronym for AIDS was WOG – for Wrath of God – suggesting the illness was a righteous punishment. Surgeon General C. Everett Koop was one of the first public officials to embrace the fight against AIDS, sending out brochures across the nation in 1988 promoting strategies to prevent transmission, including condom use [25]. While many protested President Reagan's slow response to the epidemic, he was still the first sitting president to use the word gay in a public speech, marking a huge turning point both in the nation's acceptance of LGBT issues and in the fight against AIDS.

Within the community, some rifts that had grown between lesbians, gay men, and trans communities began to heal as these groups banded together to care for the sick. Grassroots LGBT health organizations such as Gay Men's Health Crisis and AIDS Coalition to Unleash Power (ACT UP) created a new infrastructure that agitated for social change and protested government and medical inaction. Eventually, as the medical community rallied around the AIDS epidemic, generating increased funding for research on the epidemiology, treatment, and prevention of the disease, these organizations began to work with the medical community. Thus, the AIDS epidemic shaped the medical community by creating some of the first community-based participatory research partnerships, forging new leaders in public health, and catalyzing groundbreaking infectious disease research and drug development. As researchers developed drugs for AIDS, and courageous doctors, many of them members of the LGBT community, cared for AIDS patients, respect gradually grew between the LGBT and medical communities. While gay men were the main focus of this shift in public health dialogue, as they comprised the majority of the early victims of the AIDS epidemic, lesbians, bisexuals, and transgender people were affected as well. The creation of LGBT-focused health organizations allowed LGBT people to access care in ways that did not exist before AIDS. Many of those who were identified as bisexual and/or trans were also vulnerable and continue to this day to be disproportionately affected by HIV infection [26].

Current Issues in LGBT Medicine

Health Inequities

Health inequities persist for all LGBT populations compared to peer groups similar in race, ethnicity, income level, and education. Young MSM (men who have sex with men) comprise one of the few groups in the USA for whom the incidence of HIV infection continues to rise and are a focus of continued partnership between the medical and LGBT communities [26]. Trans patients continue to face poor access to general medical care, and many lack coverage for transgender-related therapies specifically. All LGBT people face extremely high rates of sexual violence, a problem that physicians should address in their patient care. Lesbians and bisexual women have higher rates of smoking and lung cancer and a higher stage at diagnosis for gynecological malignancies. However, there have also been many success stories in the arena of LGBT health, particularly with regard to public health measures. By partnering with at-risk LGBT communities, public health officials have been able to decrease transmission of meningitis, hepatitis A, and HIV. In recent years, public health advertisements have attempted to target and engage specific demographic groups, such as lesbians or young MSM of color, with regard to a range of issues including smoking, frequent screening for STIs, domestic violence, and more frequent gynecological follow-up. In large cities, we have also seen the development of LGBT-specific health centers, such as the Callen-Lorde Community Health Center in New York and Fenway Health in Boston. Therefore, while LGBT patients have historically faced significant challenges in obtaining appropriate health care, medical and public health workers are taking strides to end some of the disparities.

Sexual Orientation Change Efforts

Despite the removal of homosexuality from the DSM decades ago, and the proven ineffectiveness of reparative therapies, some psychotherapists continue to attempt to change their patients' sexual orientations. All major relevant professional organizations have now produced consensus documents condemning therapies intended to change sexual orientation. Nonetheless, such therapies continue despite ample evidence that they have deleterious effects, especially for LGBT youth [27]. The attempt to eliminate such therapies is now shifting to the courts, with some significant success in attempts to use consumer fraud and other statutes to prevent these practices [28]. Some jurisdictions have created laws banning anti-gay therapies, though even these measures generally contain loopholes, for instance for clergy providing anti-gay counseling [29].

Trans Issues

Trans issues have moved to the forefront of the LGBT political agenda in the last decade, with a focus on such issues as trans mental health, homelessness, and lack of access to care. While LGBT patients generally have less insurance and poorer access to care than their peers [30], trans people are the most marginalized group within the LGBT community, and often have even fewer resources than their lesbian, gay, and bisexual counterparts. Thus the extreme expense of hormone therapy and gender affirmation surgery weighs especially heavily on this group. While some insurers are beginning to cover these procedures, many trans people lack access to the hormones and surgeries that allow

them to pass safely in society, apply for jobs, feel secure in their identities, and in many cases alleviate intense depression. Several recent high-profile legal decisions have highlighted questions around whether trans people have the right to access gender-affirming medical and surgical care, particularly when they are incarcerated or lack insurance [31]. Because so many trans people have no legal pathway to hormones and surgery in the USA, many travel to foreign countries for cheaper and occasionally black market procedures without proper postsurgical care. Others receive sex hormones from unofficial sources, and even participate in "injection parties" where non-official providers will inject silicone for body contouring, a highly dangerous procedure that causes disfigurement as often as it results in desired cosmetic changes to facial, hip, or other anatomical structures [32].

Another battle that trans people face is the right to define their own transitions. In prior decades some clinics followed rigid guidelines regarding the use of hormones and surgery. For instance, a patient required an evaluation and permission from a physician before beginning medical and surgical steps for transition, and might need to agree in advance to have both "top" and "bottom" surgery before any intervention could begin. Today trans people prefer to tailor their choices to suit their specific needs, rather than follow one set pathway. For instance, some trans people identify with a gender that is neither male nor female and must negotiate with doctors to attain the services they seek. Because prescription medications, surgery, and insurance reimbursement all require the participation of physicians, trans people continue to work with the medical community, though now insisting that a much greater emphasis be placed on informed consent, shared decision-making, and respect for individual values and preferences. The challenge of working toward a respectful, safe, and fair approach to gender transitions is particularly evident in the emerging field of childhood and adolescent transitioning, with its complex dialogue between parents, professionals, and children about the appropriate time to transition.

Conclusion

This chapter presents an historical overview intended to help providers care more thoughtfully and sensitively for their LGBT patients. We have explored some of the historical roots that underlie changing definitions of common terms, including gender identity and sexual orientation. It is important for clinicians to grasp these concepts and to understand what they still do not know about patients' lived experiences, in order to work respectfully with LGBT patients. Consider, for instance, the task of a clinician who encounters a male-identified, masculine-presenting, natal female patient who is attracted to and sexually active with men. Currently, few providers possess the knowledge and skills needed to sensitively explore and understand such a person's gender identity and orientation. However, such competence is crucial for many aspects of health care, including assessment for pregnancy, STIs, and long-term gynecological follow-up, as well as possible trauma and sexual assault. Rather than focus on rigid classification schemes that are so much a part of medicine, we urge practitioners to follow their patients' values and preferences in exploring issues of sexual orientation and gender identity. Our goal as professionals is not to fit patients into a taxonomy but to help people attain and maintain wellness through the tools that medicine provides.

Scientific understanding of gender and sexuality continues to evolve. Because of this, it is necessary to maintain clinical humility and let our patients guide us. What is right for one patient is not necessarily correct for another; we must allow each of our patients to shape their own identities and communicate how those identities affect their lived experiences and health-care needs. While education for health-care providers on LGBT issues is increasing, to date it remains insufficient. We must do our best to address the health-care issues affecting our patients, but we must also recognize there is much we do not know and view our LGBT patients as our educators. As clinicians, we must remember medicine's historical errors and avoid making similar mistakes in our own practices. By maintaining compassion and asking honest questions, we can form effective partnerships with our patients to help us all navigate the health-care system successfully and aim for the best possible care.

Resources

Those interested in additional reading should consider the texts listed below.

1. Chauncey, G. Gay New York: Gender, Urban Culture, and the Making of the Gay Male World, 1890–1940. Basic Books; 1994.
2. D'Emilio, J. "The Homosexual Menace," in Making Trouble: Essays on Gay History, Politics and the University. New York: Routledge; 1992.

References

1. Institutes of Medicine. The health of lesbian, gay, bisexual and transgender people: building a foundation for better understanding. Washington, DC: National Academies Press; 2011.
2. Chauncey G. Gay New York: gender, urban culture, and the making of the gay male world, 1890–1940. New York: Basic Books; 1994.
3. von Krafft-Ebing R. Psychopathia sexualis, with especial reference to the antipathic sexual instinct, a medico-forensic study. Translation published by Rehman, FJ. No copyright; 1852. Available from: https://archive.org/details/psychopathiasexu00krafuoft. Accessed 30 Jan 2016.
4. Ellis H. Studies in the psychology of sex, vol II, sexual inversion. No Copyright; 1927. Project Gutenberg e-book. Available from: http://onlinebooks.library.upenn.edu/webbin/gutbook/lookup?num=13611. Accessed 30 Jan 2016.
5. Hall R. The well of loneliness, No copyright;1928. Available from Project Gutenberg e-book: http://gutenberg.net.au/ebooks06/0609021. Accessed 30 Jan 2016.
6. Freud, S. Letter to an American mother, 1935. In: E Freud, editor. The letters of Sigmund Freud. New York: Basic Books; 1975. p. 423–4. Quoted in Drescher J. A history of homosexuality and organized psychoanalysis. J Am Acad Psychoanal Dyn Psychiatry. 2008; 36(3):443–60.
7. Michael Moore F. Drag!: male and female impersonators on stage, screen and television: an illustrated world history. Jefferson: McFarland and Company Incorporated Pub; 1994.
8. Lerner B. Breast cancer wars. Oxford: Oxford University Press; 2001.
9. Mukerjee S. The emperor of all maladies. New York: Simon and Schuster; 2010.
10. Hunt S. Taking heart – cardiac transplantation past, present and future. N Engl J Med. 2006;355(3):231–5.
11. Valenstein E. Great and desperate cures: the rise and decline of psychosurgery and other radical treatments for mental illness. New York: Basic Books; 1986.
12. Donaldson v O'Connor, 422 US 563 (1975).
13. Leavitt D. The man who knew too much: Alan Turing and the invention of the computer. New York: W. W. Norton; 2006.
14. Anonymous, "Electro-shock: the agony of the years after." In: Katz J, editor. Gay American history, lesbians and gay men in the U.S.A. Meridian Books; 1992.
15. Drescher, J. A history of homosexuality and organized psychoanalysis. J Am Acad Psychoanal Dyn Psychiatry. 2008;36(3):443–60. Especially note his citation of Bergler, E. Homosexuality: disease or way of life. New York: MacMillan Publishing Company; 1956.
16. Johnson DK. The lavender scare: the cold war persecution of gays and lesbians in the Federal Government. Chicago: The University of Chicago Press; 2004.
17. D'Emilio J. The homosexual menace. In: Making trouble: essays on gay history, politics and the university. New York: Routledge; 1992.
18. Kuhn B. Gay power! The stonewall riots and the gay rights movement, 1969. Minneapolis: Twenty-First Century Books; 2011.
19. Feinberg L. Stone butch blues. Ithaca: Firebrand Books; 1993. This autobiographical novel provides a moving account of abuses, within and outside of the criminal justice system, of a young lesbian in mid-century America.
20. Kinsey P, et al. Sexual behavior in the human male. Philadelphia: Saunders; 1948. Sexual behavior in the human female. Saunders; 1953.
21. Berube A. Coming out under fire: the history of gay men and women in world war two. New York: Simon and Schuster; 2000.
22. Meyerowitz J. How sex changed: a history of transsexuality in the United States. Cambridge, MA: Harvard University Press; 2002.
23. Bayer R. Homosexuality and American psychiatry: the politics of diagnosis. Princeton University Press: Princeton; 1987.
24. CDC. HIV and AIDS: United States, 1981–2000. Morb Mortal Wkly Read. 2001; 50(21):430–4. [cited 2015 November 8].

Available from: http://www.cdc.gov/mmwr/preview/mmwrhtml/mm5021a2.htm.

25. NIH. The C. Everett Koop Papers, AIDS, the Surgeon General and the Politics of Public Health. [cited 2016 January 21]. Available from: https://profiles.nlm.nih.gov/ps/retrieve/Narrative/QQ/p-nid/87.

26. CDC. HIV among gay and bisexual men. 2015. [cited 2016 January 19]. Available from: http://www.cdc.gov/hiv/group/msm/.

27. Murphy TF. Redirecting sexual orientation: techniques and justifications. J Sex Res. 1992;29:501–23.

28. Ferguson v. JONAH, Case Number L-5473, Hudson County Superior Court, New Jersey; 2013.

29. See, for instance the California law, 2012 Cal. Legis. Serv. Ch. 835 (S.B. 1172) (codified at Cal. Bus. & Prof. Code §§ 865(a) & 865.1 (2012).

30. Lesbian, Gay, Bisexual, and Transgender Health. (n.d.). [cited 2016 January 19]. Available from: http://www.healthypeople.gov/2020/topics-objectives/topic/lesbian-gay-bisexual-and-transgender-health.

31. Sontag D. Transgender woman cites attacks and abuse in men's prison. The New York Times [Internet]. 2015. Available from: http://www.nytimes.com/2015/04/06/us/ashley-diamond-transgender-inmate-cites-attacks-and-abuse-in-mens-prison.html?_r=0.

32. Murray LR. The high price of looking like a woman. The New York Times [Internet]. 2011. Available from: http://www.nytimes.com/2011/08/21/nyregion/some-transgender-women-pay-a-high-price-to-look-more-feminine.html?_re=0.

Conceptualizing Trauma in Clinical Settings: Iatrogenic Harm and Bias

3

Tonia C. Poteat and Anneliese A. Singh

This chapter uses several frameworks to describe the types of trauma that are commonly faced by lesbian, gay, bisexual, and transgender (LGBT) people, how these experiences influence LGBT patient expectations of healthcare treatment and treatment outcomes, and how providers can offer care that is LGBT-affirmative, culturally responsive, and embeds patient advocacy within its approach. A multilevel model is used to frame the types of discrimination and trauma that LGBT people often experience (Fig. 3.1). The biopsychosocial model, trauma theory, and resilience theory are used to provide a structure for conceptualizing LGBT trauma experiences (Fig. 3.2). The chapter ends with a trauma-informed care (TIC) model that can be used to improve healthcare for LGBT patients.

Defining Trauma

Trauma has been defined as the psychological reaction occurring in response to adverse events, such as sexual violence, a car accident, or a natural disaster [1]. These experiences manifest in myriad ways. For example, many survivors experience denial and shock immediately following a traumatic event, and people who have survived trauma often do not display outward emotional symptoms, yet may experience physical symptoms such as headaches [2]. The age at which trauma occurs, type and duration of trauma experienced, and process of coping add a developmental component to trauma, and clinical outcomes are strongly

influenced by the resources available to support healthy coping [3].

Trauma experiences have been studied extensively; however, relatively little attention has examined the ways in which specific trauma experiences and coping may differ between LGBT people and those who are cisgender and/or heterosexual [4]. Because LGBT people often experience trauma in the form of micro- and macroaggressions related to multiple overlapping societal oppressive forces (e.g., cisgenderism, heterosexism, racism, classism), this unique context of discrimination influences the way in which LGBT people respond to traumatic experiences [5].

What Do We Know About Trauma and Experiences of LGBT People in Healthcare?

A national report on the healthcare experiences of LGBT people found that experiences of discrimination were widespread [6]. When asked about details of the discrimination, almost 56% of lesbian, gay, or bisexual (LGB) respondents reported at least one of the following experiences: being refused needed care, being blamed for their health status, or healthcare professionals using harsh or abusive language, refusing to touch them or using excessive precautions, or being physically rough or abusive. Seventy percent of transgender and gender-nonconforming respondents reported one or more of these experiences; respondents of color and low-income respondents experienced even higher rates of discrimination and substandard care.

These experiences of trauma can be described across multiple levels: institutional, interpersonal, and intrapersonal (see Fig. 3.1). Institutional trauma (also termed structural trauma) describes routine, repetitive exposure of LGBT people to microaggressions (e.g., heteronormative and cissexist assumptions) and macroaggressions (e.g., heterosexist and cissexist violence). These experiences can lead LGBT people to conceal their sexual orientations and/or

T.C. Poteat, PhD, MPH, PA-C (✉)
Johns Hopkins School of Public Health, 615 N. Wolfe St., Baltimore, MD 21205, USA
e-mail: tpoteat@jhu.edu

A.A. Singh
The University of Georgia, Counseling and Human Development Services, Athens, GA, USA

© Springer International Publishing AG 2017
K.L. Eckstrand, J. Potter (eds.), *Trauma, Resilience, and Health Promotion in LGBT Patients*,
DOI 10.1007/978-3-319-54509-7_3

Fig. 3.1 Examples of multilevel types of trauma experienced by LGBT people

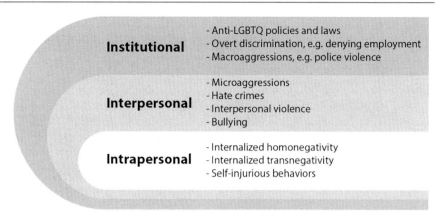

Institutional
- Anti-LGBTQ policies and laws
- Overt discrimination, e.g. denying employment
- Macroaggressions, e.g. police violence

Interpersonal
- Microaggressions
- Hate crimes
- Interpersonal violence
- Bullying

Intrapersonal
- Internalized homonegativity
- Internalized transnegativity
- Self-injurious behaviors

gender identities [7]. LGBT people also experience cumulative interpersonal trauma, defined as trauma experienced with at least one other person, such as sexual assault, intimate partner violence, and childhood sexual abuse [8]. Similar to institutional trauma, interpersonal trauma experiences can lead LGBT people to manifest distrust, hypervigilance, and other self-protective responses in their relationships with partners, family members, friends, and other people and systems in which they have experienced trauma and with whom they interact [9]. Lastly, LGBT people are at great risk for experiencing intrapersonal trauma, such as non-suicidal self-injury and suicide, often as result of experiencing multiple levels of societal discrimination. LGBT people may turn to non-suicidal self-injury – or other maladaptive behaviors – in an attempt to manage the pain, anxiety, distress, and dissociation that result from exposure to multiple levels of trauma. These multiple levels of trauma may also exacerbate maladaptive thought processes, including internalized homonegativity and/or transnegativity. For example, in a recent survey of transgender people [10], over 41% of the sample reported at least one suicide attempt, and rates of suicide attempts increased in the context of job loss and other life stressors related to being transgender.

Unfortunately, institutional, interpersonal, and intrapersonal traumas can also be enacted within healthcare. At the institutional level, the healthcare system itself may create harm. For example, a transgender man who needs cervical cancer screening may face discrimination from an insurance company that refuses to pay for Pap testing because he is identified as male. In order to get the exam, he may also face the discomfort of sitting in the waiting room of a gynecologist's office where he receives stares because he is the only male patient. These experiences may be traumatizing and deter future healthcare seeking, even though the patient's interactions with his healthcare provider are positive overall.

Qualitative research suggests that providers may unwittingly perpetuate interpersonal discrimination and trauma through well-meaning efforts to manage their lack of LGBT-specific medical knowledge [11] and/or to treat every patient the same [12] despite the existence of identity-specific needs. For example, providers may not routinely ask about a patient's sexual orientation outside of the context of sexual health, assuming that this information is not clinically relevant. Providers may feel uncomfortable asking about sexual orientation and gender identity altogether, due to fear of offending a patient. However, failure to gather this information conveys the message that these essential aspects of patients' lives are not important to the provider. Moreover, without information on sexual orientation, for example, providers may make heteronormative assumptions about who constitutes family for that person and inadvertently exclude important decision-making partners from engagement in the patient's care.

Even when aware of LGBT identities, lack of knowledge can lead providers to rely on stereotypes in the provision of care. For example, a well-meaning provider may tell a concerned lesbian with multiple partners that she does not need screening for certain sexually transmitted infections because her partners are female. The provider's lack of knowledge of same-sex sexual practices as well as assumption that lesbians have only female sexual partners may therefore result in substandard care and miss an opportunity for safer sex education.

Healthcare providers should also be aware that many LGBT people have low expectations of providers before even entering a healthcare setting [13]. For instance, lesbian women may experience significant distrust when working with healthcare providers due to societal heterosexism and interpersonal trauma experiences. Transgender people may also distrust mental healthcare providers due to the long history of pathologizing and gatekeeping perpetrated by the mental health profession, with particular regard to accessing hormone therapy [14]. LGBT individuals may anticipate that healthcare providers will not be affirming and culturally competent with regard to sexual orientation and gender identity and therefore may delay or avoid accessing care altogether.

The expectation of mistreatment or a lack of LGBT-affirmative training is not an unrealistic expectation, as research has consistently identified that healthcare settings and providers are underprepared to serve LGBT people. For instance, in a study of medical residents and their knowledge, attitudes, and skills regarding working with LGBT adolescents, Kitts [15] found that the majority of the sample of trainees did not assess sexual orientation or gender identity when conducting a sexual history with adolescents, nor did the majority correctly identify a connection between being a LGBT adolescent and suicide despite the existence of a significant body of literature identifying LGBT adolescents as the population at highest risk for suicide attempts. In addition, studies have reported that healthcare practitioners feel uncomfortable discussing sexual health concerns with their LGBT patients [16] and that disclosure of LGBT identity remains a concern for LGBT people accessing healthcare due to anticipated discrimination and prior experiences of stigma [17].

In addition to the above experiences of trauma and discrimination, LGBT people may also experience de novo trauma or trauma-related symptoms as they begin to interface with healthcare settings. For example, in a large survey of transgender adults, 24% reported being denied equal treatment, 25% reported being harassed or disrespected, and 2% reported being physically assaulted, such as being hit or punched, in a healthcare setting [10]. Sometimes trauma in the healthcare setting is enacted by lack of acknowledgment, as exemplified by inadequate options on intake and ongoing paperwork to denote gender identity (e.g., only having two options of male or female) or to denote partners (e.g., having the option of "spouse" without options of "partner" or recognizing people who are polyamorous). At other times, trauma is promulgated by micro-inequities, as when healthcare providers display nonverbal behaviors that communicate anti-LGBT bias, such as disdainful looks, avoiding eye contact, or maintaining excessive physical distance. Often, these experiences of de novo trauma in healthcare settings cause LGBT people to feel that they are being judged for who they are in terms of their sexual orientation and gender identities, as opposed to being served in an affirmative manner.

Affirmative care occurs when, for example, a transgender woman survivor of trauma meets with her gynecologist and receives both verbal and nonverbal affirmative messages welcoming her to the practice, which include being asked questions about her correct pronouns, name, and terms to use when discussing her body, and having her choices

respected throughout the encounter. Insurance coverage can also be a major source of trauma for LGBT people, as many transgender people cannot access important medical care and surgeries and LGBT people may be underenrolled in healthcare coverage. Fortunately, the Affordable Care Access Act has made affordable healthcare available to many LGBT people and prohibits discrimination on the basis of sexual orientation and gender identity [18]; for instance, transgender people's access to hormone treatment and some surgeries has been increased. Nevertheless, there are still many restrictions that transgender people face in accessing gender-specific services.

Theoretical Approaches to Understanding and Addressing Trauma with LGBT Patients

Biopsychosocial models, trauma theory, and resilience theory can assist in understanding and addressing trauma with LGBT patients. A biopsychosocial model attends to three dimensions of health: biological (e.g., physical), psychological (e.g., emotions, cognitions, behaviors), and social (e.g., cultural backgrounds, contextual environments; see Figure 3.2). This framework aids in conceptualizing how illness and health intersect with LGBT patients' mental well-being and social support (or lack thereof) in their environments.

Trauma theory can inform how healthcare providers work with LGBT people who have survived trauma, including those who have experienced mistreatment in healthcare settings. For instance, people who have had trauma

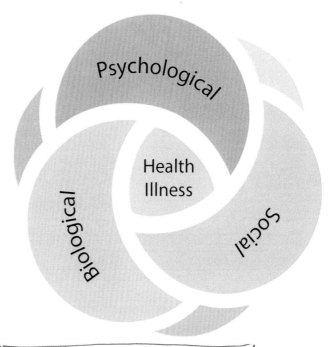

Fig. 3.2 Biopsychosocial model of health and illness

experiences may manifest hypervigilance and intrusive symptoms, such as flashbacks and nightmares [5]. Alternatively, individuals who have survived trauma may not manifest symptoms at all. For all LGBT individuals, it is important to evaluate what life experiences have been challenging or traumatic, and how these experiences continue to impact their lives. Understanding that both societal and interpersonal discrimination and violence influence how LGBT people interact with healthcare systems, providers can anticipate the likelihood of past discrimination and trauma, and assess for common symptoms within intake paperwork and patient interviews. When interacting with LGBT people who have survived trauma, providers can also be cautious not to misdiagnose trauma symptoms as clinical disorders that are not trauma-specific (e.g., anxiety disorders that are not triggered by history of a traumatic event) [9]. Such misdiagnoses may cause further stigma and lead to inappropriate interventions that compound the negative consequences of prior trauma.

Trauma theorists also note that there may be differential coping reactions based not only on the developmental age at which a major trauma occurs but also related to the amount of stress a person has experienced previously [8]. For example, Shipherd et al. [19] showed that transgender people are more likely than cisgender individuals to display trauma symptoms that impair function after experiencing discrimination or violence. Because trauma survivors often experience guilt and shame relating to the trauma, healthcare providers should be aware that LGBT people may feel reluctant to disclose their history of trauma. They may further benefit from having their experiences validated and affirmed by healthcare providers, as LGBT people live in a society that is often invalidating.

Resilience has been defined as an individual's ability to cope with adverse events [20]. A resilience model can help providers identify patient strengths and coping resources to leverage their healing. Integrating a resilience approach to working with LGBT survivors builds on understanding the impact of trauma by recognizing that LGBT people develop coping resources and strengths in response to trauma [21]. Resilience research with transgender people of color who have survived traumatic life events, for example, has identified that simultaneous development of gender and racial/ethnic identity pride as well as connection to transgender communities of color are sources of resilience for navigating oppression in society. Because resilience development can vary tremendously across communities and environmental contexts, healthcare providers should be prepared when working with members of LGBT populations to encounter individuals with a wide spectrum of coping strategies that range from maladaptive to resilient.

While healthcare providers may encounter many challenges in delivering LGBT-affirming care, a crucial starting point is to focus on the quality of the relationship they build with their patients – whether brief or long term – and work to ensure that their patients have a positive experience in this relationship. This often one-time interaction with healthcare providers, when positive, informs and assures LGBT patients that their lives are valuable and their experiences of discrimination and trauma are believed and validated. These positive experiences can encourage LGBT individuals to continue to access rather than avoid healthcare in the future and to share their positive healthcare experiences with members of the larger LGBT community, potentially encouraging these individuals to also seek care.

Trauma-Informed Care for LGBT People

Trauma-informed care for LGBT people is a unifying, culturally responsive approach that is inclusive of the multiple levels at which LGBT people can experience trauma. When healthcare providers use a trauma-informed care approach in their work with LGBT individuals, there is an opportunity to validate patients' experiences of trauma and minimize inflicting further trauma as a provider. Such validation and awareness are crucial in healthcare settings, as research has consistently shown that LGBT people have negative experiences within healthcare settings [6, 10, 22]. Trauma-informed care for LGBT patients is discussed in detail in Chap. 16; however, a succinct description of TIC will be described here given its importance when working with LGBT patients.

Identifying Trauma

Healthcare providers have a better chance of addressing trauma if they are aware of a patient's history; therefore, it is good practice to screen all patients routinely. Several screening tools are available [23]. While none of these tools have been specifically validated among LGBT patients, the Primary Care Post Traumatic Stress Disorder Screen (PC-PTSD) has been designed for use in primary care and other medical settings [24]. The PC-PTSD consists of the following questions:

In your life, have you ever had any experience that was so frightening, horrible, or upsetting that, in the past month, you:

1. *Have had nightmares about it or thought about it when you did not want to?*
2. *Tried hard not to think about it or went out of your way to avoid situations that reminded you of it?*
3. *Were constantly on guard, watchful, or easily startled?*
4. *Felt numb or detached from others, activities, or your surroundings?*

If a patient answers "yes" to any three items or more, it suggests trauma-related problems. A cut-off of three affirmative answers on the PC-PTSD has a sensitivity of 0.78, specificity of 0.85, positive predictive value of 0.65, and negative predictive value of 0.92 for PTSD [24]. Patients who meet the cut-off may benefit from referral to a mental health professional with both expertise in trauma and experience with LGBT clients. All patients who have experienced trauma should be screened for suicidal thoughts given the greater risk for suicide in this context [25].

Staying attuned to a patient's body language, tone of voice, eye contact, and level of participation can provide important clues to the existence of a trauma history. Signs of rising anxiety or emotional arousal may indicate that the patient has experienced a trigger. When this happens, it is important for the provider to remain calm and supportive, without becoming defensive or pressuring the person to talk about what may have triggered them. A key element of preventing harm and promoting resilience is empowering the patient to determine what information they want to share and what components of the physical exam they are willing to undergo. Explaining the purpose of the question and/or exam is key. For example, when asking about sexual orientation, one might begin with a statement/question such as: "I ask about the sexual orientation of all of my patients because it helps me to provide better care. Are you willing to tell me your sexual orientation today?"

Some LGBT patients may not feel safe disclosing or discussing traumatic experiences with a healthcare provider, especially if the healthcare setting itself has been a site of trauma. For some LGBT patients, simply entering a medical facility may be triggering. Moreover, healthcare providers may unintentionally participate in interactions that can cause retraumatization due to lack of awareness, implicit bias, and their own reactivity [26].

Addressing Implicit Bias

Implicit bias results from subtle cognitive processes that operate without awareness or intent. The underlying implicit attitudes and stereotypes responsible for implicit bias are automatic beliefs or associations that are ascribed to a specific sociocultural group [27]. Most research on implicit bias has been conducted with racial/ethnic minority groups; however, recent studies suggest that implicit bias toward LGBT people is also common [28] and may influence clinical care in a similar fashion [11, 29].

Although automatic, implicit bias can be changed [30]. According to a recent review [30, 31], providers can take a number of actions to reduce implicit bias, including:

1. Consciously affirming egalitarian goals and considering specific implementation strategies;

2. Considering "gut" reactions to specific individuals or groups as potential indicators of implicit bias and reflecting on the potential effect of these reactions on professional interactions;

3. Acknowledging and reappraising rather than suppressing uncomfortable feelings and thoughts;

4. Considering the situation from the patient's perspective;

5. Considering changing situations that increase negative or stereotypical responses, for example, removing images that associate all gay men with STIs.

In addition, consistent exposure to counter-stereotypic examples of people can inhibit negative implicit attitudes [32, 33]. Professional development opportunities that provide training in cultural sensitivity and foster the acquisition of egalitarian communication strategies (e.g., asking every patient what pronoun they use) may be useful in reducing bias. *Trauma-Informed Medical Care (TI-Med)* is one example of a continuing medical education course designed to enhance trauma-informed, patient-centered communication [34]. This curriculum is not specific to LGBT survivors of trauma; rather it focuses on building self-awareness, respect, empowerment, collaboration, and connection into any provider-patient relationship.

Reducing Reactivity

It is common and normal for healthcare providers to feel uncomfortable and uncertain when faced with clinical situations that are unfamiliar and or even contradict their core values. Acknowledging those feelings as well as understanding and validating their source are important steps toward reducing reactivity. When feeling reactive, providers should make sure to pause before responding so as to recenter and assess what they need both for self-care and to provide the best care for the patient. If necessary, a provider may want to let the patient know they need to gather more information or make a consultation in order to obtain the most up-to-date and helpful information, then schedule a visit in the near future at which to follow-up. Reducing reactivity allows the provider to approach the patient encounter feeling clear and calm, and reduces the likelihood of inadvertently contributing to the patient's trauma burden [26].

Preventing Harm to LGBT People in Healthcare Settings

Harm prevention includes addressing both the clinical environment and the quality of interpersonal interactions [35, 36]. Welcoming environments include images and patient information that include diverse LGBT people and families, mission statements and policies that explicitly preclude discrimination on the basis of gender identity and sexual orientation, and forms and electronic health records that allow patients to identify themselves as they wish, regardless of the legal status of their relationships or gender [37]. Ideally, the clinical setting will permit disclosure of LGBT identities in a private and confidential manner to avoid exposing the patient to potential discrimination by other patients or providers. For example, transgender patients should be able to designate the appropriate name and pronoun on clinical forms at registration and have these used during all interactions with clinical staff, both administrative and medical.

Development of a trusting patient-provider relationship is key to preventing harm. Such a relationship is facilitated by respectful communication that honors the identity and relationships of LGBT patients and avoids making assumptions about sexual relationships, partners, and family structures. Open-ended, nonjudgmental questions and active listening strategies are the best strategies to promote effective communication and trust. Ensuring that every member of the healthcare staff has basic education in cultural competency, including an understanding of how LGBT identities intersect with other identities such as race, ethnicity, and class, is integral to avoiding iatrogenic harm. Opportunities for such training are available both online and in person. The National LGBT Health Education Center (http://www.lgbthealtheducation.org) provides webinars and publications that address LGBT cultural competency. The Human Rights Campaign (www.hrc.org) and discipline-specific organizations such as the American Medical Association (http://www.ama-assn.org/ama/pub/about-ama/our-people/member-groups-sections/glbt-advisory-committee/glbt-resources.page) provide LGBT cultural competency benchmarks for organizations and providers.

Promoting Resilience

Incorporating resilience promotion into clinical practice is part of a providing trauma-informed care. Engagement, empowerment, and collaboration are key elements of trauma-informed care that promote resilience [25]. Providers should strive to ensure that clinical systems are transparent, healthcare personnel are trustworthy, care is collaborative, and that LGBT patients feel emotionally and physically safe in the clinical setting and have both voice and choice in their care. Subsequent chapters will focus on the specifics of trauma-informed care.

Advocacy on Behalf of LGBT People in Clinical Settings

Because of the multiple levels of trauma many LGBT people have experienced over the lifespan, healthcare providers can play a crucial role by supporting or participating in advocacy efforts for LGBT trauma survivors. Advocacy entails working to reduce instances of oppression encountered by LGBT people both within and outside of clinical settings [38], as well as using the privilege accorded healthcare providers to enact social change to affirm the human rights of LGBT people. Healthcare providers can engage in advocacy in two ways: *with* LGBT people and *on behalf of* LGBT people [39]. For example, advocacy might entail teaching LGBT survivors of trauma on how to advocate for their own affirmative care. This might include making sure that the survivors are aware of and able to describe their trauma symptoms when interfacing with healthcare providers in order to set the stage for more responsive treatment, in addition to being able to identify when healthcare provision is not affirmative or appropriate. Alternately, advocacy on behalf of LGBT people includes advocacy actions that healthcare providers can take when LGBT people are not present, such as beginning a working group or committee to ensure that intake processes and other clinical documentation are LGBT-affirming.

Healthcare providers can engage in advocacy collaboratively with LGBT people and on behalf of LGBT people within three domains: micro level, meso level, and macro level [39] (Fig. 3.3). The micro level includes individual interactions within healthcare settings, such as physician assistant and patient or mental health counselor and patient. In these micro-level interactions, healthcare providers can advocate collaboratively with LGBT people to recognize barriers they face within and outside the healthcare setting, and advocate on behalf of LGBT people by identifying potential LGBT-allies within the healthcare setting. The meso level of advocacy includes the healthcare setting itself and the community. Within the meso level, healthcare providers can advocate collaboratively with LGBT people to develop action teams within the healthcare setting to address how to provide more affirmative treatment to LGBT survivors of trauma, while advocating on behalf of LGBT people might include developing and implementing an LGBT-affirming treatment plan in the healthcare setting that anticipates potential barriers and challenges and works to address these proactively. The third level of advocacy is the macro level, referred to as the public arena. Healthcare providers can collaboratively advocate with LGBT people by writing publications (e.g., newsletter articles, letters to the editor) about a particular healthcare barrier faced by LGBT survivors of trauma, and advocating on behalf of LGBT people could include lobbying legislators at the local, state, and national level for LGBT-affirming policy changes (e.g., insurance coverage of transgender surgeries). See Table 3.1 for more examples of opportunities for healthcare provider advocacy with LGBT patients.

Fig. 3.3 Strategies for healthcare providers to advocate for LGBT people

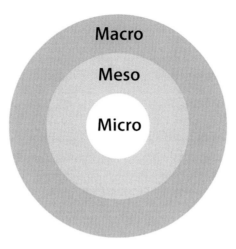

Collaborative Advocacy

Macro
- advocacy opportunities for clinicians
- lobbying legislators
- organizational and institutional efforts

Meso
- collaborative action teams
- implementing LGBT-affirmative treatment plans

Micro
- patient-provider interactions
- leadership training

Table 3.1 Opportunities for healthcare provider advocacy

Levels of advocacy	Types of advocacy activities
Micro level	Advocating on behalf of individual patients and addressing cissexist and heterosexist bias from fellow healthcare providers
	Teaching LGBT patients self-advocacy skills in working with healthcare providers
Meso level	Organizing education and training opportunities for healthcare providers on working with LGBT patients
	Leading an action team identifying how to make the healthcare environment and paperwork more LGBT-affirmative
Macro level	Advocating for healthcare professional organizations to lead on LGBT-affirming policy change
	Lobbying legislators and other local, state, or national leaders to create LGBT-affirming healthcare laws and increase access to LGBT-affirmative healthcare

When engaging as advocates for LGBT patients, healthcare providers can expect to encounter resistance at micro, meso, and macro levels. Heterosexism is a deeply embedded structural feature of healthcare systems, which reflect the values of society at large; therefore, providers who engage in change efforts may experience frustration and dismay as they face challenges in making healthcare settings more affirmative to LGBT survivors of trauma. Although it is impossible to eradicate these challenges, healthcare providers can leverage their efforts through consultation and collaboration with a wide variety of community stakeholders that already provide and/or support LGBT-affirming healthcare. For example, before embarking on development of a new community health clinic program for LGBT patients experiencing homelessness and intimate partner violence, one might consider forming a task force that includes not only healthcare providers and administrators from the clinic but also representatives from local organizations that serve people in the community affected by these issues. In these instances, collaboration can not only bolster healthcare provider advocacy efforts but also expand the influence of their LGBT-affirming advocacy and assure that the voices and choices of LGBT patients and their supporters are heard and incorporated.

Clinical Scenario

Tierra is an 18-year old trans woman whose parents immigrated to the United States from Trinidad before she was born. She socially transitioned at a young age and grew up in a community where her gender identity was respected. She excelled academically, engaged in multiple extracurricular activities, and was elected president of the student council during her senior year in high school. She has now enrolled in a college far from home and comes to see you at the student health center for routine medication refills. When you enter the room, you notice that she jumps a bit and looks startled. During the medical history, she repeatedly glances toward the door. When you ask her about this, she quickly asserts that everything is fine. As you introduce the sexual history, she becomes irritable and refuses to respond to any questions, stating: "You think all transgender girls are good for is sex!"

While her response comes as a surprise, you stay calm and warm in your demeanor. You let her know that you ask sexual history questions of all of your patients and reassure her that she doesn't have to answer any questions that make her uncomfortable. You then ask if there's anything she'd like to talk with you about. She says no and asks if she can come back later to finish the encounter. A week later, she calls and asks to speak only with you. During the conversation, she discloses that she was recently taunted and sexually assaulted on campus by a group of boys who locked her in a classroom where she was studying. Until now, she was reticent to tell anyone about this experience because she was ashamed and didn't want to disappoint her parents.

Discussion Questions

1. What are signs that an LGBT patient may have experienced prior trauma?
2. What role do providers play in identifying and responding to trauma among their LGBT patients?
3. How do intersectional factors impact an LGBT person's experience of trauma?
4. What strategies can health professionals use to provide a safe and empowering experience for LGBT patients?
5. What community resources are available to support LGBT patients who have experienced trauma?

Summary Practice Points

- Hyperarousal is common among people who have experienced trauma.
- Staying very busy by taking on extra activities may be one way that people avoid experiencing feelings and thoughts related to the trauma.
- Creation of a calm and empowering environment facilitates engagement in care for people who have survived trauma.
- Health professionals play a key role in identifying and responding to trauma among LGBT patients and connecting them with appropriate resources.

Resources

1. FORGE. *Transgender Sexual Violence Survivors: A Self-Help Guide to Healing and Understanding.* September 2015. Available at http://forge-forward.org/2015/09/trans-sa-survivors-self-help-guide/
2. Substance Abuse and Mental Health Services Administration. Trauma-Informed Approach and Trauma-Specific Interventions. Available at http://www.samhsa.gov/nctic/trauma-interventions. Includes
   (a) Key principles of a trauma informed approach
   (b) Links to trauma-specific interventions
3. American Academy of Family Physicians. AAFP Reprint No. 289D. Recommended Curriculum Guidelines for Family Medicine Residents: Lesbian, Gay, Bisexual, Transgender Health, 2015. Available at: http://www.aafp.org/dam/AAFP/documents/medical_education_residency/program_directors/Reprint289D_LGBT.pdf
4. University of California, San Francisco. LGBT Resource Center. Available at: https://lgbt.ucsf.edu/lgbt-education-and-training. The site includes links to articles, publications, and online trainings.
5. The Fenway Institute. The National LGBT Health Education Center On-Demand Webinars. Available at: http://www.lgbthealtheducation.org/training/on-demand-webinars/
6. Green BL, Saunder PA, Power E, et al. Trauma-Informed Medical Care: A CME Communication Training for Primary Care Providers. *Family Medicine.* 2015 January; 47 (1): 7–14.
7. Reeves E. A Synthesis of the Literature on Trauma-Informed Care. *Issues in Mental Health Nursing.* 2015; 36(9): 698–709.

References

1. American Psychological Association. Trauma. 2015. Available from: www.apa.org/topics/trauma.
2. Courtois CA, Ford JD. Treatment of complex trauma: a sequenced, relationship-based approach. New York: Guilford Press; 2013.
3. Freyd JJ, DePrince AP, Gleaves DH. The state of betrayal trauma theory: reply to McNally-conceptual issues and future directions. Memory. 2007;15(3):295–311.
4. Richmond K, Burnes T, Carroll K. Lost in trans-lation: interpreting systems of trauma for transgender clients. J Trauma. 2012;18(1):45–57.
5. Brown LS. Cultural competence in trauma therapy: beyond the flashback. Washington, DC: American Psychological Association; 2008.
6. Legal L. When health care isn't caring: Lambda Legal's survey of discrimination against LGBT people and people living with HIV. New York: Lambda Legal; 2010.
7. Meyer I. Prejudice, social stress, and mental health in lesbian, gay, and bisexual populations: conceptual issues and research evidence. Psychol Bull. 2003;129:674–97.
8. Briere J, Scott C. Principles of trauma therapy: a guide to symptoms, evaluation, and treatment. Sage: Thousand Oaks; 2014.
9. Mizock L, Lewis TK. Trauma in transgender populations: risk, resilience, and clinical care. J Emot Abus. 2008;8:335–54.
10. Grant JM, Mottet LA, Tanis J, Harrison J, Herman JL, Kiesling M. Injustice at every turn: a report of the national transgender discrimination survey. Washington, DC: National Center for Transgender Equality & National Gay and Lesbian Task Force; 2011.
11. Poteat T, German D, Kerrigan D. Managing uncertainty: a grounded theory of stigma in transgender health care encounters. Soc Sci Med. 2013;84:22–9.

12. Willging CE, Salvador M, Kano M. Brief reports: unequal treatment: mental health care for sexual and gender minority groups in a rural state. Psychiatr Serv. 2006;57(6):867–70.

13. Heck JE, Sell RL, Gorin SS. Health care access among individuals involved in same-sex relationships. Am J Public Health. 2006;96(6):1111–8.

14. Singh AA, Burnes TR. Shifting the counselor role from gatekeeping to advocacy: ten strategies for using the competencies for counseling with transgender clients for individual and social change. J LGBT Issues Couns. 2010;4(3–4):241–55.

15. Kitts RL. Barriers to optimal care between physicians and lesbian, gay, bisexual, transgender, and questioning adolescent patients. J Homosex. 2011;57:730–47.

16. Hinchliff S, Gott M, Galena E. 'I daresay I might find it embarrassing:' general practitioners' perspectives on discussing sexual health issues with lesbian and gay patients. Health Soc Care Community. 2005;13(4):345–53.

17. Mattocks KM, Sullivan JC, Bertrand C, Kinney R, Sherman MD, Gustason C. Perceived stigma, discrimination, and disclosure of sexual orientation among a sample of lesbian veterans receiving care in the Department of Veterans Affairs. LGBT Health. 2015;2(2):147–53.

18. Progress CfA. The Affordable Care Act and LGBT families: everything you need to know 2013. Available from: https://www.americanprogress.org/issues/lgbt/report/2013/05/23/64225/the-affordable-care-act-and-lgbt-families-everything-you-need-to-know/.

19. Shipherd JC, Maguen S, Skidmore WC, Abramovitz SM. Potentially traumatic events in a transgender sample: frequency and associated symptoms. Traumatology. 2011;17:56–67.

20. Masten AS. Ordinary magic: resilience processes in development. Am Psychol. 2001;56(3):227–38.

21. Singh AA. Transgender youth of color and resilience: negotiating oppression, finding support. Sex Roles J Res. 2012;68:690–702.

22. Fredriksen-Goldsen KI, Kim H-J, Emlet CA, Muraco A, Erosheva EA, Hoy-Ellis CP, et al. The aging and health report: disparities and resilience among lesbian, gay, bisexual, and transgender older adults. Seattle: Caring And Aging With Pride; 2011.

23. US Department of Veterans Affairs. PTSD: National Center for PTSD. 2015. Available from: http://www.ptsd.va.gov/professional/provider-type/doctors/screening-and-referral.asp.

24. Prins A, Ouimette P, Kimerling R, Cameron RP, Hugelshofer DS, Shaw-Hegwer J, et al. The primary care PTSD screen (PC-PTSD): development and operating characteristics. Prim Care Psychiatry. 2003;9:9–14.

25. Substance Abuse and Mental Health Services Administration. Trauma-informed approach and trauma-specific interventions. 2015. Available from: www.samhsa.gov/nctic/trauma-interventions.

26. Potter J. Self-discovery: a toolbox to help clinicians communicate with clarity, curiosity, creativity, and compassion. In: Makadon H, Mayer K, Potter J, Goldhammer H, editors. Fenway guide to lesbian, gay, bisexual, and transgender health. 2nd ed. Philadelphia: American College of Physicians; 2015.

27. Banaji M, Heiphetz L. Attitudes. In: Fiske S, Gilbert D, Lindzey G, editors. Handbook of social psychology. 5th ed. New York: Wiley; 2010. p. 348–88.

28. Dorsen C. An integrative review of nurse attitudes towards lesbian, gay, bisexual, and transgender patients. Can J Nurs Res. 2012;44(3):18–43.

29. Carabez R, Pellegrini M, Mankovitz A, Eliason M, Scott M. Does your organization use gender inclusive forms? Nurses' confusion about trans* terminology. J Clin Nurs. 2015;24(21–22):3306–17.

30. Blair I. The malleability of automatic stereotypes and prejudice. Personal Soc Psychol Rev. 2002;6:242–61.

31. Blair IV, Steiner JF, Havranek EP. Unconscious (implicit) bias and health disparities: where do we go from here? Perm J. 2011;15(2):71–8.

32. Dasgupta N, Rivera LM. When social context matters: the influence of long-term contact and short-term exposure to admired outgroup members on implicit attitudes and behavioral intentions. Soc Cogn. 2008;26(1):112–23.

33. Dovidio JF, Fiske ST. Under the radar: how unexamined biases in decision-making processes in clinical interactions can contribute to health care disparities. Am J Public Health. 2012;102(5):945–52.

34. Green BL, Saunders PA, Power E, Dass-Brailsford P, Schelbert KB, Giller E, et al. Trauma-informed medical care: CME communication training for primary care providers. Fam Med. 2015;47(1):7–14.

35. Wilkerson JM, Rybicki S, Barber CA, Smolenski DJ. Creating a culturally competent clinical environment for LGBT patients. J Gay Lesbian Soc Serv. 2011;23(3):376–94.

36. Makadon HJ, Mayer KH, Potter J, Goldhammer H, editors. The Fenway guide to lesbian, gay, bisexual and transgender health. 2nd ed. Philadelphia: American College of Physician; 2015.

37. Cahill S, Bradford J, Grasso C, Makadon H. How to gather data on sexual orientation and gender identity in clinical settings. Boston: Fenway Institute, Fenway Health; 2012.

38. Singh AA. It takes more than a rainbow sticker!: advocacy on queer issues in counseling. In: Ratts MJ, Toporek RL, Lewis JA, Ratts MJ, Toporek RL, Lewis JA, editors. ACA advocacy competencies: a social justice framework for counselors. Alexandria: American Counseling Association; 2010. p. 29–41.

39. Lewis J, Arnold M, House R, Toporek R. Advocacy competencies 2003 [cited 2016 Jan 30]. Available from: http://www.counseling.org/docs/default-source/competencies/advocacy_competencies.pdf.

Impact of Stress and Strain on Current LGBT Health Disparities

Robert-Paul Juster, Jennifer A. Vencill, and Philip Jai Johnson

Introduction

Health inequalities are experienced by sexual and gender minority populations as a consequence of stigma and represent a national public health priority [1]. Despite social progress in North America, perceived discrimination attributable to sexual orientation is reported by 29–78% of lesbian, gay, bisexual, and transgender (LGBT) Canadians [2] and 42% of LGBT Americans [3]. Further, violence against gender nonconforming lesbian, gay, bisexual, and transgender people remains "alarmingly high," with approximately 20–25% of lesbian and gay people reporting some form of violence within their lifetimes. Indeed, these figures likely underestimate the experience of violence and discrimination against LGBT people, as the US federal survey on violence does not commonly contain questions on sexual orientation or gender identity [4].

These distinct experiences of violence and discrimination, which create cumulative stress and strain for LGBT individuals, are referred to as *minority stress* [5, 6]. Minority stress can be defined as the enduring stress that sexual minority individuals experience as a result of their minority status within a pervasively stigmatizing social climate [5, 7]. Meyer [8] identified three overarching characteristics: (1) minority stress is *uniquely* experienced by LGBT individuals and is different from mundane stressors encountered by people from majority or nonstigmatized backgrounds; (2) minority stress is *chronic*, ranging from mundane offenses to extreme instances of harassment and

violence; and finally (3) minority stress is *socially based* and caused by other people, groups, institutions, and political processes. It should be noted that much of the data in support of this model is derived from research on gay men or men who have sex with men (MSM), although recent research has supported the applicability of the model for lesbian/bisexual women's experiences [9–14] as well as those of transgender individuals [15, 16]. Moreover for transgender individuals, "sexual minority" does not necessarily apply as stigma is related to gender identity.

The experience of minority stress can be thought of as the consequence of experiencing a combination of specific processes: (i) enacted, (ii) felt, and (iii) internalized stigma. Specifically, (i) *enacted stigma* comprises the objective or external events of discrimination and stigma people experience; (ii) *felt stigma* is the expectation of rejection and vigilance that arises in response to such events; and (iii) *internalized stigma* is the internalization of negative attitudes, feelings, and internal representations of a sexual minority identity [6, 12]. As defined by Stuenkel and Wong [17], enacted stigma refers to the hostile behaviors and perceptions, also known as bias and discrimination, of majority group individuals toward an individual stigmatized or seen as different [18]. However, the experience of stigma can occur in the absence of overt discrimination. For example, felt stigma represents the internalization of perceived stigma that leads people to engage in concealment to avoid rejection, bias, and discrimination.

Similarly, LGBT individuals will often engage in identity concealment behaviors so as to avoid being "outed" and potentially becoming the target of prejudicial reactions. Unlike heterosexual individuals for whom stigma tends to be salient when sexual orientation becomes personally relevant [19], among LGBT individuals for whom sexual orientation forms an inextricable component of identity, stigma becomes an ever-present phenomenon, with concealment, expectations of rejection, and hypervigilance being understandable (but not always inevitable) consequences.

R.-P. Juster, PhD (✉) • P.J. Johnson, PhD
Program for the Study of LGBT Health, Division of Gender, Sexuality, and Health, Columbia University, 722 W 168th Street, Room 337, New York, NY 10031, USA
e-mail: robertpauljuster@gmail.com

J.A. Vencill, PhD
Program in Human Sexuality, Department of Family Medicine & Community Health, University of Minnesota Medical School, Minneapolis, MN, USA

© Springer International Publishing AG 2017
K.L. Eckstrand, J. Potter (eds.), *Trauma, Resilience, and Health Promotion in LGBT Patients*, DOI 10.1007/978-3-319-54509-7_4

For bisexual and transgender individuals, the experience of stigma comes from both heterosexual individuals and within the LGBT community [19–21]. Although little research has examined attitudes toward bisexual and transgender individuals within the commonly and perhaps erroneously perceived "monolithic" LGBT community, lesbians and gay men often see the issues experienced by bisexual and transgender people as completely separate from their own [20], and transphobic attitudes have been shown to be particularly prevalent among gay men [22]. Thus, divisions within the LGBT community can generate unique forms of minority stress.

Minority stress processes affect the psychological, physical, and behavioral health of LGBT individuals [1]. Many of the health consequences, such as anxiety and mood disorders, physical complaints, maladaptive substance use, and cardiovascular disease, are catalyzed and/or exacerbated by psychosocial stress (Fig. 4.1). However, additional research is urgently needed to elucidate the biological mechanisms that explain how minority stress "gets under the skin" to affect the health and well-being of LGBT individuals [23].

This chapter will outline the neurobiology linking chronic stress to health outcomes, as well as recent research developments applying biological approaches to describe LGBT health disparities as they relate to minority stress and trauma. Our focus will be on stress physiology and the development of the allostatic load model used to describe "wear and tear" on the brain and body caused by chronic stress and unhealthy behaviors. We will also discuss how healthcare providers can incorporate this knowledge to deliver LGBT healthcare in a competent and sensitive manner. The next section will begin with a brief introduction to stress physiology and explain how initial adaptive mechanisms can become maladaptive when chronically activated under stressful circumstances.

Biological Stress

Stress is broadly defined as a real or interpreted threat to an individual that results in biological and behavioral responses. The stress-disease literature includes three broad perspectives with regard to measurement of stress and subsequent coping: environmental, psychological, and biological. As a multidimensional construct, stress involves interactions among *inputs* (environmental stressors), *processes* (subjective psychological distress), and *outputs* (objective biological stress responses). Though often investigated separately [24, 25], these elements of stress and coping are best studied in conjunction with one another, as each dimension can impact the others. For example, the release of stress hormones as part of the biological response

to environmental and psychological stress mobilizes energy to promote adaptation (e.g., behaviors that function to distance a person from an environmental stressor or damp down maladaptive psychological processes).

Absolute stressors (e.g., natural disasters, sexual assault) that threaten survival lead invariably to acute stress responses and, potentially, to posttraumatic distress. By comparison, *relative stressors* (e.g., negotiating traffic, public speaking) threaten one's well-being only if the person deems them stressful. As is principally the case for relative stressors, situations that are novel, unpredictable, threaten self-preservation, and/or diminish one's sense of control contribute additively to biological stress responses [26, 27]. Cumulative exposure to multiple relative stressors can render an individual more susceptible to traumatic symptoms (e.g., hypervigilance) in the face of an absolute stressor or accumulated relative stressors that "break the camel's back," so to speak. Based on the minority stress model outlined earlier, chronic internal and external stressors – and subsequent stress responses – may be more pernicious and emotionally salient among LGBT individuals.

Biological stress responses are activated whenever real or interpreted threats are detected via neural systems. The interpretation of a "threat" triggers the *sympathetic-adrenal-medullary (SAM)* axis to release *catecholamines* (e.g., adrenalin) within seconds from the adrenal medulla. This response system is fast-acting and reflexive, preparing the body to respond almost immediately to threat. Similarly, the neural interpretation of "threat" activates the paraventricular nucleus of the hypothalamus to release *corticotropin-releasing factor* (CRF), which in turn activates the *hypothalamic-pituitary-adrenal* (HPA) axis. Specifically, CRF travels through a portal system linking the hypothalamus to the pituitary gland, where it signals the secretion of *adrenocorticotropic hormone* (ACTH) from the capillary-rich environment of the anterior pituitary. Systemic ACTH then travels to the adrenal glands, where it precipitates cellular activities in the zona fasciculata region of the adrenal cortex to produce the glucocorticoid *cortisol*, which in turn is responsible for transforming fat into sugar to fuel biobehavioral responses [28]. Compared to the SAM axis, the HPA cascade is slower, occurring within minutes after the perception of a threat. Thus, the SAM and HPA axes synergistically mobilize energy necessary for adaptation; however, this comes at the cost of acute and/or chronic recalibration of many biological functions that ensure health of the whole organism [29] (Fig. 4.2).

The brain's ultimate role during stress is to detect threat and promote adaptation. In addition to the pituitary and hypothalamic control of the HPA axis, there are three major brain structures involved in the regulation of stress responses: (i) the *hippocampus*, which is linked to memory and cognition, in addition to being implicated in negative

Fig. 4.1 Biological effects of stress on the brain and body

Effects of Stress Over Time

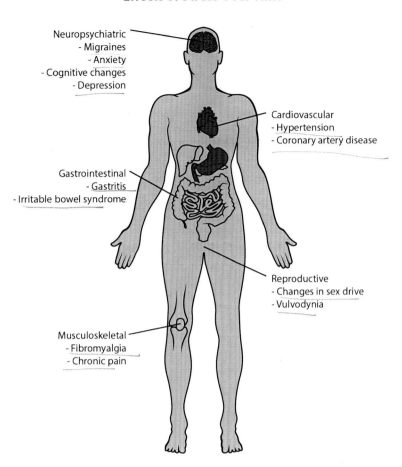

Neuropsychiatric
- Migraines
- Anxiety
- Cognitive changes
- Depression

Cardiovascular
- Hypertension
- Coronary artery disease

Gastrointestinal
- Gastritis
- Irritable bowel syndrome

Reproductive
- Changes in sex drive
- Vulvodynia

Musculoskeletal
- Fibromyalgia
- Chronic pain

feedback regulation that shuts down the HPA axis; (ii) the *amygdala*, which is responsible for threat perception and emotional processing with outputs to SAM axis and neuroendocrine regulatory systems; and (iii) the *frontal cortex*, which is involved in cognition and exerting top-down control over subcortical structures and the development of coping responses [30–35]. With regard to HPA-axis regulation, the hippocampus is inhibitory, the amygdala is excitatory, and the frontal cortex can be both. Neural regulation of allostatic mechanisms is further shaped by individual differences in constitutional (genetics, development, experience), behavioral (coping and health habits), and historical (trauma/abuse, major life events, stressful environments) factors that ultimately determine one's vulnerability and/or resilience to stress.

Life Cycle Model of Stress

Lupien et al. [36] proposed that the consequences of chronic stress and/or trauma depend on age of exposure and, accordingly, brain development of specific regions regulating the HPA axis. Environmental stress in the prenatal period affects the development of the hippocampus, prefrontal cortex, and amygdala, and shapes the neural development of these regions. After birth, the effects of postnatal stress vary according to environmental exposures: for instance, maternal separation during childhood generally leads to *increased* secretion of cortisol, whereas exposure to severe abuse is associated with *decreased* levels of cortisol. It is important to note that, from the prenatal period onward, all developing brain areas are sensitive to the effects of stress hormones; however, some areas undergo rapid growth during key critical windows. From birth to 2 years old, for example, the developing hippocampus is most vulnerable to the effects of stress. By contrast, exposure to stress that persists over a longer duration between birth through late childhood can lead to changes in volume of the amygdala, which continues to develop until the late 20s.

During adolescence, the rapid development of the hippocampus slows down but continues to show marked plasticity as evidenced by perpetual neurogenesis of the dentate gyrus [37]. Other stress-regulatory regions, including the frontal cortex, continue to mature into adulthood. Consequently, stress exposure during the transition into emerging adulthood can have major effects on the frontal cortex. Studies

Fig. 4.2 Hypothalamic-
pituitary-adrenal (HPA) axis
contributing to biological stress
response

Biological Stress Response

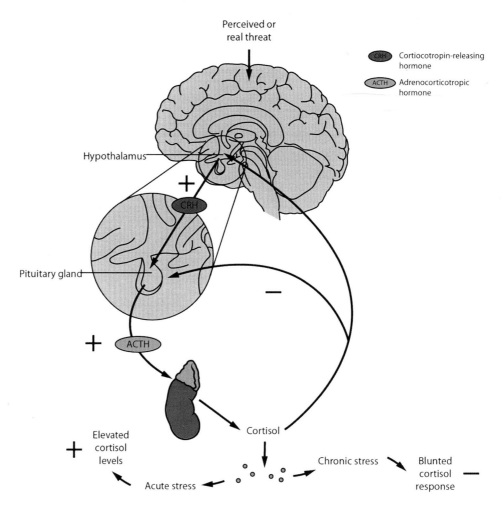

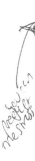

show that adolescents are highly vulnerable to stress because of pubertal changes in gonadal hormones and sensitivities of the HPA axis that can persist into adulthood. In adulthood and into older age, the brain regions that undergo the most rapid decline as a result of aging are once again highly vulnerable to the effects of stress hormones, including the manifestation of effects from earlier life [36].

Lifelong brain changes ultimately diminish a person's ability to adapt, leading to subtle recalibrations in stress responsivity that could be used to detect disease trajectories [38]. According to the life cycle model of stress and a growing body of preclinical research, regional volumes of these neurological structures in conjunction with biological signatures (e.g., hypercortisolism vs. hypocortisolism) can be used to predict differential risk profiles for specific psychopathologies (e.g., depression vs. PTSD) in adulthood as well as predict that traumatic experiences might have occurred in early life [36]. From a clinical perspective, however, direct measurement of central nervous system substrates is costly and potentially invasive, while indirect

assessment using peripheral biomarkers routinely collected in blood draws (e.g., glucose, cholesterol) could be compiled with stress biomarkers (e.g., adrenalin, cortisol).

Life stressors resulting from stigma are believed to render LGBT individuals more vulnerable to a variety of mental health conditions [39]. We believe that specific psychopathological trajectories can be demarcated by distinct biological signatures related to stress hormones and stress-related biomarkers. While extant literature on LGBT health has focused on psychosocial questionnaires and population surveys, few interdisciplinary studies have assessed physiological measures of biopsychosocial stress among LGBT individuals [40]. Moreover, with the exception of research focused on the HIV/AIDS pandemic among sexual minority men [41–46], biological stress mechanisms have not been extensively investigated among healthy LGBT populations. The following sections will provide the reader with emerging literature that applies measures of stress biology to understanding health inequities experienced by LGBT individuals.

Reactive Cortisol

Stress responses are adaptive in the short term, while long-term activations can result in physiological dysregulation. The *reactivity hypothesis* [47] proposes that exaggerated physiological and behavioral reactivity to stressors is a risk factor for stress-related diseases such as cardiovascular disease, among others [48, 49]. Such pathophysiological reactivity is potentially discernable by examining the magnitude of physiological stress responses in controlled laboratory settings.

Stress reactivity has traditionally been defined according to increases in stress biomarkers from baseline and upon stressor exposure; however, the prolongation and total duration of stress responses persisting after the stressor ceases are also critical to consider [50, 51]. Indeed, the reactivity hypothesis has been criticized for often ignoring or dismissing physiological *recovery*, a period after exposure that is characterized by much individual variability [52–54] and that may have significant clinical implications for LGBT individuals. For instance, rumination is associated with delayed cortisol recovery [55] and evidence suggests that sexual minorities may experience more ruminative processes than heterosexuals [23, 56, 57].

Stress reactivity and recovery could also extend clinically to treatments aimed at addressing psychological, emotional, and physiological responses to minority stress (e.g., systematic desensitization, biofeedback, and ecological momentary assessment (EMA)). EMA refers to methods that ask participants to repeatedly self-report their affective, behavioral, and cognitive states in naturalistic setting and has been used, for example, to demonstrate a relationship between a lifetime history of discrimination and current smoking status among Black and Latino men living in the USA [58]. We believe that using such tools to examine dynamic changes in stress reactivity and related phenomena that occur in response to gender and sexual minority stress processes would significantly expand our understanding of the factors that contribute to resilience and health among LGBT individuals.

A body of emerging research is assessing stress reactivity in LGBT populations. The first study on this topic was conducted by Hatzenbuehler and McLaughlin [59], who reported that LGB individuals growing up in less socially tolerant states evidenced blunted cortisol reactivity and hypothesized that this dampened HPA-axis pattern might indicate a pathophysiological profile associated with trauma and fatigue [60]. A novel study comparing LGB men and women to heterosexual individuals of both sexes demonstrated that sexual orientation modulates endocrine stress reactivity [61]. Eighty-seven participants were exposed to a psychosocial stressor involving public speech and mental arithmetic. Results revealed that lesbian/bisexual women demonstrated higher cortisol levels 40-min poststressor than heterosexual women, while gay/bisexual men demonstrated lower cortisol levels throughout testing compared to heterosexual men who peaked 20-min poststressor, as is usually observed [26].

The latter study showed that gay/bisexual men demonstrate stress reactivity profiles more closely aligned with those of heterosexual women, while lesbian/bisexual women show patterns more akin to those of heterosexual men. Although speculative, the delayed peak observed among lesbian/bisexual women could be indicative of ruminative processes. This would be consistent with reports by Hatzenbuehler and colleagues [23, 56, 57] who showed that lesbians and gay men are more ruminative than heterosexuals in response to stigma-related stressors. Importantly, rumination is associated with delayed poststressor cortisol recovery [55]. While ruminative cognitive-behavioral processes were not assessed, this approach represents a promising avenue for future inquiry, especially in the context of further understanding mental health.

In contrast to findings among women and consistent with a gender-based reversal in male-typical HPA-axis hyper-reactivity [62], lower overall cortisol concentrations were observed throughout testing among gay/bisexual men relative to heterosexual men. From a sexual minority stress perspective and in light of Hatzenbuehler and McLaughlin's [63] findings showing a blunted cortisol response among young sexual minority adults exposed to high-structural stigma environments as adolescents, this suggests that gay/bisexual men may be displaying HPA-axis downregulation. Indeed, an expanding literature is examining the relationship between hypocortisolism and severe stressors early in development [64, 65] or in the face of traumatic experiences [66], both of which are ubiquitous among sexual minority men [1]. The functional significance of this blunted cortisol stress reactivity to a psychosocial stressor must be further delineated since it is not clear whether this hormonal profile represents an adaptive or maladaptive process among sexual minority men. As will become evident in the following section, assessing circadian variations in stress hormone levels may prove to be a valuable technique that can be used to discern an individual's level of vulnerability and/or resilience.

Diurnal Cortisol

Stress hormones can be measured diurnally to capture naturalistic variation. For instance upon awakening, the *cortisol awakening response* (CAR) represents a normal surge in cortisol levels reaching maximal concentrations approximately

STRESS [ASSOCIATED] [↓ w/ coming out]

30 min after awakening [67]. This surge is followed by gradually declining cortisol concentrations throughout the day as pulsatile secretion decreases in amplitude and frequency [68]. The nadir usually occurs around midnight, after which cortisol levels start to rise again during the early morning hours [69]. These dynamics are normal mechanisms that help ensure adaptive functioning of metabolism, cognition, and so on. Measuring diurnal cortisol can be complemented by ecological momentary assessment of emotional and social processes occurring throughout the day that can have clinical applications.

Like stress reactivity, diurnal HPA-axis functioning can be used to identify disease vulnerabilities. A meta-analysis of 62 studies concluded that while the CAR is positively associated with workplace stress and general life stress, it is negatively associated with symptoms of burnout, fatigue, and exhaustion [70]. Hypocortisolism is a phenomenon that occurs in approximately 20–25% of patients suffering from stress-related diseases like chronic fatigue syndrome, fibromyalgia, PTSD, burnout [71, 72], and atypical depression, to name a few [60]. By contrast, increased HPA-axis functioning during the afternoon and evening has been strongly associated with depressive symptoms [73, 74]. Figure 4.3 illustrates how psychopathological conditions can be hypothetically conceptualized to differ in terms of distinct biological signatures that we believe can one day be applied in clinical practice to differentiate conditions with otherwise overlapping symptomatologies.

Diurnal cortisol is beginning to be applied in LGBT research with particular regard to stigma and "coming out." Benibgui [75] found that LGB emerging adults (ages 17–27) from Montréal with low social support experienced increased psychosocial stress that corresponded to increased

depressive symptoms and decreased self-esteem. While the majority of the sample (77–88%) had disclosed their sexual orientation to family members, LGB youth with increased internalized homophobia had flatter cortisol profiles that corresponded to an increased vulnerability to adverse mental health conditions [75]. Another study showed that compared to those who did not disclose their sexual orientation at work, disclosure was unexpectedly associated with higher cortisol levels and negative affect among LGB individuals [40]. Shedding light on this nonintuitive finding is another study showing that gay men who disclosed their sexual orientation to supervisors reported significantly higher hostility in their work environments, significantly lower perceived promotion opportunities, and significantly higher turnover intentions as evidenced by their desires to quit [76].

In contrast, disclosure of sexual orientation can also have positive effects on diurnal cortisol and mental health [77]. Using the same sample described earlier vis-à-vis stress reactivity [61], LGB individuals who had completely disclosed their sexual orientation to family and friends demonstrated lower morning cortisol levels and fewer symptoms of depression, anxiety, and burnout than those who had not completed the disclosure process. Future research would do well to also correlate disclosure to persons outside one's immediate interpersonal network.

Allostasis and Allostatic Load

Thus far, we have focused on stress hormones in a cortisol-centric manner that does not consider other related biological systems. As an inherently adaptive mechanism in reactive and diurnal contexts, physiological dynamics in

Fig. 4.3 Hypothetical diurnal cortisol profiles in normal and psychopathological conditions

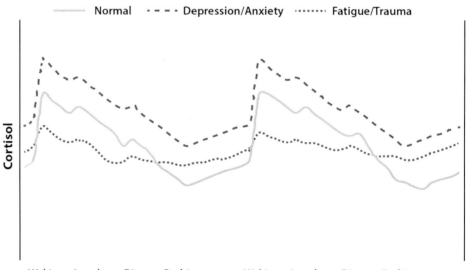

Diurnal cortisol variation in mental health conditions

―― Normal   - ‑ ‑ Depression/Anxiety   ········ Fatigue/Trauma

Cortisol

Waking Lunch   Dinner Bedtime   Waking Lunch   Dinner Bedtime

stress hormone functions are examples of *allostasis*, defined as adaptive biological processes that preserve "stability through change" [78]. The neurobiologist Sterling and the epidemiologist Eyer coined the term *allostasis* to describe dynamic, multifaceted biological processes that maintain physiological stability by recalibrating homeostatic parameters and matching them appropriately to meet environmental demands [78]. Analogous to our understanding of resilient systems that have the capacity to dynamically adjust and stabilize when faced with perturbations [79], allostatic processes likewise alter metabolic functioning via compensatory and anticipatory mechanisms in both reactive and diurnal contexts. Compensatory alterations during acute stress include, for example, decreased digestive and bodily growth/repair processes that are adjusted to accommodate increased neurological, cardiovascular, respiratory, and immunological activities that are metabolically taxing. Under these circumstances, allostasis becomes taxing and differs from normal responsivity as an allostatic state.

Four potential pathophysiological profiles representing allostatic states have been outlined [39]. First, *repeatedly activated responses* refer to simply too much stress in the form of repeated, novel events that cause cumulative elevations of stress mediators over sustained periods of time. Second, *nonhabituating responses* refer to failure to habituate or adapt to the same stressor that leads to the overuse of stress mediators because of the failure of the body to dampen or eliminate the hormonal stress response to a repeated event. Third, *prolonged responses* represent a failure to shut off either the hormonal stress response or to display the normal trough of the circadian patterns. Fourth, *inadequate responses* represent hypoactive stress responses that may involuntarily allow other systems, such as inflammation, to become hyperactive. In essence, allostatic states reflect response patterns in which physiological systems become over or underactive, leading to multisystemic physiological dysregulations.

The multisystemic strain attributable to chronic stress, adversity, and trauma is referred to as allostatic load [80]. *Allostatic load* (AL) is defined as the multisystemic "wear and tear" the brain and the rest of the body experience when repeated allostatic responses exact their noxious toll when exposed to chronic stress. Under such conditions, stress hormones like adrenaline and cortisol first become misbalanced and induce an interconnected cascade of interdependent biological processes that sequentially collapse as individual biomarkers become dysregulated and lead to disease outcomes [81]. AL can be indexed using combinations of stress-related biomarkers to represent physiological dysregulation [82].

Validation using longitudinal data from the MacArthur Studies of Successful Aging cohort led to a *count-based AL index* representing the following ten biomarkers [82]: 12-h urinary cortisol, adrenaline, and noradrenaline output; serum dehydroepiandrosterone-sulfate (DHEA-S), high-density lipoprotein (HDL), and HDL-to-total cholesterol ratio; plasma glycosylated hemoglobin; aggregate systolic and diastolic blood pressures; and waist-to-hip-ratio. Participants' values falling within high-risk quartiles (clinical and preclinical ranges based on percentiles) with respect to the sample's biomarker distributions are dichotomized as "1" and those within normal ranges as "0." Once tabulated, these are summed to yield an AL index ranging from a possible 0 to 10 which can then be used to predict health outcomes.

The thematic advantages of applying an elevated-risk-zone system when scoring AL are fivefold as they represent (1) *early warning signals*, since cutoffs are anchored at subclinical thresholds; (2) *multi-finality*, in that similar AL algorithms predict different tertiary outcomes; (3) *flexibility*, since calculations are based on different biomarker combinations; (4) *synergism* that captures the cumulative interaction of numerous biomarkers; and finally (5) *antecedents* that powerfully predict individual variation in AL [83]. In sum, AL algorithms are objective reflections of biological functioning that are intricately interconnected with genetic, neurological, developmental, behavioral, cognitive, and social factors.

Clinical Allostatic Load Index

The AL index is thus far a research measure that may become useful as a clinical tool in the future; however, it is not yet ready for prime time, as clinical norms have yet to be established. In cases where medical professionals currently measure other stress-related biomarkers in standard blood tests (e.g., fibrinogen, cytokines, cortisol), attention is typically placed on values reaching clinically significant levels based on population norms if these exist for any given novel biomarker. For readers interested in knowing how to determine an AL index for clinical and research investigative purposes, a simple formulation can be used to calculate the index based on clinical reference ranges used in current practice for diagnostic purposes. For each biomarker value included, a subclinical cutoff can be easily calculated based on normative clinical ranges. Note that for some emerging biomarkers, like cortisol, clinical norms have yet to be established.

For example, consider total cholesterol, with a normal range between 3.3 and 5.2 nmol/L. First, to determine the *range*, subtract the lower limit from the upper limit (5.2 − 3.3 = 1.9). Second, to determine the *quartile*, divide the range by four (1.9/4 = 0.475). Finally, to determine the *cutoff*, either subtract the quartile from the upper limit for the upper cutoff (5.2 − 0.475 = 4.725) or add the quartile to the lower limit for the lower cutoff (3.3 + 0.475 = 3.775) in the case of biomarkers such as HDL cholesterol, DHEA-S, and albumin where lower levels may be associated with health risk. Based on this example, a patient with total cholesterol of 4.725 nmol/L or higher would receive a score of "1," while values below this cutoff would be scored as "0." A clinical AL index is therefore the sum of subclinically dysregulated biomarkers for a given individual. Previous work demonstrated that a clinical AL index was associated with increased subjective reports of chronic stress, frequency of burnout symptoms, and hypocortisolemic profiles characteristic of fatigue states [72].

A review by Juster et al. [84] of nearly 60 empirical studies suggests that AL indices incorporating subclinical ranges for numerous biomarkers (mean = 10; range = 4–17) predict clinical outcomes better than traditional biomedical methods that address only clinical thresholds for single biomarkers. Importantly, AL inclusion of neuroendocrine and/or immune biomarkers is stronger than metabolic syndrome parameters or systemic clusters in the prediction of stress-related conditions like cardiovascular disease and psychopathology. The most consistent causes of AL are increased age, low socioeconomic status, non-white race/ethnicity, workplace stress, and involvement in emotionally taxing activities such as caregiving. In the context of LGBT health, Fig. 4.4 illustrates how sexual minority stress relates to stress physiology and AL that are in turn predictive of both physical and mental health conditions.

Sexual orientation and developmental aspects related to sexual identity formation are related to AL. In the same study that assessed diurnal cortisol described above [77], analyses examined 21 biomarkers related to neuroendocrine, immune, metabolic, and cardiovascular functioning and teased apart between-group (sexual orientation) and within-group (disclosure processes) differences. Results showed no between-group differences as a function of sexual orientation except that gay/bisexual men evidenced fewer depressive symptoms and AL driven by lower triglycerides, BMI, and cytokine levels than heterosexual men. While no overall AL differences were found as a function of full disclosure, a follow-up analysis found that retrospective coping strategies during sexual identity formation were critical. Specifically, retrospective avoidance coping strategies (e.g., trying to forget everything, keeping one's emotions to one's self, using medication to feel better) during sexual identity formation and disclosure were associated with current elevations in perceived stress, daily hassles, and AL [85]. By contrast, seeking social support was associated with less perceived stress. Taken together, these preliminary findings suggest that the coping strategies enacted during key developmental periods unique to LGBT individuals could help protect against AL and poorer mental health.

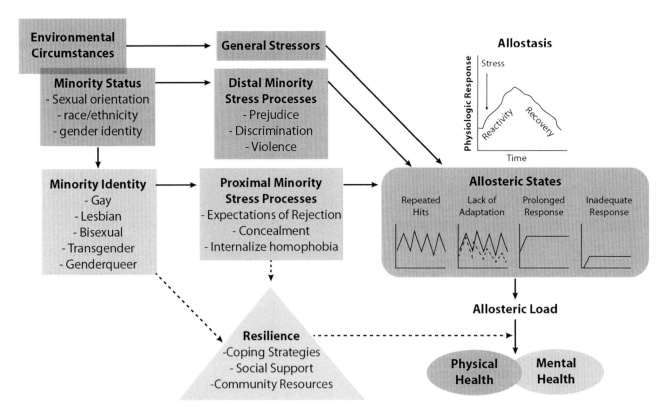

Fig. 4.4 Conceptual model of sexual minority stress and allostatic load (Adapted from Refs. [6, 36])

Psychosocial Implications and Clinical Perspectives

While further research is needed to explore and delineate the potential pathways to resilience for LGBT individuals, a growing body of research points to the benefits of establishing identity-related social support for LGBT individuals [7, 86–87]. DiFulvio and colleagues [86] specifically note the value of *social connectedness* for LGBT youth, which refers to the perception of individuals that they belong, are cared for, and can feel empowered within a given context. In a qualitative study utilizing in-depth interviews with 15 sexual minority youth, these authors outlined a process of negotiating an identity seen as different and defective with family and friends and, in the face of rejection, developing the ability to reclaim this identity and derive empowerment through connections with similar peers.

The importance of having accepting others in one's support network and the benefits conferred by eliminating individuals who might be critical or unsupportive of one's sexual identity is also critical for older LGBT adults [88]. Surprisingly, Snapp and colleagues did not find any impact of community support on development of self-esteem among LGBT young adults, whereas both family and peer support were found to be strong predictors [87]. Perhaps more worrisome, exposure to similar others increases sexual risk-taking among LGBT young adults [89]. Thus, healthcare providers must be sensitive to the fact that mere exposure to similar others and including them in one's support network does not guarantee positive effects on mental health and health behaviors. The key feature is that support network members be included because they are aware of the individual's sexual identity and can provide acceptance and affirmation.

One vital way in which healthcare providers can provide affirmation and acceptance for an LGBT person's sexual and/or gender identities is by identifying and normalizing the impact of minority stress and trauma on the individual's lived experience. This normalization process involves providing psychoeducation to LGBT individuals regarding the multifaceted effects of family, societal, and peer rejection and violence, as well as assurance that it is common and understandable to develop a plethora of thoughts, feelings, physiological reactions (e.g., heart racing, sweating, etc.), and behaviors in response to threats to one's identity and safety. Indeed, the hypervigilance that some individuals develop in response to stigma-related stressors can in fact be adaptive in encouraging avoidance of situations in which safety might be compromised.

Normalizing these experiences can help provide LGBT individuals with avenues to form more supportive connections (particularly in a group-based context), and derive empowerment by attributing their distress to stigma rather than personal failings and recognizing that their emotional, cognitive, and physiological responses make sense in light of the hostility of their social environments [90]. Psychoeducation can also include providing information on the psychobiology of stress reactivity in the context of stigma, as has been discussed by Fisher [91] in the context of responding to past trauma. Specifically, Fisher [91] suggests that providing psychoeducation on the psychobiology of self-injurious behaviors in the midst of a traumatic experience might help decrease an individual's experience of shame and encourage exploration of more adaptive coping strategies [91]. Unfortunately, no published research has examined the effect of psychoeducation on the psychobiology of response to identity-based stigma and trauma or the psychological well-being and coping strategies of LGBT individuals. While psychoeducation may be a therapeutically useful tool, providers must utilize this strategy with caution and only when the individual has developed a sense of security and trust in the relationship with the provider.

It should be noted that we have, for the most part, discussed responses to stress and treatment approaches as uniform among LGBT individuals, perhaps inadvertently reiterating the perceived monolithic nature of the LGBT community. In actuality, it is important for researchers and practitioners to note that experiences of sexual minority stress can differ widely on the basis of an individual's gender, gender identity, and sexual orientation. These experiences can also differ vastly when the intersections of race, physical ability, age, and other identity categories are taken into account. For example, the prejudicial experiences directed at *genderqueer* individuals (i.e., those who do not identify with the gender binary as male nor female or who may view their identity as beyond gender or in-between) may be significantly different from those directed toward male-to-female or female-to-male transgender individuals [21]. Therefore, responses demonstrated by individuals in response to minority stressors must be examined within the diversity of their identities and lived experiences.

In order to maximize the ability of an intervention to foster resilience, psychoeducation may be most effective when it includes opportunities to build supportive networks and a strong emphasis on identifying an individual's strengths and positive coping strategies in response to both past and ongoing stigma- and trauma-based stressors [92]. Healthcare providers can demonstrate affirmation of their LGBT individuals' lived experiences by pointing out that the very resources utilized to adapt to minority stress can be the very same resources used during recovery from the effects of enacted and felt stigma.

Social Policy Implications

Knowledge generated in the stress-disease literature expands our understanding of health inequalities that carry critical conceptual implications for social policy. Social justice focuses on the philosophy of equality of opportunity. For example, *gender relations* refers to expectations related to etiquette and understanding how we relate to each other, while *institutionalized gender* refers to the ways that gender is constructed within large social systems that dictate value systems, social class, and hierarchies of privilege [93]. Institutionalized stigma and heterosexism include, for example, the denial of marriage rights, disadvantaged treatment in schools and workplaces, and disenfranchisement of sociocultural resources like religion and spirituality that often dehumanize LGBT individuals and contribute to further distress [1, 94]. These macro-level factors have important conceptual implications for scientist-practitioners. For example, the use of stress biomarkers could be used to discern the existence of LGBT healthcare inequalities before and after social policy changes trickle down into systems more proximate to the individual.

Social inequalities have health consequences [95]. Compelling research shows that LGBT Americans living in states without policies that protect against hate crimes and employment discrimination experience significantly higher rates of mental distress than those living in states with protective policies [96]. Likewise, LGBT individuals living in states with constitutional amendments banning same-sex marriage experience increased rates of generalized anxiety disorder, depressive disorders, and alcohol abuse. Geopolitical strata with antigay prejudice are associated with increased rates of all-cause mortality among sexual minorities [97]. By contrast, those living in states that recognize same-sex marriages show no increased development of these conditions [98].

Social policy changes can affect the health of sexual minorities. A pioneering study documented significant decreases in general medical and mental healthcare visits and costs among gay men 12 months after Massachusetts legalized same-sex marriage [99]. This study demonstrates how changes in distal policies can progressively eliminate institutionalized stigma and promote public health benefits [99]. Given ongoing debate in the United States and worldwide concerning, for example, same-sex marriage, a fascinating social experiment would be to assess biological stress indices as a function of American states with and without protective policies over time to further understand the relation between social policy and biological processes. In theory, LGBT Americans exposed to less structural stigma should evidence different biological signatures than LGBT individuals from less progressive geo-political strata.

Structural stigma experienced by sexual and gender diverse minorities is modifiable. North America is undergoing geo-political changes that necessitate research evidence to help inform, for instance, the remaining American states without protective legislations and many nations worldwide that still criminalize homosexuality. This makes the comprehensive measurement of stress biomarkers a crucial endeavor, providing us with an objective biometric of macro-level effects that can inform policy makers of the pernicious effects of institutionalized gender and how to improve the health of marginalized groups. The health and well-being of sexual minorities is not a matter of political debate but a matter of public health.

Practitioners can help LGBT clients identify their internal strengths and foster resilience by creating support networks and engaging in advocacy efforts for public policy change and social reform. Thus, practitioners must become informed about local resources in order to refer their clients to advocacy groups, activist events, panel discussions, and pride marches where it is possible to speak out against the experiences of stigma and violence and receive community support [86]. Commitment to and participation in such community engagement can, as DiFulvio eloquently states, "serve as a way for [LGBT individuals] to make meaning of an identity that has been silenced and allows them to regain a sense of power over their lives" (p. 616). At the same time, in light of the identity-based violence that has, through pervasive societal stigma, become an inextricable part of the social fabric of LGBT lived experience, recommendations to engage in community advocacy efforts must be made collaboratively with LGBT clients and following a thorough assessment of the extent of their support network and safety.

Case Scenario

Ashlee is a 19-year-old White female who grew up in the rural Midwest and is just completing her first year of college (Fig. 4.5). She presents to the campus health clinic complaining of significant fatigue, irritability, and recent pain with urination. Ashlee reports that she has been oversleeping, missing her classes, and generally feeling "kinda blah." During the visit, she indicates to you that this is her first time at the campus health clinic and inquires whether her parents might find out about the appointment or have access to her records. She seems nervous about being at the clinic and you notice her tendency to keep an eye on the exit. During the intake, Ashlee looks surprised when you ask her about recent sexual partners as part of the routine intake process. She thanks you for not assuming her partners' genders and shares that during a recent visit to

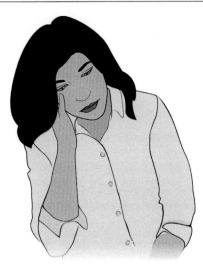

Fig. 4.5 Ashlee is a 19-year-old white female who grew up in the rural Midwest and is just completing her first year of college

her family physician, she was asked "how many men" she had been sexual with over the past year. Ashlee disclosed that she has recently come out to herself and her college friends that she is a lesbian. She is tearful in describing her expectation that her family will "disown" her if they learn about her sexual orientation. She also fears that her parents may become physically violent towards her, as they have hit her in the past when they didn't like decisions she'd made.

Discussion Questions

1. How can healthcare agencies and institutions ensure inclusivity of sexual and gender minorities when it comes to forms/paperwork, screening questions, and routine intake procedures?
2. What additional information might you want or need to gather from this patient? Why or how might that information be useful in your assessment and treatment of Ashlee?
3. How might the trauma of being rejected by one's family impact biomarkers and AL?
4. How can healthcare agencies and institutions communicate that they are safe and affirming environments for LGBT individuals?
5. What are a healthcare provider's legal and ethical responsibilities when a patient discloses feeling at risk of violence?

Summary Practice Points

- Patients like Ashlee who have trauma histories commonly present with "garden variety," stress-related symptoms and concerns of somatic health. Arriving at an accurate diagnosis can be challenging and necessitates an integrated approach with diverse professionals.
- It is important to screen all patients for trauma, and particularly those who, like Ashlee, appear to be triggered when asked about sexual contact. Screening should include specific questions about sexual assault, abuse, coercion or harassment, and intimate partner violence.
- In addition to considering the contribution of Ashlee's sexual identity to her lived experience, it is important to inquire about other, overlapping stigmatized identities (e.g., rural background, history of sexual abuse, etc.), as research suggests that multiple stressors can produce additive effects.

Key issues to explore with patients like Ashlee include sexual health, self-acceptance of sexual minority identity, and disclosure, including a consideration of the differential mental health impact of nondisclosure versus active concealment of identity. Additionally, it is important to learn more about Ashlee's current coping mechanisms (positive and negative), particularly the presence or absence of supportive interpersonal connections. As noted throughout this chapter, enhancing one's engagement with affirming and accepting social networks is an important predictor of health and well-being among LGBT populations.

References

1. IOM. The health of lesbian, gay, bisexual, and transgender people: building a foundation for better understanding. Washington, DC: The National Academies Press; 2011.
2. Beauchamp D. Sexual orientation and victimization, 2004. In: Statistics CCfJ, editor. . Ottawa: Statistics Canada. p. 2004.
3. Mays VM, Cochran SD. Mental health correlates of perceived discrimination among lesbian, gay, and bisexual adults in the United States. Am J Public Health. 2001;91(11):1869–76.
4. National Coalition of Anti-Violence Programs. 2013 report on lesbian, gay, bisexual, transgender, queen and HIV-affected hate violence. 2014. Accessed 6 April 2017. Available at: http://www.avp.org/storage/documents/2013_ncavp_hvreport_final.pdf.
5. Meyer IH. Minority stress and mental health in gay men. J Health Soc Behav. 1995;36(1):38–56.
6. Meyer IH. Prejudice, social stress, and mental health in lesbian, gay, and bisexual populations: conceptual issues and research evidence. Psychol Bull. 2003;129(5):674–97.

7. Grossman AH, D'Augelli AR, Hershberger SL. Social support networks of lesbian, gay, and bisexual adults 60 years of age and older. J Gerentol. 1999;55:171–9.

8. Meyer IH. Prejudice and discrimination as social stressors. In: Meyer IH, Northridge ME, editors. The health of sexual minorities: public health perspectives on lesbian, gay, bisexual, and transgender populations. New York: Springer; 2007. p. 242–67.

9. Abercrombie HC, Speck NS, Monticelli RM. Endogenous cortisol elevations are related to memory facilitation only in individuals who are emotionally aroused. Psychoneuroendocrinology. 2006;31(2):187–96.

10. Bjorkman M, Malterud K. Lesbian women coping with challenges of minority stress: a qualitative study. Scand J Public Health. 2012;40(3):239–44.

11. Frost DM, Lehavot K, Meyer IH. Minority stress and physical health among sexual minority individuals. J Behav Med. 2015;38(1):1–8.

12. Lingiardi V, Baiocco R, Nardell N. Measures of internalized sexual stigma for lesbians and gay men: a new scale. J Homosex. 2012;59:1191–210.

13. Mason TB, Lewis RJ. Minority stress and binge eating among lesbian and bisexual women. J Homosex. 2015;62(7):971–92.

14. Szymanski DM, Chung YB. The lesbian internalized homophobia scale: a rational/theoretical approach. J Homosex. 2001;41(2):37–52.

15. Bockting WO, Miner MH, Swinburne Romine RE, Hamilton A, Coleman E. Stigma, mental health, and resilience in an online sample of the US transgender population. Am J Public Health. 2013;103(5):943–51.

16. Gamarel KE, Reisner SL, Laurenceau JP, Nemoto T, Operario D. Gender minority stress, mental health, and relationship quality: a dyadic investigation of transgender women and their cisgender male partners. J Fam Psychol. 2014;28(4):437–47.

17. Stuenkel D, Wong V. "Stigma" 8thChronic illness: Impact and interventions. 2013.

18. Stueknel DL, Wong VK. Stigma. In: Larsen PD, Lubkin IM, editors. Chronic illness: impact and intervention. Boston: Jones and Bartlett; 2009.

19. Herek GM, Chopp R, Strohl D. Sexual stigma: putting sexual minority health issues in context. In: Meyer IH, Northridge ME, editors. The health of sexual minorities: public health perspectives on lesbian, gay, bisexual, and transgender populations. New York: Springer Science and Business Media; 2007. p. 171–208.

20. Weiss JM. GL vs. BT: the archaeology of biphobia and transphobia within the U.S. gay and lesbian community. J Bisexuality. 2004;3:25–55.

21. Worthen M. An argument for separate analyses of attitudes towards lesbian, gay, and bisexual women, MtF and Ftm transgender individuals. Sex Roles. 2013;68:703–23.

22. Warriner K, Nagoshi CT, Nagoshi JL. Correlates of homophobia, transphobia, and internalized homophobia in gay or lesbian and heterosexual samples. J Homosex. 2013;60:1297–314.

23. Hatzenbuehler ML. How does sexual minority stigma "get under the skin"? A psychological mediation framework. Psychol Bull. 2009;135(5):707–30.

24. Levine S. Developmental determinants of sensitivity and resistance to stress. Psychoneuroendocrinology. 2005;30(10):939–46.

25. Levine S, Ursin H. What is stress? In: Brown MR, Koob GF, Rivier C, editors. Stress neurobiology and neuroendocrinology. New York: Marcel Dekker; 1991. p. 3–21.

26. Dickerson SS, Kemeny ME. Acute stressors and cortisol reactivity: a meta-analytic review. Psychosom Med. 2002;54:105–23.

27. Lupien SJ, Ouelle-Morin, I., Hupback, A., Walker, D., Tu, M.T., Buss, C., Pruessner, J, McEwen, B.S. Beyond the stress concept: allostatic load – a developmental biological and cognitive perspective. In: Cicchetti D, editor. Handbook series on developmental psychopathology. Wisconsin 2006. p. 784–809.

28. Sapolsky RM, Romero LM, Munck AU. How do glucocorticoids influence stress responses? Integrating permissive, suppressive, stimulatory, and preparative actions. Endocr Rev. 2000;21(1):55–89.

29. McEwen BS, Wingfield JC. The concept of allostasis in biology and biomedicine. Horm Behav. 2003;43:2–15.

30. McEwen BS, Weiss JM, Schwartz LS. Selective retention of corticosterone by limbic structures in rat brain. Nature. 1968;220(5170):911–2.

31. Gray TS, Bingaman EW. The amygdala: corticotropin-releasing factor, steroids, and stress. Crit Rev Neurobiol. 1996;10(2):155–68.

32. Reul JM, de Kloet ER. Two receptor systems for corticosterone in rat brain: microdistribution and differential occupation. Endocrinology. 1985;117(6):2505–11.

33. Sanchez MM, Young LJ, Plotsky PM, Insel TR. Distribution of corticosteroid receptors in the rhesus brain: relative absence of glucocorticoid receptors in the hippocampal formation. J Neurosci. 2000;20(12):4657–68.

34. Thayer JF, Lane RD. Claude Bernard and the heart-brain connection: further elaboration of a model of neurovisceral integration. Neurosci Biobehav Rev. 2009;33(2):81–8.

35. McEwen BS. Protection and damage from acute and chronic stress: allostasis and allostatic overload and relevance to the pathophysiology of psychiatric disorders. Ann N Y Acad Sci. 2004;1032:1–7.

36. Lupien SJ, McEwen BS, Gunnar MR, Heim C. Effects of stress throughout the lifespan on the brain, behaviour and cognition. Nat Rev Neurosci. 2009;10(6):434–45.

37. Gould E, McEwen BS, Tanapat P, Galea LA, Fuchs E. Neurogenesis in the dentate gyrus of the adult tree shrew is regulated by psychosocial stress and NMDA receptor activation. J Neurosci. 1997;17(7):2492–8.

38. McEwen BS. Protective and damaging effects of stress mediators. N Engl J Med. 1998;338(3):171–9.

39. Herek GM. Sexual stigma and sexual prejudice in the United States: a conceptual framework. In: Hope DA, editor. Contemporary perspectives on lesbian, gay, and bisexual identities. New York: Springer Science + Business Media; 2009. p. 65–111.

40. Huebner DM, Davis MC. Gay and bisexual men who disclose their sexual orientations in the workplace have higher workday levels of salivary cortisol and negative affect. Ann Behav Med. 2005;30(3):260–7.

41. Leserman J, Petitto JM, Golden RN, Gaynes BN, Gu H, Perkins DO, et al. Impact of stressful life events, depression, social support, coping, and cortisol on progression to AIDS. Am J Psychiatry. 2000;157(8):1221–8.

42. Kertzner RM, Goetz R, Todak G, Cooper T, Lin SH, Reddy MM, et al. Cortisol levels, immune status, and mood in homosexual men with and without HIV infection. Am J Psychiatry. 1993;150(11):1674–8.

43. Hengge UR, Reimann G, Schafer A, Goos M. HIV-positive men differ in immunologic but not catecholamine response to an acute psychological stressor. Psychoneuroendocrinology. 2003;28(5):643–56.

44. Greeson JM, Hurwitz BE, Llabre MM, Schneiderman N, Penedo FJ, Klimas NG. Psychological distress, killer lymphocytes and disease severity in HIV/AIDS. Brain Behav Immun. 2008;22(6):901–11.

45. Antoni MH, Schneiderman N, Klimas N, LaPerriere A, Ironson G, Fletcher MA. Disparities in psychological, neuroendocrine, and immunologic patterns in asymptomatic HIV-1 seropositive and seronegative gay men. Biol Psychiatry. 1991;29(10):1023–41.

46. Gorman JM, Kertzner R, Cooper T, Goetz RR, Lagomasino I, Novacenko H, et al. Glucocorticoid level and neuropsychiatric

symptoms in homosexual men with HIV infection. Am J Psychiatry. 1991;148(1):41–5.

47. Manuck SB. Cardiovascular reactivity in cardiovascular disease: "once more unto the breach". Int J Behav Med. 1994;1(1):4–31.

48. Lovallo WR. Cardiovascular responses to stress and disease outcomes: a test of the reactivity hypothesis. Hypertension. 2010;55(4):842–3.

49. Lovallo WR, Gerin W. Psychophysiological reactivity: mechanisms and pathways to cardiovascular disease. Psychosom Med. 2003;65(1):36–45.

50. Brosschot JF, Pieper S, Thayer JF. Expanding stress theory: prolonged activation and perseverative cognition. Psychoneuroendocrinology. 2005;30(10):1043–9.

51. Brosschot JF. Markers of chronic stress: prolonged physiological activation and (un)conscious perseverative cognition. Neurosci Biobehav Rev. 2010;35(1):46–50.

52. Rutledge T, Linden W, Paul D. Cardiovascular recovery from acute laboratory stress: reliability and concurrent validity. Psychosom Med. 2000;62(5):648–54.

53. Earle TL, Linden W, Weinberg J. Differential effects of harassment on cardiovascular and salivary cortisol stress reactivity and recovery in women and men. J Psychosom Res. 1999;46(2):125–41.

54. Linden W, Earle TL, Gerin W, Christenfeld N. Physiological stress reactivity and recovery: conceptual siblings separated at birth? J Psychosom Res. 1997;42(2):117–35.

55. Stewart JG, Mazurka R, Bond L, Wynne-Edwards KE, Harkness KL. Rumination and impaired cortisol recovery following a social stressor in adolescent depression. J Abnorm Child Psychol. 2013;41 (7):1015–26.

56. Hatzenbuehler ML, McLaughlin KA, Nolen-Hoeksema S. Emotion regulation and internalizing symptoms in a longitudinal study of sexual minority and heterosexual adolescents. J Child Psychol Psychiatry. 2008;49(12):1270–8.

57. Hatzenbuehler ML, Nolen-Hoeksema S, Dovidio J. How does stigma "get under the skin"?: the mediating role of emotion regulation. Psychol Sci. 2009;20(10):1282–9.

58. Brondolo E, Monge A, Agosta J, Tobin JN, Cassells A, Stanton C, et al. Perceived ethnic discrimination and cigarette smoking: examining the moderating effects of race/ethnicity and gender in a sample of Black and Latino urban adults. J Behav Med. 2015;38 (4):689–700.

59. Hatzenbuehler, M.L. and McLaughlin, K.A., 2014. Structural stigma and hypothalamic–pituitary–adrenocortical axis reactivity in lesbian, gay, and bisexual young adults. Ann Behav Med, 47 (1), pp.39–47.

60. Fries E, Hesse J, Hellhammer J, Hellhammer DH. A new view on hypocortisolism. Psychoneuroendocrinology. 2005;30(10):1010–6.

61. Juster RP, Hatzenbuehler ML, Mendrek A, Pfaus JG, Smith NG, Johnson PJ, et al. Sexual orientation modulates endocrine stress reactivity. Biol Psychiatry. 2015;77(7):668–76.

62. Kirschbaum C, Wust S, Hellhammer D. Consistent sex differences in cortisol responses to psychological stress. Psychosom Med. 1992;54(6):648–57.

63. Hatzenbuehler ML, McLaughlin KA. Structural stigma and hypothalamic-pituitary-adrenocortical axis reactivity in lesbian, gay, and bisexual young adults. Ann Behav Med. 2013;47:39–47.

64. Gunnar MR, Frenn K, Wewerka SS, Van Ryzin MJ. Moderate versus severe early life stress: associations with stress reactivity and regulation in 10–12-year-old children. Psychoneuroendocrinology. 2009;34(1):62–75.

65. MacMillan HL, Georgiades K, Duku EK, Shea A, Steiner M, Niec A, et al. Cortisol response to stress in female youths exposed to childhood maltreatment: results of the youth mood project. Biol Psychiatry. 2009;66(1):62–8.

66. Yehuda R, Halligan SL, Golier JA, Grossman R, Bierer LM. Effects of trauma exposure on the cortisol response to dexamethasone administration in PTSD and major depressive disorder. Psychoneuroendocrinology. 2004;29(3):389–404.

67. Pruessner JC, Wolf OT, Hellhammer DH, Buske-Kirschbaum A, von Auer K, Jobst S, et al. Free cortisol levels after awakening: a reliable biological marker for the assessment of adrenocortical activity. Life Sci. 1997;61(26):2539–49.

68. Clow A, Hucklebridge F, Stalder T, Evans P, Thorn L. The cortisol awakening response: more than a measure of HPA axis function. Neurosci Biobehav Rev. 2010;35(1):97–103.

69. Loucks E, Juster RP, Pruessner JC. Neuroendocrine biomarkers, allostatic load, and the challenge of measurement: a commentary on Gersten. Soc Sci Med. 2008;66:525–30.

70. Chida Y, Steptoe A. Cortisol awakening response and psychosocial factors: a systematic review and meta-analysis. Biol Psychol. 2009;80(3):265–78.

71. Marchand A, Juster RP, Durand P, Lupien SJ. Burnout symptom sub-types and cortisol profiles: what's burning most? Psychoneuroendocrinology. 2014;40:27–36.

72. Juster RP, Sindi S, Marin MF, Perna A, Hashemi A, Pruessner JC, et al. A clinical allostatic load index is associated with burnout symptoms and hypocortisolemic profiles in healthy workers. Psychoneuroendocrinology. 2011;36(6):797–805.

73. Muhtz C, Zyriax BC, Klahn T, Windler E, Otte C. Depressive symptoms and metabolic risk: effects of cortisol and gender. Psychoneuroendocrinology. 2009;34(7):1004–11.

74. Deuschle M, Schweiger U, Weber B, Gotthardt U, Korner A, Schmider J, et al. Diurnal activity and pulsatility of the hypothalamus-pituitary-adrenal system in male depressed patients and healthy controls. J Clin Endocrinol Metab. 1997;82(1):234–8.

75. Benibgui M. Mental health challenges and resilience in lesbian, gay, and bisexual young adults: biological and psychological internalization of minority stress and victimization. Montreal: Concordia University; 2010.

76. Tejeda M. Nondiscrimination policies and sexual identity disclosure: do they make a difference in employee outcomes? Empl Responsib Rights J. 2006;18(1):45–59.

77. Juster RP, Smith NG, Ouellet E, Sindi S, Lupien SJ. Sexual orientation and disclosure in relation to psychiatric symptoms, diurnal cortisol, and allostatic load. Psychosom Med. 2013;75(2):103–16.

78. Sterling P, Eyer J. Allostasis: a new paradigm to explain arousal pathology. In: Fisher S, Reason J, editors. Handbook of life stress, cognition and health. New York: Wiley; 1988. p. 629–49.

79. Cicchetti D. Annual Research Review: resilient functioning in maltreated children – past, present, and future perspectives. J Child Psychol Psychiatry. 2013;54(4):402–22.

80. McEwen BS, Stellar E. Stress and the individual. Mechanisms leading to disease. Arch Intern Med. 1993;153(18):2093–101.

81. Juster RP, Bizik G, Picard M, Arsenault-Lapierre G, Sindi S, Trepanier L, et al. A transdisciplinary perspective of chronic stress in relation to psychopathology throughout life span development. Dev Psychopathol. 2011;23(3):725–76.

82. Seeman E, Singer BH, Rowe J, Horwitz RI, McEwen B. Price of adaptation – allostatic load and its health consequences. Arch Intern Med. 1997;157:2259–68.

83. Singer B, Ryff CD, Seeman T. Operationalizing allostatic load. In: Schulkin J, editor. Allostasis, homeostasis, and the costs of psychological adaptation. New York: Cambridge University Press; 2004. p. 113–49.

84. Juster RP, McEwen BS, Lupien SJ. Allostatic load biomarkers of chronic stress and impact on health and cognition. Neurosci Biobehav Rev. 2010;35(1):2–16.

85. Juster RP, Ouellet E, Lefebvre-Louis JP, Sindi S, Johnson PJ, Smith NG, et al. Retrospective coping strategies during sexual identity formation and current biopsychosocial stress. Anxiety Stress Coping. 2016;29(2):119–38

86. DiFulvio GT. Sexual minority youth, social connection and resilience: from personal struggle to collective identity. Soc Sci Med. 2011;72(10):1611–7.

87. Snapp S, Watson RJ, Russell ST, Diaz RM, Ryan C. Social support networks for LGBT young adults: low cost strategies for positive adjustment. Fam Relat. 2015;64:420–30.

88. D'Augelli AR, Hershberger SL, Pilkington NW. Lesbian, gay, and bisexual youth and their families: disclosure of sexual orientation and its consequences. Am J Orthopsychiatry 1998;68(3):361–371; discussion 72–5.

89. Wright ER, Perry BL. Sexual identity distress, social support, and the health of gay, lesbian, and bisexual youth. J Homosex. 2006;51 (1):81–110.

90. Pachankis JE, Hatzenbuehler ML, Hickson F, Weatherburn P, Berg RC, Marcus U, et al. Hidden from health: structural stigma, sexual orientation concealment, and HIV across 38 countries in the European MSM Internet Survey. AIDS. 2015;29 (10):1239–46.

91. Fisher J, editor. The work stabilization in trauma treatment. Paper presented at Trauma Center Lecture Series, Boston; 1999.

92. Howard JM, Goelitz A. Psychoeducation as a response to community disaster. Brief Treat Crisis Intervent. 2004;4:1–10.

93. Johnson JL, Greaves L, Repta R. Better science with sex and gender: a primer of health research. Ottawa: Canadian Institutes for Health Research Institute of Gender and Health; 2007.

94. Herek GM, Garnets LD. Sexual orientation and mental health. Annu Rev Clin Psychol. 2007;3:353–75.

95. Hatzenbuehler ML. Social factors as determinants of mental health disparities in LGB populations: implications for public policy. Soc Issues Policy Rev. 2010;4(1):31–62.

96. Hatzenbuehler ML, Keyes KM, Hasin DS. State-level policies and psychiatric morbidity in lesbian, gay, and bisexual populations. Am J Public Health. 2009;99(12):2275–81.

97. Hatzenbuehler ML, Bellatorre A, Lee Y, Finch BK, Muennig P, Fiscella K. Structural stigma and all-cause mortality in sexual minority populations. Soc Sci Med. 2014;103:33–41.

98. Hatzenbuehler ML, McLaughlin KA, Keyes KM, Hasin DS. The impact of institutional discrimination on psychiatric disorders in lesbian, gay, and bisexual populations: a prospective study. Am J Public Health. 2010;100:452–9.

99. Hatzenbuehler ML, O'Cleirigh C, Mayer K, Safren SA, Bradford J. Effects of same-sex marriage laws on health care use and expenditures in sexual minority men: a quasi-natural experiment. Am J Public Health. 2012;102(2):285–91.

The Role of Resilience and Resilience Characteristics in Health Promotion

Laura Erickson-Schroth and Elizabeth Glaeser

Introduction

Despite how commonly it is used, the term resilience is surprisingly difficult to define. Is resilience a characteristic of particularly adaptable people or an everyday trait that unites many of us? Is it a process or an outcome? How do we measure resilience? Does resilience-building require the same steps for everyone? Resilience as a concept is of particular interest among marginalized communities because of the often repeated episodes of adversity that these groups face. Defining and designing robust measures of resilience would therefore be helpful in identifying factors that contribute to resilience and in creating resilience-building interventions. Although there is much still to be learned, research to date has identified a number of strategies that can be used by individual clinicians, in clinical practice settings, and at the health policy level to promote resilience development in lesbian, gay, bisexual, and transgender (LGBT) people. These strategies often differ when taking into account other aspects of LGBT individuals' identity (such as race, social class, or ability status). The best outcomes result when organizations and providers work with community members to provide spaces and systems that support resilience, rather than attempting to fit community members into existing models of care that do not take their voices into account.

What Is Resilience and How Does It Develop?

Resilience is a concept that originated in developmental psychology to help understand why some children and adolescents who face adversity early in life go on to do well when others do not. The American Psychological Association defines resilience as "the process of adapting well in the face of adversity, trauma, tragedy, threats or significant sources of stress [1]." Resilience researcher Ann Masten argues that resilience is ordinary and that it involves behaviors, thoughts, and actions that can be learned and developed in anyone. Similarly, researcher Froma Walsh defines resilience as the ability to not only overcome or survive adversity but to grow and flourish as a result of one's experience [2, 3]. Many scholars have attempted to operationalize resilience in order to develop ways to measure and then promote resilience factors; however, there remain various definitions of resilience and multiple ways in which it can be operationalized.

Experts generally agree that the development of resilience requires an interaction between an individual (e.g., intrapersonal factors such as genetic loading, personality traits) and their environment (e.g., interpersonal and structural factors), but debate continues as to whether resilience is an outcome or a process. Figure 5.1 presents an oversimplified model for factors impacting the development of resilience, each of which will be discussed in detail.

Factors affecting the development of resilience may include genetic, epigenetic, individual, interpersonal, and environmental influences. Studies demonstrate that it is possible for vulnerability to posttraumatic stress disorder to be passed from one generation to another [4]. Reduced cortisol levels, which have been linked with vulnerability to posttraumatic stress disorder (PTSD), were more likely in both mothers who developed PTSD in response to the events of September 11 and those who did not [4]; the reduced cortisol levels were also noticed in infants born shortly after

L. Erickson-Schroth, MD, MA (✉)
Mount Sinai Beth Israel, Hetrick Martin Institute, 10 Nathan D. Perlman Place, New York, NY 10003, USA
e-mail: Erickson.schroth@gmail.com

E. Glaeser, BS
The Department of Child and Adolescent Psychiatry, NYU Langone Medical Center, New York, NY, USA

© Springer International Publishing AG 2017
K.L. Eckstrand, J. Potter (eds.), *Trauma, Resilience, and Health Promotion in LGBT Patients*,
DOI 10.1007/978-3-319-54509-7_5

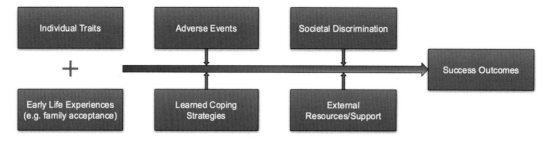

Fig. 5.1 Factors impacting the development of resilience among LGBT individuals

September 11 of the mothers with PTSD. Research also illustrates the epigenetic aspects of resilience. Epigenetic changes are those that alter gene expression rather than the DNA sequence itself. Studies demonstrate that early life adversity can cause epigenetic variability. For example, intimate partner violence and parental stress pre- and post-partum predict DNA methylation in offspring. In turn, loving and nurturing behaviors have been found to lower stress levels in young mice [5, 6]. These data not only highlight the biologic effects of adverse experiences, they suggest that behavior and environmental changes may be instrumental in promoting adaptation and recovery from adversity, although just how this may occur remains poorly understood.

Studies conducted in the general population reveal a number of individual, interpersonal, and environmental factors that appear to contribute to resilience. For example, in a seminal study looking at children of parents with mental illness, approximately half of the children experienced positive developmental outcomes and did not become mentally ill or exhibit maladaptive behaviors despite having been raised in adverse conditions [7]. Resilience or relative success later in life in these children was attributed to an individual process involving multiple factors, including school environments, sporting or musical achievement, responsibility in school, having a relationship with a teacher, and social success [7, 8]. Similarly, in a large-scale study performed after the September 11 World Trade Center attacks, resilience or lack of posttraumatic stress was predicted by gender, age, race/ethnicity, education, level of trauma exposure, income change, social support, frequency of chronic disease, and recent and past life stressors. Resilience was more likely in men than women, older people than younger people, Asians than Caucasians, and those without a college education [9]. These studies suggest that there are some potentially mutable factors that can be targeted to promote a patient's successful adaptation to adversity. Importantly, while some aspects of resilience are global, others may apply to specific cultures and situations, making research into LGBT-specific resilience an important next step [10].

LGBT Resilience Research

Scholars and practitioners have long been working toward putting theories of resilience into practice to improve the lives of marginalized populations. While little is known about the specific biological and epigenetic aspects of resilience for this population, much of the prior work on resilience can be adapted and applied to the LGBT population [11]. For many individuals, an LGBT identity may be only one aspect of marginalization and it is important to consider each person's path to overcoming adversity individually.

Essential to an understanding of resilience in LGBT populations is the minority stress model, formulated by Meyer [12], who argues that "stigma, prejudice, and discrimination create a hostile and stressful social environment that causes mental health problems." Since Meyer's original article, numerous researchers have investigated the ways in which environmental factors affect mental health in LGBT populations. Initially validated in gay men, the minority stress model has now been studied in sexual minority women [13] and in transgender populations [14]. The model has also been expanded to include factors such as shame, which can mediate between minority stressors and distress [15].

Other researchers studying specific resilience factors in LGBT populations have identified a number of factors that may contribute to positive coping, greater life satisfaction, and fewer maladaptive behaviors – outcomes defined as resilience by the academic literature broadly. Factors that correlate with these resilience outcomes include peer and more general social support, family acceptance, and community connectedness [14, 16–21]. Specifically, in further research into social support for youth, Hatzenbuehler and Ryan, among others, have found that growing up in a supportive environment is protective against suicide and predicts later life satisfaction. Clinicians looking to use a "treatment-as-prevention" approach should consider the impact of supportive families and communities on later resilience for LGBT individuals.

Investigators have also found that LGBT people use both internal and external resilience strategies to deal with discrimination. For example, many LGBT people have developed internal coping strategies that include defining themselves, embracing their self-worth, recognizing gender- and race-based oppression, and taking pride in LGBT and racial status. They also engage in health-promoting processes such as facilitative coping with techniques like positive reframing, self-sufficiency, use of metaphors, responsibility to others, spirituality, and enacting healthy behavioral practices such as seeking social support, seeking professional support, acting "as if," engaging in hobbies, using humor, and exercising agency when possible [16, 21–29]. Additional strategies demonstrated among youth include: acceptance and resistance of stereotypes, connectedness with supportive adults, intentional self-care behaviors, social activism, and cognitive and behavioral flexibility [30].

In addition to looking for strength internally, LGBT people also reach out to others in the broader social context, seeking out connections to LGBT-affirming communities and supportive non-LGBT friends and family members [21, 23, 24]. They can also seek opportunities to provide service to fellow community members as advisors and mentors, helping both themselves and others in the process. As subsequent chapters will explore, resilience can vary based on age, gender identity, race, ethnicity, and other demographic measures.

Research into LGBT resilience is beginning to focus on the need to examine the effectiveness of specific interventions in promoting resilience [24, 31, 32]. For example, a pilot study at a high school gay-straight alliance introduced students to a trauma-informed cognitive behavioral therapy (CBT) curriculum that included identification of minority and general stressors, discussion of coping strategies, and then development of cognitive coping, affect regulation, and problem-solving skills [33]. Although the author did not test changes in resilience after the intervention, he did emphasize the role that this type of program could play in the development of resilience. Many other researchers have developed interventions whose primary goal is behavioral change or improvement in health outcomes, but are likely to have impacted resilience as well [34–38]. Many of these interventions target the systems around individuals (families, teachers, schools, health-care settings) rather than individuals themselves in order to reduce isolation and marginalization and thus increase general resilience by promoting acceptance and reducing minority stress.

Importantly, while the minority stress model provides a framework to understand how health disparities develop in LGBT populations, many LGBT individuals develop adaptive coping and resilience despite exposure to psychosocial stressors. Stall et al. showed that even in the context of high levels of sexual minority stress, the majority of men who have sex with men did not participate in high-risk sexual behaviors and were not HIV infected [39]. Those who were diagnosed with HIV had more co-occurring psychosocial risk factors. Switching from a deficit-based approach (i.e., implementing an intervention after individuals have suffered adversity), many interventionists are now using a "treatment-as-prevention" approach for LGBT individuals. Examples of such interventions include focusing on the uptake of pre-exposure prophylaxis (PrEP) to help individuals like those in the Stall study prevent another adverse event and/or increasing coping skills around an HIV diagnosis [39].

LGBT Resilience in the Context of Health Promotion

While there has been little formal research into interventions that promote resilience in LGBT populations, clinics and other health-care settings routinely employ interventions believed to be effective in promoting resilience. Both individual client encounters and clinic-wide programs can provide opportunities for resilience promotion. Due to a number of built-in limitations, health-care settings tend to employ certain types of strategies (individual sessions, therapy groups) and not others (peer-based programming, family interventions), despite the fact that these less common types of approaches may be just as beneficial in promoting resilience, if not more so [40–44].

On an individual level, there are a number of strategies clinicians can use to encourage the development of resilience in their patients (see Table 5.1). Most importantly, providers should attempt to create a good rapport with clients, promoting a sense of trust and establishing themselves as safe to seek out. Listening to clients and asking open-ended questions, while respecting their identities, helps to build a supportive relationship (see Chap. 17). From there, providers can help clients to understand that their experiences are part of a larger system of oppression (see Box 5.1. Sample Script) and give them a sense of shared community with others who are resilient within this system (see Fig. 5.2).

Table 5.1 Clinic-wide strategies to promote client resilience

Create a safe physical space
Provide warmth in the reception area by assuring that reception staff are trained in LGBT-affirming practices
Ensure privacy in areas where it is needed
Have gender-neutral bathrooms
Adapt medical records to allow for appropriate names and pronouns
Create Human Resources policies that make staff feel safe
Provide resources for the whole person
Hire staff knowledgeable about community resources
Refer clients to non-medical resources (employment, housing, internships)
Facilitate insurance and prescription access
Embed mental health services (such as support groups) that focus on trauma and resilience
Hire providers with experience in trauma work
Make the clinic a part of the community and the community a part of the clinic
Hire from within the community
Involve community members as part of a patient and/or a community advisory board that meets regularly
Offer peer-run services
Encourage clients to take on leadership roles
Involve clients' families and friends in their care
Host community events
Show up at community events run by other organizations
Send your providers to teach in the community
Send your providers to learn from the community (trainings)
Run staff trainings within your clinic focussed on learning about clients' experiences (so clients do not have to educate providers)

Box 5.1 Sample Script

Sample script for clinicians to discuss resilience with LGBT clients:

Clinician	You've told me about a number of difficult experiences you've had dealing with discrimination. Often, you end up feeling very alone.
Client	Yes, I feel like I'm being targeted and like no one understands.
Clinician	Why do you think you, in particular, have been targeted?
Client	I don't know. I'm ugly. I'm dumb. Maybe they bother me because I dress girly.
Clinician	Do you think they target other people who dress the way you do?
Client	Yeah, I guess. They don't like people who look different.
Clinician	Why do you think that is?
Client	They're scared of difference. They don't like gay people or trans people.
Clinician	What makes them feel uncomfortable?
Client	I don't know, maybe seeing a guy who's more feminine makes them feel vulnerable, like they don't know what it means to be a man anymore.

Box 5.1 (continued)

Clinician	It sounds like it's probably about their own problems dealing with their internal struggles.
Client	Yeah, they take it out on us but really it's about them.
Clinician	I wonder if other LGBT people talk about similar things with their clinicians.
Client	They must.
Clinician	Do you think other people feel depressed or lonely because they're targeted?
Client	Yeah, there are probably a lot of people who feel like me.
Clinician	Are there place where LGBT people can talk to each other about discrimination?
Client	Yeah, I've heard there are groups at the LGBT Center. They probably work together on ways to deal with things and fight the system.
Clinician	Have you ever been to one of those groups?
Client	No, but maybe I'll try it. . .

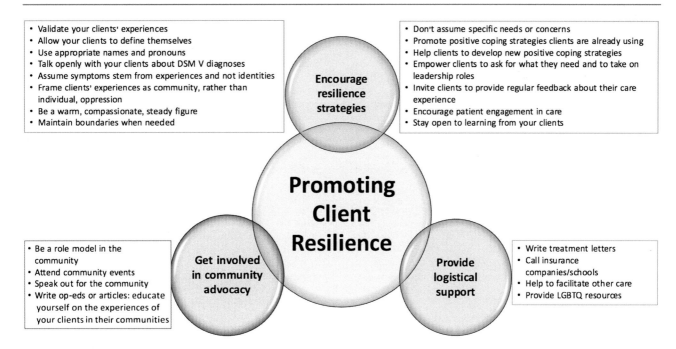

Fig. 5.2 Strategies promoting client resilience

Within the context of a larger clinical practice, there are also many ways to create an environment that promotes resilience (see Table 5.1). Just as important as the physical environment of clinics is their investment in involving LGBT community members in the development of their programs and policies, even in those clinics that are not LGBT specific. Hiring from within LGBT communities and encouraging staff to learn as much as they can about these communities will build strength and resilience, as will including LGBT people on boards and patient advisory committees.

Conclusions

Resilience in LGBT populations remains a fertile field for investigation, as many unknowns remain. Because resilience itself is difficult to define, research into resilience, both among LGBT and non-LGBT populations, is just beginning to come into its stride. Within LGBT populations, research to identify specific interventions that build resilience and promote health is urgently needed. However, using the wide variety of tools we have discussed above, resilience-building strategies can begin to be implemented intentionally in clinical practice settings and during individual client encounters.

References

1. Association AP. The road to resilience 2016. Available from: http://www.apa.org/helpcenter/road-resilience.aspx.
2. Walsh F. Family resilience: a framework for clinical practice. Fam Process. 2003;42(1):1–18.
3. Masten AS. Ordinary magic: resilience processes in development. Am Psychol. 2001;56(3):227.
4. Yehuda R, Engel SM, Brand SR, Seckl J, Marcus SM, Berkowitz GS. Transgenerational effects of posttraumatic stress disorder in babies of mothers exposed to the World Trade Center attacks during pregnancy. J Clin Endocrinol Metab. 2005;90(7):4115–8.
5. Radtke KM, Ruf M, Gunter HM, Dohrmann K, Schauer M, Meyer A, et al. Transgenerational impact of intimate partner violence on methylation in the promoter of the glucocorticoid receptor. Transl Psychiatry. 2011;1(7):e21.
6. Mueller BR, Bale TL. Sex-specific programming of offspring emotionality after stress early in pregnancy. J Neurosci. 2008;28 (36):9055–65.
7. Rutter M. Protective factors in children's responses to stress and disadvantage. In: Rolf MWKJE, editor. Primary prevention in psychopathology: social competence in children. Hanover: University Press of New England; 1979.
8. Rutter M. Resilience in the face of adversity. Protective factors and resistance to psychiatric disorder. Br J Psychiatry. 1985;147:598–611.
9. Bonanno GA, Galea S, Bucciarelli A, Vlahov D. What predicts psychological resilience after disaster? The role of demographics, resources, and life stress. J Consult Clin Psychol. 2007;75(5):671.
10. Ungar M. Nurturing hidden resilience in at-risk youth in different cultures. J Can Acad Child Adolesc Psychiatry. 2006;15(2):53.

11. Herrick AL, Lim SH, Wei C, Smith H, Guadamuz T, Friedman MS, et al. Resilience as an untapped resource in behavioral intervention design for gay men. AIDS Behav. 2011;15(Suppl 1):S25–9.

12. Meyer IH. Prejudice, social stress, and mental health in lesbian, gay, and bisexual populations: conceptual issues and research evidence. Psychol Bull. 2003;129(5):674.

13. Kaysen D, Kulesza M, Balsam KF, Rhew IC, Blayney JA, Lehavot K, et al. Coping as a mediator of internalized homophobia and psychological distress among young adult sexual minority women. Psychol Sex Orientat Gend Divers. 2014;1(3):225–33.

14. Bockting WO, Miner MH, Swinburne Romine RE, Hamilton A, Coleman E. Stigma, mental health, and resilience in an online sample of the US transgender population. Am J Public Health. 2013;103(5):943–51.

15. Mereish E, Poteat VP. Effects of heterosexuals' direct and extended friendships with sexual minorities on their attitudes and behaviors: intergroup anxiety and attitude strength as mediators and moderators. J Appl Soc Psychol. 2015;45(3):147–57.

16. Budge SL, Katz-Wise SL, Tebbe EN, Howard KA, Schneider CL, Rodriguez A. Transgender emotional and coping processes facilitative and avoidant coping throughout gender transitioning. Couns Psychol. 2013;41(4):601–47.

17. Grant J, Mottet L, Tanis JE, Harrison J, Herman J, Keisling M. Injustice at every turn: a report of the national transgender discrimination survey. Washington, DC: National Center for Transgender Equality : National Gay and Lesbian Task Force; 2011.

18. Koken JA, Bimbi DS, Parsons JT. Experiences of familial acceptance–rejection among transwomen of color. J Fam Psychol. 2009;23(6):853.

19. Mizock L, Lewis TK. Trauma in transgender populations: risk, resilience, and clinical care. J Emot Abus. 2008;8(3):335–54.

20. Ryan C, Russell ST, Huebner D, Diaz R, Sanchez J. Family acceptance in adolescence and the health of LGBT young adults. J Child Adolesc Psychiatr Nurs. 2010;23(4):205–13.

21. Singh AA, Hays DG, Watson LS. Strength in the face of adversity: resilience strategies of transgender individuals. J Couns Dev. 2011;89(1):20–7.

22. Eyre SL, de Guzman R, Donovan AA, Boissiere C. 'Hormones is not magic wands' ethnography of a transgender scene in Oakland, California. Ethnography. 2004;5(2):147–72.

23. Gray NN, Mendelsohn DM, Omoto AM. Community connectedness, challenges, and resilience among gay Latino immigrants. Am J Community Psychol. 2015;55(1–2):202–14.

24. Harper A, Singh A. Supporting ally development with families of trans and gender nonconforming (TGNC) youth. J LGBT Issues Couns. 2014;8(4):376–88.

25. McFadden SH, Frankowski S, Flick H, Witten TM. Resilience and multiple stigmatized identities: lessons from transgender persons' reflections on aging. In: Positive Psychology. New York: Springer; 2013. p. 247–67.

26. Reisner SL, Gamarel KE, Dunham E, Hopwood R, Hwahng S. Female-to-male transmasculine adult health: a mixed-methods community-based needs assessment. J Am Psychiatr Nurses Assoc. 2013;19(5):293–303.

27. Bradford J, Reisner SL, Honnold JA, Xavier J. Experiences of transgender-related discrimination and implications for health: results from the Virginia transgender health initiative study. Am J Public Health. 2012;103(10):1820–9.

28. Singh A. "Just getting out of bed is a revolutionary act": the resilience of transgender people of color who have survived traumatic life events. Traumatology. 2010.

29. Singh AA, Meng S, Hansen A. "It's already hard enough being a student": developing affirming college environments for trans youth. J LGBT Youth. 2013;10(3):208–23.

30. Meichenbaum D. Ways to bolster resilience in LGBTQ youth The Melissa Institute for Violence Prevention and Treatment Conference; Miami, 2015.

31. Herrick AL, Lim SH, Wei C, Smith H, Guadamuz T, Friedman MS, et al. Resilience as an untapped resource in behavioral intervention design for gay men. AIDS Behav. 2011;15(1):25–9.

32. McElroy J, Wintemberg J, Haller K. Advancing health care for lesbian, gay, bisexual, and transgender patients in Missouri. Mo Med. 2015;112(4):262.

33. Heck NC. The potential to promote resilience: piloting a minority stress-informed, GSA-based, mental health promotion program for LGBTQ youth. Psychol Sex Orientation Gend Divers. 2015; 2(3):225.

34. Collier KL, Colarossi LG, Hazel DS, Watson K, Wyatt GE. Healing our women for transgender women: adaptation, acceptability, and pilot testing. AIDS Educ Prev. 2015;27(5):418–31.

35. Hergenrather KC, Geishecker S, Clark G, Rhodes SD. A pilot test of the HOPE intervention to explore employment and mental health among African American gay men living with HIV/AIDS: results from a CBPR study. AIDS Educ Prev. 2013;25(5):405.

36. Logie CH, Lacombe-Duncan A, Weaver J, Navia D, Este D. A pilot study of a group-based HIV and STI prevention intervention for lesbian, bisexual, queer, and other women who have sex with women in Canada. AIDS Patient Care STDs. 2015;29(6):321–8.

37. Nyamathi A, Reback CJ, Shoptaw S, Salem BE, Zhang S, Yadav K. Impact of tailored interventions to reduce drug use and sexual risk behaviors among homeless gay and bisexual men. Am J Mens Health. 2015. pii: 1557988315590837.

38. Pachankis JE, Hatzenbuehler ML, Rendina HJ, Safren SA, Parsons JT. LGB-affirmative cognitive-behavioral therapy for young adult gay and bisexual men: a randomized controlled trial of a transdiagnostic minority stress approach. 2015.

39. Stall R, Mills TC, Williamson J, Hart T, Greenwood G, Paul J, et al. Association of co-occurring psychosocial health problems and increased vulnerability to HIV/AIDS among urban men who have sex with men. Am J Public Health. 2003;93(6):939–42.

40. Goodman LA, Pugach M, Skolnik A, Smith L. Poverty and mental health practice: within and beyond the 50-minute hour. J Clin Psychol. 2013;69(2):182–90.

41. Williams AR, McDougall JC, Bruggeman SK, Erwin PJ, Kroshus ME, Naessens JM. Estimation of unreimbursed patient education costs at a large group practice. J Contin Educ Heal Prof. 2004;24 (1):12–9.

42. Brindis CD, Klein J, Schlitt J, Santelli J, Juszczak L, Nystrom RJ. School-based health centers: accessibility and accountability. J Adolesc Health. 2003;32(6):98–107.

43. Senderowitz J. Involving youth in reproductive health projects. Washington, DC: FOCUS on young adults; 1998.

44. South J, Bagnall A-M, Hulme C, Woodall J, Longo R, Dixey R, et al. Findings of the review of effectiveness: what are the effects of peer-based interventions on prisoner health? (review question 1). 2014.

Childhood and Adolescence

Shelley L. Craig and Ashley Austin

Epidemiology and Healthcare Needs

Diverse Sexual Orientations in Childhood and Adolescence

The healthcare needs of sexually diverse (SD) children and adolescents (or all those who are not heterosexual) exist in a developmental context of emergent and shifting identities. Although population approximations vary widely, an estimated 2–11% of all adolescents are sexual orientation minorities [1, 2]. While awareness of gender identity [one's internal sense of identity (e.g., male, female, or something else)] emerges in early childhood, adolescence is the developmental stage during which sexual orientation (romantic or sexual attraction to people of a specific gender) plays an increasingly important role [3]. It should be noted that the average ages of (1) awareness of an SD identity (or nonheterosexual identity) and (2) disclosure of that SD identity to others are decreasing, having recently been assessed at ages 12 and 18, respectively [4]. Definitions of sexual orientation typically include three facets: sexual attraction, sexual behavior, and sexual identity (e.g., heterosexual, bisexual, lesbian/gay) [5]. These three components exist on continuums that can evolve or change across the lifespan [6–8]. The terms used to describe sexual orientation identities are continuously changing, ranging from more traditional labels such as gay, lesbian, and bisexual, to more contemporary labels such as pansexual, graysexual,

and queer[1] [9]. During the marked identity development of adolescence, sexual orientation can be conceptualized as complex and somewhat dynamic. For varying reasons, some adolescents prefer not to adopt SD labels, yet engage in SD behavior, experience same-sex attraction, or identify with a variety of SD communities [10]. Such identity development is considered normative [11] and is reflective of the diversity of sexual identities among adolescents.

Diverse Gender Identities in Childhood and Adolescence

The healthcare needs of gender diverse (GD) children and adolescents (e.g., transgender, gender variant, gender nonconforming, a gender identity or expression that does not conform exactly to biological sex or societal expectations) may vary considerably based on many factors. Biological sex refers to biological and physical anatomy and is used to assign gender at birth. Gender refers to the attitudes, feelings, and behaviors that are associated with an individual's biological sex. Behavior that is compatible with cultural expectations is referred to as gender-normative, while behavior viewed as incompatible with these expectations is perceived as gender nonconforming. A clear understanding of gender identity development and the range of gender experiences among children and adolescents, as well as the associated terminology, is a prerequisite for all discussions of gender identity-specific healthcare needs and potential interventions.

S.L. Craig, PhD, RSW, LCSW (✉)
Factor-Inwentash Faculty of Social Work, University of Toronto, 246 Bloor Street West, Toronto, ON, Canada M5S 1A1
e-mail: shelley.craig@utoronto.ca

A. Austin, PhD, LCSW
School of Social Work, Barry University, 11300 NE 2nd Avenue, Miami Shores, FL 33161-6695, USA
e-mail: AAustin@barry.edu

[1] Definitions: Pansexual refers to not being limited in sexual choice with regard to biological sex, gender, or gender identity. Queer is often an umbrella term and includes many who feel somehow outside of the societal norms in regards to gender or sexuality. Graysexual refers to an individual that is generally asexual but is capable of sexual desire under certain conditions (e.g., love or romance). Asexual refers to a person who has no sexual feelings or desires.

© Springer International Publishing AG 2017
K.L. Eckstrand, J. Potter (eds.), *Trauma, Resilience, and Health Promotion in LGBT Patients*,
DOI 10.1007/978-3-319-54509-7_6

It is increasingly clear that experiences of gender are not binary (either male or female); rather, gender identity comprises a multidimensional spectrum of experiences [12]. Contemporary gender identities beyond the male/female binary include, but are certainly not limited to, bigender, genderqueer, gender creative, gender fluid, gender expansive, gender neutral, and transgender. Terms such as gender fluid, genderqueer, and gender creative convey a broad, flexible range of gender expression, with interests and behaviors that are not limited by restrictive boundaries of stereotypical expectations of girls or boys. Moreover, gender fluidity may suggest that adolescents experience themselves as both a boy and a girl at the same time, that their gender identity varies from day to day or across circumstances, or that neither the term boy or girl describes them accurately [5]: While the term transgender (often abbreviated as trans*) is frequently used as an umbrella term to encompass the full range of GD identities, it is most often applied more specifically to adolescents whose experiences of gender dysphoria (i.e., emotional distress associated with a gender identity that is not aligned with biological sex) and cross-gender play, activities, and appearance are insistent, persistent, and consistent [13]. Awareness of gender identity occurs relatively young, as children can typically identify themselves as boys or girls by age 3 and gender identity is generally stable by age 4 [10, 14].

Of children who present to health professionals with gender nonconforming behaviors, self-expression, or identities, research suggests that a transgender, gender nonconforming, or GD identity does not persist for the majority into adolescence [10, 15]. Yet, there is increasing speculation that these percentages may be underestimated as a result of skewed research processes, as well as the possibility that participants, as a result of the implicit and explicit pressure to conform to gender-normative behavioral expectations associated with biological sex, are reluctant to share persisting experiences of gender dysphoria [16]. To date, the correlates of persisting or desisting gender nonconformity remain unknown [10], but emerging research suggests that it is likely the result of a complex interplay between biological, environmental, and psychological factors [17]. It appears that dysphoria that arises during childhood and intensifies during adolescence is very unlikely to abate, and gender identification during puberty (10–12 for natal females and 12–14 for natal males) is likely to remain stable throughout the lifespan [15, 18, 19]. However, the presentation and expression of gender presentation associated with one's gender identity may continue to develop over time (Fig. 6.1).

As the emergence and stability of GD identities vary across the developmental lifespan of children and adolescents, the healthcare needs of these adolescents also vary. For example, reversible pubertal suppression

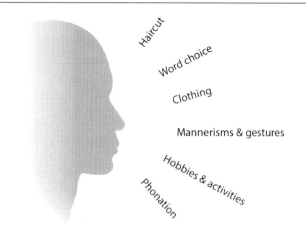

Ways to Express Gender

Fig. 6.1 Ways for individuals to express aspects of their gender

(i.e., hormone blockers) for GD adolescents is identified as an important and often critical medical intervention for children during but not prior to onset of puberty [18, 20]. Similarly, for adolescents interested in transitioning physically, hormone therapy to regulate pubertal development of the desired gender can be initiated during adolescence, but never prior to puberty onset. The recommended age for hormone initiation is 16 years old [21, 22]; however, this may vary between providers.

The Context of Healthcare for Sexual and Gender Diverse Children and Adolescents: An Affirmative Trauma-Informed Perspective

Health Risks and Vulnerabilities

Sexual and gender diverse (SGD) children and adolescents experience significant health disparities that may have severe and enduring consequences [23]. The Centers for Disease Control (CDC) reports that compared to students who are not SD, "a disproportionate number of... [SD] students engage in a wide range of health risk behaviors" [24 p. 49]. Another recent study found SGD adolescents are at increased risk in multiple areas beyond sexual health; SGD adolescents experience additional risk in an average of nine areas such as school/family environment, behavioral health, and mental health [25], which may have daunting consequences on well-being.

A meta-analysis determined that the risk for increased suicidality (thoughts and behavior) was three times greater among SD adolescents than heterosexual adolescents, with greatest risk among bisexual adolescents [26]. General risk factors such as depression and substance use, as well as identity-based risks such as homophobic discrimination, are associated with high rates of suicidal behavior [5]. SD adolescents have higher rates of suicidal "ideation, planning and attempts" [27] at 22.8%, compared to 6.6% for non-SD adolescents. Risks may be particularly exacerbated among certain subgroups of SGD adolescents. For example, White Latino and American Native/Pacific Islander SD adolescents have been found to have a higher prevalence of suicide attempts compared to Black and Asian SD adolescents, often attributed to negative cultural views of suicide in the latter groups [27]. However, other studies of SGM youth have not found differences in suicidality by race or ethnicity [28]. Research suggests that GD adolescents have an exceptionally high risk of suicidality [29–31]; among transgender young adult respondents (18–24) to the National Transgender Discrimination Survey, 45% reported having attempted suicide [29].

SGD adolescents also experience elevated rates of depression compared to their non-SGD counterparts [26, 32, 33]. One large-scale community-based study of SGD adolescents found that 30% reported clinical levels of psychosocial distress and 15% met criteria for major depressive disorder [28]. Depressive disorders are particularly troubling, with some research suggesting SGD adolescents may be four times more likely than non-SGD adolescents to meet diagnostic criteria for major depressive disorder [34]. While gender differences among SGD children and adolescents remain understudied, females have been found to have higher rates of depression at younger ages [35, 36].

SGD adolescents have conspicuously high rates of sexual risk behaviors resulting in disproportionate rates of sexually transmitted infections (STIs), such as HIV, and unintended pregnancy. Young SGD males comprise 72% of new HIV infections among all young people (ages 13–24) in the United States, and new infections increased by 22% for this group between 2008 and 2010 [37]. Young ethnic and racial minority SGD were at particular risk, with African Americans comprising 55% of new infections among young SGD males [38]. Transgender adolescents, particularly racial and ethnic minorities, also account for a troubling proportion of new HIV infections [24]. Transfeminine (i.e., transgender individuals with a male biological sex who identify with femininity to a greater extent than masculinity) adolescents are especially vulnerable, with HIV seroprevalence as high as one in four among this subgroup [39]. While few studies have assessed female SGD adolescents, emerging research suggests that this hidden population experiences higher rates of sexual risk behaviors than non-SGD peers, including sex with multiple partners, unprotected vaginal intercourse, and substance use [40, 41]. SGD adolescents are 2–10 times more likely to become pregnant or cause a pregnancy than their non-SGD peers [42–44].

In contrast to misperceptions that female SGD adolescents have few risks for HIV and other STI's, some female SGD adolescents may actually face greater risks than both male SGD and non-SGD adolescents [45].

According to studies based on the Youth Risk Behavior Survey (YRBS), substance use and related risks are higher among SGD adolescents [46]. A meta-analysis [47, 48] found that SGD adolescents report earlier onset and heightened rates of substance use nearly twice those of their non-SGD peers and determined that certain subgroups experience even greater disparities. For example, bisexual adolescents demonstrate rates of substance use three times higher than heterosexual adolescents. Ziyadeh and colleagues [49] found that compared to girls who described themselves as "heterosexual," girls describing themselves as "mostly heterosexual" or "lesbian/bisexual" evidenced greater rates of alcohol risk behaviors, including number of alcoholic drinks in the past month, incidents of binge drinking in the past year, and consuming alcohol prior to age 12. It appears that a significant proportion of SGD adolescents are on a high-risk substance use trajectory that extends into adulthood beginning at an early age [50]. While research focused on substance use risk specifically among GD adolescents is sparse, existing studies suggest elevated rates of substance use, particularly among those who have experienced bullying [51], family rejection, victimization, and homelessness [52]. SGD adolescents residing in rural areas may have exceptionally high rates of substance use compared to those in urban locales [53].

SGD children and adolescents comprise a disproportionate number of the adolescent homeless population, with estimates ranging from 9 to 45% [54–57]; a few studies have found that GD or racial/ethnic minority SGD adolescents are particularly overrepresented in this population [54]. Using data from the Massachusetts YRBS, Corliss et al. [58] found that SGD students experienced homelessness 4–13 times more often than their non-SGD counterparts, even when controlling for other demographic factors. Conflict with parents and victimization (e.g., sexual or physical abuse) contribute to the increased likelihood of SGD youth homelessness [52, 55, 59].

SGD children and adolescents are also overrepresented in the child welfare and foster care systems, often due to the disproportionate rates of sexual and physical victimization experienced by SGD youth [60]. In Los Angeles County, which has the largest population of foster care adolescents in the United States, approximately one in five foster care adolescents are SGD identified. Certain subgroups are particularly overrepresented; 86% of SGD children and adolescents in foster care are Latino, Black, or Asian/Pacific Islander, and nearly 6% are transgender [61]. SGD adolescents are twice as likely to experience less stable and more frequent foster care or residential group home placements than their non-SGD counterparts [61, 62]. SGD adolescents in child welfare and foster care experience high levels of harassment, isolation, and rejection [63–65], and worry about providers violating their confidentiality – specifically the disclosure of their SGD identities without consent [66]. Such violations increase risk for discrimination and rejection by foster families, including increased risk of adolescents being kicked out of foster homes or becoming homeless. SGD adolescents are significantly more likely to state that they were not treated well by the foster care system. Many (18%) report identity-based discrimination, with almost 14% requiring inpatient care for emotional reasons, compared to only 4% for non-SGD adolescents [61].

Identity-Based Stigma, Discrimination, and Victimization

SGD adolescents are disproportionately exposed to stigma, discrimination, and victimization. Research consistently demonstrates that SGD adolescents are significantly more likely to experience multiple forms of victimization (e.g., verbal, physical, sexual), as well as endure pervasive stigma and marginalization (e.g., isolation, ostracization, pathologization), than their non-SGD peers [7, 29, 67–69]. While schools are the settings for staggering amounts of SGD-based bullying and mistreatment, the victimization of SGD children and adolescents is not limited to "any particular social context as it pervades their school, family, religious, and community environments" [70 p. 228]. In a sample of SGM adolescents ($n = 350$; ages 14–21), Dragowski et al. [70] found that nearly three quarters were verbally victimized (72%), and many had objects thrown at them (13%), and/or were physically attacked (11%) because of their SGD status. These findings support D'Augelli and colleagues' earlier work [71], which found that victimization was pervasive in a sample of SGD adolescents ($n = 528$), with 80% reporting verbal harassment, 11% reporting physical harassment, and nearly 9% reporting sexual harassment. SGD adolescents are often victimized in public places, as well as in their own families. Victimization by family members often begins in childhood for SGD, particularly when children exhibit gender nonconformity at an early age [71].

Research from lifetime victimization studies finds that childhood abuse and maltreatment by parents/guardians are more frequent in SGD populations than among their non-SGD counterparts [72]. Burgeoning research with SGD adolescents suggests that they experience disparate rates of physical and sexual victimization by parents or caretakers [73, 74]. A meta-analysis of 37 studies conducted by Friedman and colleagues [73] determined that SGD adolescents were 3.8 times more likely to experience childhood sexual abuse and 1.2 times more likely to be physically abused by a parent or caretaker compared to non-SGD peers. Subgroup analysis revealed that physical abuse was higher for bisexual adolescents compared to lesbian or gay adolescents, and males experienced greater rates of sexual victimization than their female counterparts. Research indicates that GD adolescents are at higher risk for all forms of victimization (i.e., physical, sexual, verbal, and psychological abuse) by family members [71, 75] than adolescents whose presentation and behavior are more gender-normative. Importantly, these increased risks have not been found to contribute to increased SGD identification.

Mounting research demonstrates the onslaught of SGD-based bullying experienced by SGD adolescents in schools. The 2011 National School Climate Survey [76] explored feelings of safety and experiences of school-based victimization among 8534 SGD students (ages 13–20). An overwhelming majority experienced verbal harassment as a result of SD (82%) or GD (64%). Over half (55.2%) were cyberbullied or victimized through online formats (e.g., text messages, postings on social media). Moreover, a disturbing number were physically harassed (38.3%) or physically assaulted (18.3%) at school based on their SGD status [76]. These experiences may have devastating consequences. Goldblum et al. [69] demonstrated that adults who had experienced identity-based discrimination in school were four times more likely to have a history of suicide attempts than those who had not. School victimization appears to be even more severe among SGD adolescents who transgress gender norms. Individuals who were gender nonconforming experienced alarming rates of harassment (78%), physical assault (35%), and sexual violence (12%) in schools [29]. In a sample of 290 GD young adults, 44.9% reported experiencing in-school gender-based violence during their adolescent years [69].

In addition to experiencing a disproportionate risk for violence and victimization, SGD adolescents are also exposed to incessant homophobic and transphobic stigma and microaggressions which exist across multiple life domains and may manifest as family rejection, lack of inclusive legal protections, absence of safe and inclusive school and community spaces, and discrimination by school personnel, religious institutions, and healthcare providers [29, 77–80]. Microaggressions are "brief and commonplace daily verbal, behavioral, or environmental indignities, whether intentional or unintentional, that communicate hostile, derogatory, or negative slights and insults toward members of oppressed groups" [81 p. 23]. SGD individuals experience multiple types of microaggressions, such as an assumption of sexual pathology or abnormality, discomfort with SGD, invisibility of SGD identities and experiences, denial or minimization of experiences of SGD-based discrimination and stigma, the absence of safety and inclusivity in contemporary societal social institutions, and the use of homophobic and transphobic language [78–80] across a variety of social contexts (e.g., media, schools, religious institutions). Research has begun to demonstrate that exposure to microaggressions (whether intentional or not) may have detrimental impacts on the health and well-being of the minority groups subjected to them [82, 83].

It is argued that persistent experiences of homophobic and transphobic microaggressions and enacted stigma (e.g., actual experiences of discrimination) contribute to internalized homophobic/transphobic stigma [84–86]. Internalized stigma refers to the personal acceptance of the stigmatization of one's own identity as part of one's own value system, and the adaptation of one's self-concept to be congruent with such societal stigma [87]. Emerging studies suggest experiences of external or public stigma such as discrimination, victimization, and rejection from others appear to result in the internalization of homophobic and transphobic stigma [84, 88, 89]. SGD adolescents are at risk of internalizing implicit and explicit messages of homophobic and transphobic hate experienced on a daily basis. This is of notable concern as internalized homophobia and transphobia have been linked with poor health outcomes, such as suicide [88, 90, 91].

Etiology of Health Risk: A Trauma-Informed Approach

Given the severity and enduring nature of victimization and stigmatization experienced by SGD adolescents, health disparities among this population must be understood through a minority stress lens [92–94] that acknowledges the impact of minority identity-based trauma on subsequent well-being. Minority stress theory (MST) provides a framework to describe and explain the impact of stress associated with the persistent and pervasive devaluation, marginalization, and pathologization of one's minority identity [92, 94]. An elaboration of stress and coping theory [95], MST proposes that individuals from marginalized populations experience a unique form of stress due to conflict between their internal sense of self and their experiences of majority social norms and expectations [96]. As SGD children and adolescents generally do not share SGD stigma with their families, they do not learn identity-specific coping strategies as adolescents in many other minority communities do [67, 97], leaving them more vulnerable to health and mental health threats [98] and at increased likelihood of engaging in risky behaviors [99]. A manifestation of minority stress, internalized homophobia is associated with serious health consequences, including high-risk sexual behaviors [100], depression [35], and substance use in SD adolescents.

Originally developed to aid in understanding and explaining the stress experiences of SD populations, research increasingly supports the notion that the MST model also applies to GD individuals [101, 102]. A recent study of cross-sectional data from a large ($n = 1093$) and diverse online sample of transgender persons in the United States found that psychological distress was associated with enacted (i.e., actual experiences of rejection and discrimination) and felt (i.e., perceived rejection and expectations of being stereotyped or discriminated against) transphobic stigma [103]. Existing studies suggest higher levels of internalized stigma are associated with poorer coping skills [88] and greater psychological distress [90] in GD adolescents.

For SGD adolescents the often daily exposure to homophobic and transphobic stereotypes, experiences of identity-based stigma and rejection, discriminatory treatment, and exposure to victimization result in pervasive minority stress that may contribute to the development of mental, emotional, and behavioral health issues during adolescence and adulthood. An informed, affirmative clinical approach recognizes the disproportionate exposure to traumatic identity-based stressors among SGD adolescents and assesses health and corresponding healthcare needs of SGD adolescents through the lens of the MST model.

Healthcare for Sexual and Gender Diverse Children and Adolescents

While safe and affirming clinical services can be pivotal in supporting the long-term health and well-being of SGD adolescents, historically these adolescents face notable barriers to effective healthcare. SGD adolescents are less likely to have regular sources of healthcare [104] and, when they are able to access healthcare, some SGD adolescents report provider discrimination or unmet health and mental health needs [105]. This may be due to (1) an overt bias in refusal of services, (2) a lack of provider knowledge regarding SGD-specific recommendations, and/or (3) structural oppression toward SGD clients in healthcare systems (e.g., policies that do not cover SGD-specific healthcare, sex-segregated services, or practices that are heteronormative). Barriers to healthcare may be particularly salient for GD adolescents. Research indicates that transgender individuals routinely experience discrimination, as well as a lack of competent and affirmative care in healthcare settings [29, 106]. The National Transgender Discrimination Survey found that 19% of transgender individuals were denied medical care due to their transgender identity [29]. Children and adolescents with nonconforming experiences of gender are often pathologized and stigmatized, receiving treatments which reject their experience or expression of gender, discourage them from living in a manner consistent with their gender identity when different from their sex assigned at birth, and coerce them into presenting and behaving within binary gender norms. Nevertheless, the utilization of pathologizing "reparative" approaches is perpetuated by some of the most well-known and widely cited professionals working with GD children and adolescents [107]. Further, the paucity of clinical evidence to guide treatment approaches may contribute to care that is not fully inclusive of patients' and families' needs and perspectives, relying on a provider-centered approach to care rather than a patient-centered approach.

Despite a recommendation by the American Medical Association [108] that providers nonjudgmentally recognize diverse sexual orientations and behaviors, many do not apply this in practice. Kitts [3] found that physicians ($n = 184$) do not routinely discuss sexual orientation, sexual attraction, or gender identity with adolescents, even when adolescents are sexually active. Most physicians do not inquire about sexual orientation even if an adolescent reports depression or suicidality [3]. Suicide attempts often occur prior to voluntary disclosure of sexual orientation [109], yet only 57% of providers recognize that SGD adolescents have increased mental health risks [3]. An early study by Allen and colleagues [110] found that a majority of SGD adolescents (approximately 75%) did not disclose their sexual orientation to their providers because they were not asked any psychosocial questions. Providers can play a crucial role in encouraging disclosure by asking direct questions about SGD identities [111]. A study of SGD adolescents ages 13–21 ($n = 733$) found that adolescents desire a competent provider with some knowledge of SGD issues; moreover, provider interpersonal and communication skills, respect for the adolescent, and ability to discuss preventative healthcare and wellness, nutrition, safe sex, and family are critical [105]. Therefore, emerging approaches to comprehensive healthcare delivery for SGD adolescents recommend that providers acknowledge and affirm adolescent identities, screen for health risks, and communicate effectively.

Cultivating Resilience

Understanding Factors that Support Resilience

Although the majority of SGD children and adolescents make it to adulthood without significant disability, the persistent disproportionate health burden faced by SGD adults combined with the adversity encountered by SGD adolescents necessitates a focus on the factors that support development of resilience at a young age [112]. Resilience, defined as the ability to adapt constructively to risk

exposure [113], includes minimization of perceived threats to well-being [114], as well as creating meaning out of challenges [115]. Resilience and healthy coping skills are associated with better overall health, healthy decision-making, and lower likelihood of risky behaviors in adolescence [10, 116]. For SGD children and adolescents, factors that enhance resilience include individual, interpersonal, and environmental factors – such as family connectedness, caring adults and role models, and positive school environments [113, 117–121].

Family support and acceptance are considered particularly critical in protecting SGD children and adolescents against adverse health consequences, and are associated with positive outcomes related to self-esteem, social support, and general health [67, 97, 122]. Needham and Austin [123] found that (1) SGD young adults experience lower levels of parental support than their non-SGD counterparts; (2) parental support is inversely related to health outcomes including depression, substance use, and suicidal thoughts; and (3) parental support partially mediates associations between sexual orientation and marijuana and/or hard drug use among young lesbian women. Similarly, in a sample of transgender adolescents (ages 12–24) receiving care associated with medically transitioning, parental support was correlated with greater life satisfaction and less depression [122].

Social support, feeling cared for, social connectedness, and a feeling of belonging [124] are significant predictors of well-being for SGD children and adolescents [125] and have been found to positively influence self-esteem and decrease mental health symptoms [126, 127]. Grossman and Kerner [128] found that high self-esteem and social support may moderate SGD-related stressors, while Mustanksi, Newcomb, and Garofalo [113] found that high levels of social support contribute to better mental health but do not moderate the negative impact of victimization. In addition to these critical elements, emerging factors that have the potential to promote resilience among SGD children and adolescents include information and communication technologies (ICTs), affirmative programs and interventions, and affirmative healthcare.

Information and Communication Technologies

Due to their rapid uptake and wide accessibility, information and communication technologies (ICTs; e.g., internet, social media, smartphones and related apps) have the potential to promote resilience among SGD children and adolescents. Emerging research has found that adolescents in crisis turn to ICTs for support before clinical interventions or social services [129]. The impact of resilience enhancers such as ICTs may be disproportionately greater for SGD adolescents faced with multiple minority stressors due to the potential to reach adolescents that may be geographically or socially excluded, such as those in rural areas or without access to affirmative families, resources, or healthcare providers [130]. Individuals who utilize self-guided support apps (e.g., for diet, mood, stress management) are essentially using ICTs to solve their problems faster and at lower cost than is feasible with traditional behavioral interventions [131]. SGD children and adolescents commonly report barriers in offline contexts to accessing identity-specific information and support [110]. ICTs facilitate resilience by providing opportunities for SGD children and adolescents to form community, build individualized support networks, develop coping skills, engage in identity development activities, increase perceived support, and seek information in an environment that is notably safer and more accessible than their daily lives [132]. Further, both online peer support [133] and structured online programs [134] are effective ways to use in-home technology in conjunction with in-person support to bolster resilience.

As a result of the dearth of competent and affirmative healthcare providers and organizations for GD populations, social media and accessibility to online health information and resources represent particularly critical avenues for support and well-being for GD individuals and their families [135]. The internet may be utilized to gain education, explore identity, freely share feelings, socialize with others who are coping with similar situations, obtain mutual aid (for parents and adolescents), and locate affirmative providers with expertise in adolescent-specific GD issues [132]. Affirmative practices may include linking patients with online resources and virtual communities (e.g., trans-specific YouTube channels, transgender social networking groups) relevant to gender diversity [135]. Given emerging research suggesting that seeing and engaging with other GD individuals is an important aspect of positive gender identity development [102, 136], ICTs may be particularly valuable resources for GD adolescents and their families who have logistical barriers to accessing resources in their communities.

Affirmative Interventions and Programs

Affirmative approaches to care for SGD adolescents have markedly different outcomes than damaging and unethical practices that attempt to change sexual orientation and/or gender identity. Harms associated with "reparative" or "conversion" therapies are well documented [137]. Accordingly, recent Substance Abuse and Mental Health Services Administration (SAMHSA) [16] guidelines eschew these practices with SGD adolescents; such therapies should not be a part of provider practice or referral mechanisms. An accumulating evidence base suggests that affirmative interventions, which support and validate the identities, strengths, and experiences of SGD individuals, are effective in promoting health and well-being [138]. Specific examples of such interventions include: *AFFIRM*, a brief, affirmative group cognitive-behavioral coping (CBT) skills training for SGD adolescents to reduce depression and enhance stress appraisal and coping [139]; *Strengths First*, an individualized strengths-based case management program for SGD adolescents at risk of homelessness or needing a personalized approach to accessing services and resources [140, 141]; and *ASSET*, an affirmative school-based discussion-based group (not CBT) for increasing resilience and decreasing risk among SGD youth [142, 143].

Affirmative Healthcare for SGD Children and Adolescents: An Emerging Framework

Articulate Affirmation

The Society for Adolescent Health and Medicine (SAHM) [11] recommends that healthcare providers affirm the multiple dimensions of SGD identities. Such affirmation includes both acknowledging and countering the oppressive contexts in which patients may have previously experienced care by creating a welcoming and supportive environment at the onset of the clinical relationship [144]. A first step is to help children and adolescents overcome reticence or distrust by clearly articulating an affirmative and inclusive perspective of SGD identities. For example, the provider might say: "Welcome, I want to let you know that we accept all patients here, including people with all gender identities, sexual orientations, and experiences. What do you feel is important that I know about you?" Despite the dynamic nature of SD and GD identities for many individuals throughout the lifespan, it is important that providers avoid suggesting that SGD adolescent experiences are "just a phase," as such statements presume that the "provider knows best" and undercut patient/provider trust. Assurance should be provided to questioning adolescents regarding the validity and value of SGD identities along with reassuring and supportive statements [145] such as: "Every person I meet with is different. Some are gay, some are bisexual, or straight, or transgender, or combinations of the above, and I enjoy learning about how wonderful and unique each person is. When I learn about what makes you special it helps me understand you so I can help you better." Providers can provide environmental confirmation of their affirmative approach by having posters or handouts that embrace SGD identities and intake forms that affirm identities by including a wide range of possible SD and GD identities and a write-in section [10].

Particular Considerations for Gender Diverse Children and Adolescents

Affirmative approaches to healthcare for GD adolescents recognize the importance of facilitating "the child's authentic gender journey" [146 p. 339] and allowing the child to drive the process in a manner that is consistent with their developmental stage (early childhood, prepuberty, adolescence). For example, when working with children, Edwards-Leeper and Spack [21] encourage family recognition and acceptance of a child's emerging gender expression and identity while simultaneously emphasizing the importance of remaining open to the fluidity and evolution of gender identity. Affirmative best practices for GD pubertal adolescents (with consistent and persistent gender dysphoria) include prescription of hormone blockers to suppress puberty, often in conjunction with living in the social role consistent with one's identified gender [21, 147]. Postponement of puberty with accompanying unwanted physical changes is often critically important to the well-being of GD adolescents, by reducing feelings of gender dysphoria and associated psychological trauma, and facilitating development of a positive sense of self [21, 147].

Despite differences in the desire for specific interventions that may be elected to accomplish medical transitioning, it is important to recognize that the healthcare provider may be the first point of contact for adolescents and their families as they attempt to identify and understand GD identities. GD adolescents may often see many medical providers and having at least one affirmative provider as a support to process more challenging visits, multiple visits, etc. can be beneficial. As illustrated in Table 6.1, it is recommended that providers adopt an affirming clinical position that acknowledges all experiences of gender as equally healthy and valuable [148]. This affirmative approach is consistent with SAMHSA [16] guidelines that condemn as unethical and harmful any practices that coerce or support coercion of gender conformity among GD children and adolescents. These guidelines are consistent with years of practice-based knowledge about the importance of affirmative approaches, as illustrated by the following quote:

"Repeatedly, the children I work with tell me, in words and actions, that when allowed to express their gender as they feel it rather than as others dictate it, they become enlivened and engaged; when prohibited from that expression, they show symptoms of anxiety, stress, distress, anger, and depression" [146 p. 338].

In sum, unconditional positive regard for all SGD identities and expressions is fundamental to affirmative practice with SGD children and adolescents.

Consider Language

Affirmative care includes explicitly eliciting and discussing sexual orientation, attraction, and gender identity [3]. However, adolescents are unlikely to voluntarily disclose their SGD identities on their own, so providers should ask direct questions about these identities [111, 149, 150]. As the range and terminology describing SGD identities is ever expanding and evolving within adolescent cultures, providers should ask adolescents how they self-identify rather than making assumptions and/or imposing labels that may be inaccurate or that may change over time [10, 11].

Table 6.1 Particular considerations for gender diverse children and adolescents

Affirmative Providers Should	Suggested phrasing
Help facilitate gender authenticity and allow the child to articulate this journey	Many children I see feel like they are not the same as other kids their age who are boys or girls. Do you have any examples of this in your life…school, etc.?
Encourage family recognition and acceptance of a child's emerging gender expression and identity	Like many children, your child is still coming to an understanding of their own identities around gender. It is best to remain open to these explorations and evolution
For GD pubertal adolescents (with consistent and persistent gender dysphoria) prescribe hormone blockers to suppress puberty and suggest socially transitioning to living as their identified gender	We would like to help your child adjust to their identity as a (insert gender identity) and recommend blocking their hormones (fully explain this process) and ensuring they live as (insert gender identity) with clothes, shoes and hair, etc. This is how it has worked for some other families. How do you think this might work in your family?
Recognize that the healthcare provider may be the first point of contact for adolescents and their families as they attempt to understand GD identities. GD adolescents may often see many medical providers and having at least one affirmative provider as a support to process more challenging visits, multiple visits, etc. can be beneficial	I understand that you might be nervous to talk to me as a (insert doctor or other health professional) and you might have to talk to different people during the course of your care, but I want you to know that you can talk to me about anything, even about how it goes with the other providers
Adopt an affirming clinical position that acknowledges all experiences of gender as equally healthy and valuable (Austin and Craig 2015). SAMHSA (2015) guidelines that condemn as unethical and harmful practices that coerce gender conformity	I want you to know we believe that gender is different for many youth and any way that you experience gender is valuable and important. We will not pressure you to act in any way that is not comfortable to you

As some adolescents may not identify with a particular sexual orientation, asking questions about sexual attraction may be more easily understood [6, 23]. For example, a provider could ask the broad question: "What type of person are you attracted to?" Sometimes the more concrete question: "Have you ever been attracted to girls or boys, both, none, or a trans or gender nonconforming person?" may be required to ascertain the desired information. These can be followed by: "Are you attracted to anyone now?" in order initiate discussion of current relationships. Engaging in direct, open, inclusive, and nonjudgmental assessment of the romantic and sexual health experiences of SGD adolescents may facilitate an affirming and trustworthy relationship between the adolescents and the provider, leading to open and honest communication and ultimately better health outcomes.

Providers should be careful to use gender-neutral language and/or language that reflects the patient's preferred terminology [151]. This can be accomplished by introducing oneself by name and preferred gender pronoun. For example: "My name is Beth and I go by she or her. Tell me a bit about you." Avoid heteronormatively biased language throughout all interactions to facilitate SGD child and adolescent safety and comfort, and explore romantic and sexual interests in gender-neutral terms that eliminate the potential of heteronormative bias. For example, one might ask "Are you attracted to or dating anyone?" rather than "Do you have a girlfriend?" Similarly, "What have you and your partner (s) done sexually?" might be used instead of "Have you had intercourse?" and "In what ways do you protect your sexual health when sexually active?" in place of "Does your boyfriend wear a condom?" This latter question can be important for youth that may be sexually active but not in a relationship. Providers should be available to answer questions, correct misinformation, and normalize SGD identities and experiences.

Orient to the Setting and Process

Clearly explaining the setting, the provider's role, the roles of other members of the interdisciplinary team, and the treatment process can empower SGD children and adolescents and increase engagement. Providers should discuss their roles as advocates for the health of SGD adolescents and provide assurance that youth voices and choices are important. Explanations should utilize terms familiar to children and adolescents so they can make informed choices about their treatment [152].

Despite the frequent presence of family members at provider visits, in order to build trust between the SGD patient and the provider, it is critical to speak one-to-one, ensuring that the adolescent is seen alone for most of the visit and always present when reviewing the psychosocial and health history with parents or caregivers. With adolescent patients in particular, confidentiality is key and should be fully explained, with ample opportunity provided for the adolescents to ask questions (e.g., "Everything you tell me is confidential and stays between us. I will not share anything with your parents or anyone else without your permission unless you tell me that you want to seriously harm yourself or anyone else. Do you have any questions about that?"). Trust is also developed when providers use nonjudgmental and sensitive approaches and active listening [153].

Comprehensively Assess for Discrimination and Coping Strategies

Assessment clarifies the patient's needs and informs the direction of treatment. Providers should assess for discrimination in the lives of SGD children and adolescents and consider its impact on well-being [135, 154, 155]. Instead of waiting for SGD adolescents to disclose victimization, providers should routinely screen for bullying and victimization as part of the assessment (e.g., "Some patients tell me about other kids or adults who bully or pick on them. Is this something that has ever happened to you?") [11]. Part of affirmative care is validating the patients' self-reported experiences of discrimination. For example, when a child or adolescent reports an incident of discrimination, the provider should not automatically universalize it (e.g., "all kids have a hard time getting along with their classmates") or search for alternative reasons for the bully's behavior (e.g., "doesn't he call everyone those names?"). Instead, an affirming and validating provider might say: "It sounds like he picks on you." It is important to not dismiss the discrimination or accept it when one is different. Attempts to explain the abuse may be perceived by SGD adolescents as minimizing, dismissive, or a subtle form of bias, thereby undermining the provider-patient relationship. Further, this will prevent discussion of coping strategies and perceived resilience, a key part of the medical encounter. Acknowledging the biological effects of discrimination may allow for a more cogent understanding of the ways in which these issues contribute to SGD patients' healthcare needs. This is particularly important for adolescents who may struggle with situations outside of their control (e.g., bullying, family rejection). Above all, it is important to express that you are sorry the victimization happened, and that it is not the adolescent's fault.

Considering that many patterned thoughts and behaviors are developed in adolescence, providers should assess for adaptive and maladaptive coping strategies developed in response to discrimination, exploring the benefits and harms of each one and the patient's motivation to engage or disengage in these behaviors. Given the serious health and mental health consequences experienced by SGD adolescents, screening for common SGD health risks is insufficient. If serious mental or behavioral health issues such as substance use, depression, or suicidality are identified, the provider can follow up with a brief intervention (e.g., motivational interviewing) or referral to an affirmative treatment program (e.g., CBT or coping skills training). For GD adolescents, appropriate interventions might include psychoeducation regarding the World Professional Association for Transgender Health (WPATH) Standards of Care [20], discussing options and processes associated with various gender-affirming strategies (e.g., changing hair or dress, legal name changes) or medical interventions (e.g., puberty blockers, hormone therapy), and referral to knowledgeable and GD-sensitive clinicians or other healthcare professionals, when appropriate. Although more detail falls outside the scope of this chapter, additional resources can be found at: http://www.trans-health.com/clinics and http://www.transequality.org/know-your-rights/healthcare. Local resource guides are also available, such as: http://www.eqfl.org/news/TransResourceGuide.

When discussing a mutually identified health behavior change, it is important to clarify the patient's goals, potential barriers, and strategies for success and monitoring. Effective assessment should involve exploration of the utility of "risky" coping behaviors and their utility for the SGD adolescent even when simultaneously causing harm. For example: "So describe how you deal with discriminatory experiences? How does (insert behavior) help you? How is (insert behavior) less helpful to you?" Understanding interpersonal and environmental supports should include questions about the patient's family of origin as well as family of choice (e.g., partner's family, best friend's family), informal supports (e.g., friends, partners) and formal peer supports (e.g., gay-straight alliances), community groups (e.g., SGD support or social action groups), and participation in events that help celebrate SGD identities (e.g., pride festivals). To assess the strengths and resilience of SGD adolescents, providers should ask patients to list positive feelings about identifying with SGD identities. Providers should reflect on the initial assessment with children and adolescents to examine the extent to which they demonstrated affirmation of the patient's SGD identity and how this impacts the healthcare visit. Increasingly, recognition of affirmative care is being provided in health professional school curricula as a means of enhancing care for SGD adolescents. For example, the Association of American Medical Colleges [156] resource for medical educators has guidelines to promote effective care.

Support and Educate Family

Although family support is a protective factor, not all adolescents have disclosed their SGD identities to their families. When appropriate, providers should work with families to better accept and understand their children [11]. Family support and education include providing information about SGD-specific issues and needs, the impact of family acceptance and support on health outcomes, and helping parents become more supportive and affirming of their adolescents' needs. Exploring parents' inevitable feelings of guilt, fear, and/or anger about their child's identities and correcting any misconceptions are also important tasks for providers. Reinforcing with parents that their SGD child or adolescent is the same child despite disclosure of SGD status can reduce family conflict [145].

Providers should also be aware of local and national resources. Connecting with the national advocacy and support organization, Parents Families and Friends of Lesbians and Gays (PFLAG) and Trans Youth Family Allies can enable family members to learn from others how to better support their child. Encouraging families to find online information and support may also be beneficial, such as directing parents of GD children and adolescents to YouTube channels that document the lives and experiences of transgender individuals who fall within various stages of the transition process (e.g., prehormone replacement therapy, changes related to hormone usage, postsurgery, family reactions). There are also transgender-specific social networking websites (Genderspectrum.org) and conferences (www.genderodysseyfamily.org) that specifically provide support to family members of GD adolescents.

Strengthen Organizational Capacity

Organizational-level efforts such as advocacy, education, and policy change are important elements of affirmative care. Advocacy can include sustained involvement of providers in encouraging the interprofessional team to consider the specific needs of the SGD adolescent, leading efforts aimed at adopting SGD affirmative policies at the organizational level, as well as championing professional development opportunities aimed at promoting SGD competency in clinical care. Adopting affirmative organizational policies that prohibit identity-based discrimination against patients and staff creates a context and organizational culture that values and supports affirmative care [11]. Committing to educational interventions, such as trainings in affirmative practices for SGD populations, is often a critical first step [157]. Trainings need to be tailored to the specific needs and knowledge levels of providers. There is often a need for knowledge and training on the range of SGD identities, a nonbinary understanding of gender, and the important distinctions between sexual orientation and gender identity/expression. Encouragingly, Kitts [3] found that providers would like to build skills to work with SGD children and adolescents, particularly with regard to discussing sensitive issues such as SGD identities. These strategies for creating a competent and affirming organizational context can have a tremendous impact on the delivery of SGD affirmative care to youth.

Case Scenario

Case Description and Presenting Issues

Jordan is an 8-year-old Hispanic child in the third grade being raised by a single, working-class mother in a relatively large suburban area outside of a major US city (Fig. 6.2). Jordan is a biological male who is gender nonconforming in many ways: Jordan generally likes wearing dresses and skirts that are pink, purple, and sparkly; Jordan prefers wearing his hair long with bows or headbands; and Jordan primarily enjoys playing dolls, Barbies, stuffed animals, gymnastics, and soccer. Since preschool, Jordan has had several friends, mostly girls but also some boys, both at school and in the neighborhood. Over the last 2 years, however, it seems Jordan has had trouble forming new friendships, and some of Jordan's old friends, particularly

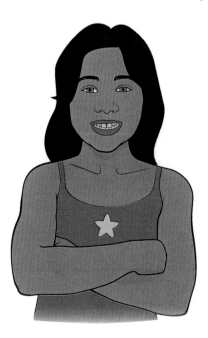

Fig. 6.2 Jordan is an 8-year-old Hispanic child in the third grade being raised by a single, working-class mother

the boys, have disappeared from his social circle. Jordan is brought to the clinic by his mother for gender identity concerns and is described by his mother as being "transgender." Jordan's mother indicates that she loves her child but is uncomfortable with Jordan's gender nonconformity and would prefer if he would pick a side – boy or girl. She is seeking help from the clinic because she wonders if Jordan needs to begin to fully transition (e.g., socially, medically, and legally) as soon as possible in order to prevent possible social, mental health, or behavioral health issues during adolescence or young adulthood. She is also hoping that if Jordan transitions early, it will prevent ongoing ostracization by peers and family members who have started to become more verbal about their discomfort with Jordan's gender fluidity.

Clinical Considerations

There are several factors to attend to when striving to engage in competent and affirmative clinical care with GD adolescents and their families. When assessing a young GD patient's clinical needs, it is important to consider the patient's age and developmental stage, as well as the persistence and consistency of experiences of gender nonconformity within a framework that acknowledges and affirms nonbinary experiences of gender. In this case, Jordan is only 8 years old and because research suggests that gender nonconformity prior to puberty is not necessarily indicative of a transgender identity in adolescence or adulthood, it is most appropriate to support (and help the family support) the child's current and potentially evolving experiences of gender. Moreover, given that puberty is not rapidly approaching for Jordan, medical interventions associated with transitioning (e.g., hormone blockers) are premature and generally not appropriate at this developmental stage.

In this case, an in-depth gender assessment reveals that Jordan has preferred wearing gender nonconforming clothing (e.g., clothing more typical of biological female children) since a relatively young age (3 years old), although recently there have been an increasing number of days where Jordan likes to wear more gender-neutral clothing (e.g., basketball shorts and a plain t-shirt), even at home alone. From a young age, Jordan always cried about getting haircuts, and has had long hair since kindergarten, but often wears it in a low pony tail with a baseball cap, because it "always gets in the way." While Jordan generally prefers a physical gender presentation that is more typical of a young girl (e.g., long hair, dresses, the colors pink and purple), unlike some transgender children Jordan has never stated or affirmed that he is a girl and he appears to have little dysphoria associated with sex organs (e.g., he has never expressed distress about the existence of his penis). When

Jordan is asked about gender identity (e.g., "how do the words boy or girl fit for you?"), Jordan describes it as follows: "I am not really a boy, but I am not really a girl...there's no name for it, I am just me." Jordan has never been bothered by male pronouns (which are used at school and at home), but is also comfortable being referred to with female pronouns (which often happens in public places). Because Jordan does not explicitly reject his male identity or exclusively claim a female identity, feels little gender dysphoria associated with his body, and demonstrates some gender fluidity, Jordan's experience of gender appears to be nonbinary and potentially one that will further evolve as he approaches puberty. Thus, the specific healthcare strategies necessary to support Jordan may be different than those used to support a transgender child or adolescent whose experience of gender is binary and includes a social transition from male to female or female to male, as well as the possibility of gender confirming medical interventions in later adolescence or adulthood (e.g., hormone therapy, surgeries). Jordan and his family may benefit most from educational and advocacy-oriented resources aimed at improving his own, as well as his family's, friends', schools', and community's understanding of and support for nonbinary experiences of gender.

Affirmative Care Approaches

Because GD issues remain invisible and marginalized in society, there is a critical need for psychoeducation aimed at both broadening and deepening understanding of the range of GD experiences and needs, as well as the various strategies for supporting GD adolescents. In Jordan's case, it is important to validate and support his mother's efforts to get him the care and services he needs, while simultaneously educating her about (1) nonbinary experiences of gender, (2) considerations associated with consistent and persistent feelings of gender dysphoria, and (3) age/developmentally appropriate intervention strategies that may or may not include "transitioning." In addition to psychoeducational interventions, supportive interventions may be important for adolescents and family members dealing with stigmatizing experiences associated with GD identities. For instance, Jordan may benefit from supportive individual or group counseling if he is teased or ostracized at school, while his mother may need support from a provider when working to help family and friends understand that Jordan is not "confused" about his gender identity, but rather that his sense of gender is more fluid or diverse than some. Finally, a provider may want to provide Jordan's family with various advocacy-oriented resources aimed at ensuring that Jordan is supported in school. Such resources might include linkages with community-based care coordination services that support SGD students in school [140, 141]; published materials that help parents advocate for their children on their own [158]; or local, regional, or national legal support aimed at creating safe school climates for SGD children and adolescents (e.g., Lambda Legal, National Center for Transgender Equality).

Questions for Learner Discussion

1. How might psychoeducation be an important intervention for this family?
2. What strategies might be shared with Jordan's mother for supporting Jordan's gender identity?
3. Why is it important that the family and the provider support Jordan's gender fluidity?
4. What would be important to know about this family as a healthcare provider?
5. What kinds of advocacy might Jordan need in his community and school?

Specific Bulleted Take Home Points

- GD identity usually becomes evident in early childhood while SD identity tends to emerge during adolescence.
- SGD children and adolescents experience pervasive identity-based stigma, discrimination, and victimization that lead to minority stress.
- As a result of minority stress, SGD children and adolescents face a range of risks to health and mental health. Affirmative care refers to an approach to health assessment and treatment in which SGD identities and identity-based stressors are acknowledged, validated, and considered in all aspects of care.

References

1. Beauchamp D. Sexual orientation and victimization. Canadian Centre for Justice Statistics [Internet]. 2004 [cited 1 Oct 2013]. Available from: http://www.statcan.gc.ca/pub/85f0033m/85f0033m2008016-eng.pdf.
2. Taylor C, Peter T, Schachter K, Paquin S, Beldom S, Gross Z, et al. Youth speak up about homophobia and transphobia: the first national climate survey on homophobia in Canadian schools. Toronto: Egale Canada Human Rights Trust; 2009.
3. Kitts R. Barriers to optimal care between physicians and lesbian, gay, bisexual, transgender and questioning adolescent patients. J Homosex. 2010;57(6):730–47.
4. Pew Research Center. A survey of LGBT Americans: attitudes, experiences and values in changing times. Pew Research Center [Internet]. 2013 [cited 20 Dec 2015]. Available from: http://www.

pewsocialtrends.org/2013/06/13/the-coming-out-experience-age-when-you-first-thought-knew-told/#first-thought.

5. Institute of Medicine. The health of lesbian, gay, bisexual, and transgender people: building a foundation for better understanding. Washington: National Academies Press; 2011.

6. Austin SB, Conron KJ, Patel A, Freedner N. Making sense of sexual orientation measures: findings from a cognitive processing study with adolescents on health survey questions. J LGBT Health Res. 2007;3(1):55–65.

7. Saewyc EM, Skay CL, Hynds P, Pettingell S, Bearinger LH, Resnick MD, et al. Suicidal ideation and attempts in north American school-based surveys: are bisexual youth at increasing risk? J LGBT Health Res. 2007;3(2):25–36.

8. Savin-Williams RC, Ream GL. Prevalence and stability of sexual orientation components during adolescence and young adulthood. Arch Sex Behav. 2007;36(3):385–94.

9. McInroy L, Craig SL. Articulating identities: language and practice with multiethnic sexual minority youth. Couns Psychol Q. 2012;25(2):137–49.

10. American Academy of Pediatrics Committee on Adolescence. Position paper: office-based care for lesbian, gay, bisexual, transgender, and questioning youth. Pediatrics. 2013;132:198–203.

11. Society for Adolescent Health and Medicine. Recommendations for promoting the health and well-being of lesbian, gay, bisexual, and transgender adolescents: a position paper of the Society for Adolescent Health and Medicine. J Adolesc Health. 2013;52:506–10.

12. Gray SAO, Carter AS, Levitt H. A critical review of assumptions about gender variant children in psychological research. J Gay Lesbian Ment Health. 2012;16(1):4–30.

13. Forcier MM, Haddad E. Health care for gender variant and gender non-conforming children. R I Med J. 2013;96(4):17–21.

14. Menvielle E. Transgender children: clinical and ethical issues in prepubertal presentations. J Gay Lesbian Ment Health. 2009;13(4):292–7.

15. Zucker KJ. The DSM diagnostic criteria for gender identity disorder in children. Arch Sex Behav. 2010;39(2):477–98.

16. Substance Abuse and Mental Health Services Administration. Ending conversion therapy: supporting and affirming LGBTQ youth. Substance Abuse and Mental Health Services Administration [Internet]. 2015 [cited 20 Jan 2016]; 15–4928. Available from: http://store.samhsa.gov/shin/content/SMA15-4928/SMA15-4928.pdf.

17. Steensma TD, Kreukels BP, de Vries AL, Cohen-Kettenis PT. Gender identity development in adolescence. Horm Behav. 2013;64(2):288–97.

18. Spack NP, Edwards-Leeper L, Feldman HA, Leibowitz S, Mandel F, Diamond DA, et al. Children and adolescents with gender identity disorder referred to a pediatric clinic. Pediatrics. 2011;129(3):418–25.

19. Steensma TD, McGuire JK, Kreukels BP, Beekman AJ, Cohen-Kettenis PT. Factors associated with desistence and persistence of childhood gender dysphoria: a quantitative follow-up study. J Am Acad Child Adolesc Psychiatry. 2013;52(6):582–90.

20. World Professional Associations for Transgender Health. Standards of care for the health of transsexual, transgender, and gender nonconforming people. 7th ed. World Professional Associations for Transgender Health [Internet]. 2011 [cited 15 Dec 2015]. Available from: http://www.wpath.org/publications_standards.cfm on 10 May 2012.

21. Edwards-Leeper L, Spack NP. Psychological evaluation and medical treatment of transgender youth in an interdisciplinary "gender management service" (GeMS) in a major pediatric center. J Homosex. 2012;59(3):321–36.

22. Hembree WC, Cohen-Kettenis P, Delemarre-van de Waal HA, Gooren LJ, Meyer WJ, Spack NP, et al. Endocrine treatment of transsexual persons: an Endocrine Society clinical practice guideline. J Clin Endocrinol Metab. 2009;94(9):3132–54.

23. Coker T, Austin B, Schuster M. The health and health care of lesbian, gay, and bisexual adolescents. Annu Rev Public Health. 2010;31:457–77.

24. Centers for Disease Control and Prevention. Sexual identity, sex of sexual contacts, and health-risk behaviors among students in grades 9–12 – youth risk behavior surveillance, selected sites, United States, 2001–2009. Morbidity and Mortality Weekly Report [Internet]. 2011 [cited 30 Dec 2015];60. Available from: http://www.cdc.gov/mmwr/pdf/ss/ss60e0606.pdf.

25. Craig SL, McInroy L. The relationship of cumulative stressors, chronic illness and abuse to the self-reported suicide risk of black and hispanic sexual minority youth. J Community Psychol. 2013;41(7):783–98.

26. Marshal M, Dietz L, Friedman M, Stall R, Smith H, McGinlet J, et al. Suicidality and depression disparities between sexual minority and heterosexual youth: a meta-analytic review. J Adolesc Health. 2011;49:115–23.

27. Bostwick W, Meyer I, Aranda R, Hughes T, Birkett M, Mustanski B. Mental health and suicidality among racially/ethnically diverse sexual minority youth. The Williams Institute [Internet]. 2014 [cited 30 Dec 2015]. Available from: http://williamsinstitute.law.ucla.edu/research/safe-schools-and-youth/ajph-jul-2014/#sthash.QrLvJTwp.dpuf. p. 1129–36.

28. Mustanksi B, Garafalo R, Emerson E. Mental health disorders, psychological distress, and suicidality in a diverse sample of lesbian, gay, bisexual, and transgender youth. Am J Public Health. 2010;100(12):2426–32.

29. Grant JM, Mottet LA, Tanis J, Harrison J, Herman JL, Keisling M. Injustice at every turn: a report of the national transgender discrimination survey. National Center for Transgender Equality and National Gay and Lesbian Task Force [Internet]. 2011 [cited 30 Dec 2015]. Available from: http://endtransdiscrimination.org/report.html.

30. Grossman AH, D'Augelli AR. Transgender youth and life-threatening behaviors. Suicide Life Threat Behav. 2005;37(5):527–37.

31. Nuttbrock L, Hwahng S, Bockting W, Rosenblum A, Mason M, Macri M, et al. Psychiatric impact of gender-related abuse across the life course of male-to-female transgender persons. J Sex Res. 2010;47:12–23.

32. Martin-Storey A, Crosnoe R. Sexual minority status, peer harassment, and adolescent depression. J Adolesc. 2012;35(4):1001–11.

33. King M, Semlyen J, Tai SS, Killaspy H, Osborn D, Popelyuk D, et al. A systematic review of mental disorder, suicide, and deliberate self harm in lesbian, gay, and bisexual people. BMC Psychiatry [Internet]. 2008 [cited 30 Dec 2015];8(70). Available from: http://www.ncbi.nlm.nih.gov/pmc/articles/PMC2533652/.

34. Fergusson DM, Horwood LJ, Beautrais AL. Is sexual orientation related to mental health problems and suicidality in young people? Arch Gen Psychiatry. 1999;56(10):876–80.

35. Marshal MP, Dermody SS, Cheong J, Burton CM, Friedman MS, Aranda F, et al. Trajectories of depressive symptoms and suicidality among heterosexual and sexual minority youth. J Youth Adolesc. 2014;42(8):1243–56.

36. Craig SL, Keane G. The mental health of multiethnic lesbian and bisexual youth: the role of self-efficacy, stress and behavioral risks. J Gay Lesbian Ment Health. 2014;18(3):266–83.

37. Centres for Disease Control and Prevention. Diagnoses of HIV infection in the United States and dependent areas, 2014. HIV Surveillance Report [Internet]. 2014 [cited 20 Jan 2016];26. Available from: http://www.cdc.gov/hiv/pdf/library/reports/surveillance/cdc-hiv-surveillance-report-us.pdf.

38. Centres for Disease Control and Prevention. HIV and young men who have sex with men. Centres for Disease Control and

Prevention [Internet]. 2014 [cited 20 Jan 2016]. Available from: http://www.cdc.gov/healthyyouth/sexualbehaviors/pdf/hiv_factsheet_ymsm.pdf.

39. Herbst JH, Beeker C, Mathew A, McNally T, Passin WF, Kay LS, et al. The effectiveness of individual, group, and community-level HIV behavioral risk-reduction interventions for adult men who have sex with men: a systematic review. Am J Prev Med. 2007;32:38–67.

40. Goodenow C. Dimensions of sexual orientation and HIV-related risk among adolescent females: evidence from a statewide survey. Am J Public Health. 2008;98(6):1051–8.

41. Thoma BC, Huebner DM, Rullo JE. Unseen risks: HIV-related risk behaviors among ethnically diverse sexual minority adolescent females. AIDS Educ Prev. 2013;25(6):535–41.

42. Lindley LL, Walsemann KM. Sexual orientation and risk of pregnancy among New York City high-school students. Am J Public Health. 2015;105(7):1379–86.

43. Saewyc EM. Research on adolescent sexual orientation: development, health disparities, stigma, and resilience. J Res Adolesc. 2011;21(1):256–72.

44. Saewyc EM, Poon C, Homma Y, Skay C. Stigma management? The links between enacted stigma and teen pregnancy trends among gay, lesbian, and bisexual students in British Columbia. Can J Hum Sex. 2008;17(3):123–39.

45. Gangamma R, Slesnick N, Toviessi P, Serovich J. Comparison of HIV risks among gay, lesbian, bisexual and heterosexual homeless youth. J Youth Adolesc. 2008;37(4):456–64.

46. Kann L, Olsen EO, McManus T, Kinchen S, Chyen D, Harris WA, et al. Sexual identity, sex of sexual contacts, and healthrisk behaviors among students in grades 9–12—youth risk behavior surveillance, selected sites, United States, 2001–2009. Morbidity and Mortality Weekly Report [Internet]. 2011 [cited 30 Dec 2015];60(7):1–133. Available from: http://www.cdc.gov/mmwr/preview/mmwrhtml/ss6007a1.htm.

47. Marshal MP, Friedman MS, Stall R, King KM, Miles J, Gold MA, et al. Sexual orientation and adolescent AOD use: a meta-analysis and methodological review. Addiction. 2008;103:546–56.

48. Marshal MP, Friedman MS, Stall R, Thompson AL. Individual trajectories of AOD use in lesbian, gay and bisexual youth and heterosexual youth. Addiction. 2009;104:974–81.

49. Ziyadeh NJ, Prokop LA, Fisher LB, Rosario M, Field AE, Camargo CA, et al. Sexual orientation, gender, and alcohol use in a cohort study of U. S. adolescent girls and boys. Drug Alcohol Depend. 2007;87:119–30.

50. Austin A, Craig SL. The role of perceived discrimination in the substance use of multiethnic sexual minority youth. J Gay Lesbian Soc Serv. 2013;25(4):420–42.

51. Reisner SL, Greytak EA, Parsons JT, Ybarra ML. Gender minority social stress in adolescence: disparities in adolescent bullying and substance use by gender identity. J Sex Res. 2015;52(3):243–56.

52. Walls NE, Hancock P, Wisneski H. Differentiating the social service needs of homeless sexual minority youths from those of non-homeless sexual minority youths. J Child Poverty. 2007;13(2):177–205.

53. Poon CS, Saewyc EM. Out yonder: sexual-minority adolescents in rural communities in British Columbia. Am J Public Health. 2009;99:118–24.

54. Cray A, Miller K, Durso LE. Seeking shelter: the experiences and unmet needs of LGBT homeless youth. Washington: Center for American Progress; 2013.

55. Toro PA, Dworsky A, Fowler PJ. Homeless youth in the United States: recent research findings and intervention approaches. In: Dennis D, Locke G, Khadduri J, editors. Toward understanding homelessness: the 2007 National Symposium on homelessness research. Washington: Abt Associates; 2007.

56. Durso LE, Gates GJ. Serving our youth: findings from a national survey of service providers working with lesbian, gay, bisexual, and transgender youth who are homeless or at risk of becoming homeless. Los Angeles: Williams Institute with the True Colors Fund and The Palette Fund; 2012.

57. Cunningham M, Pergamit M, Astone N, Luna J. Homeless LGBTQ youth. Washington: Urban Institute; 2014.

58. Corliss HL, Goodenow CS, Nichols L, Austin SB. High burden of homelessness among sexual-minority adolescents: findings from a representative Massachusetts high school sample. Am J Public Health. 2011;101:1683–9.

59. Ray N. Lesbian, gay, bisexual, and transgender youth: an epidemic of homelessness. New York: National Gay and Lesbian Task Force Policy Institute and National Coalition for the Homeless; 2006.

60. Gallegos A, White CR, Ryan C, O'Brien K, Pecora PJ, Thomas P. Exploring the experiences of lesbian, gay, bisexual, and questioning adolescents in foster care. J Fam Soc Work. 2011;14(3):226–36.

61. Wilson B, Cooper K, Kastanis A, Nezhad S. Sexual and gender minority youth in foster care. The Williams Institute [Internet]. 2014 [cited 30 Dec 2015]. Available from: http://williamsinstitute.law.ucla.edu/research/safe-schools-and-youth/lafys-aug-2014/#sthash.3BX3bNHx.dpuf.

62. Dworsky A. The economic well-being of LGB youth transitioning out of foster care. Mathematica Policy Research [Internet]. 2013 [cite 20 Jan 2016]. Available from: http://www.acf.hhs.gov/sites/default/files/opre/opre_lgbt_brief_01_04_2013.pdf.

63. Berberet H. Putting the pieces together for queer youth: a model of integrated assessment of need and program planning. Child Welfare. 2006;85:361–84.

64. Mallon GP. Permanency for LGBTQ youth. Protecting Child Publ Am Humane Soc. 2011;26(1):49–57.

65. Woronoff R, Estrada R, Sommer S. Out of the margins: a report on regional listening forums highlighting the experiences of lesbian, gay, bisexual, transgender and questioning youth in care. New York: Lambda Legal Defense and Education Fund and the Child Welfare League of America; 2006.

66. Ragg DM, Patrick D, Ziefert M. Slamming the closet door: working with gay and lesbian youth in care. Child Welfare. 2006;85:243–65.

67. Ryan C, Huebner D, Diaz R, Sanchez J. Family rejection as a predictor of negative health outcomes in white and Latino lesbian, gay, and bisexual young adults. Pediatrics. 2009;123:346–52.

68. Doty ND, Willoughby BLB, Lindahl KM, Malik NM. Sexuality related social support among lesbian, gay, and bisexual youth. J Youth Adolesc. 2010;39(10):1134–47.

69. Goldblum P, Testa R, Pflum S, Hendricks M, Bradford J, Bongar B. Gender-based victimization and suicide attempts among transgender people. Prof Psychol Res Pract. 2012;43(5):465–75.

70. Dragowski EA, Halkitis PN, Grossman AH, D'Augelli AR. Sexual orientation victimization and posttraumatic stress symptoms among lesbian, gay, and bisexual youth. J Gay Lesbian Soc Serv. 2011;23(2):226–49.

71. D'Augelli AR, Grossman AH, Starks MT. Childhood gender atypicality, victimization, and PTSD among lesbian, gay, and bisexual youth. J Interpers Violence. 2006;21(11):1462–82.

72. Balsam KF, Rothblum ED, Beauchaine TP. Victimization over the life span: a comparison of lesbian, gay, bisexual, and heterosexual siblings. J Consult Clin Psychol. 2005;73:477–87.

73. Friedman MS, Marshal MP, Guadamuz TE, Wei C, Wong CF, Saewyc E, et al. A meta-analysis of disparities in childhood sexual abuse, parental physical abuse, and peer victimization among sexual minority and sexual nonminority individuals. Am J Public Health. 2011;101:1481–94.

74. Saewyc E, Skay C, Richens K, Reis E, Poon C, Murphy A. Sexual orientation, sexual abuse, and HIV-risk behaviors among adolescents in the pacific northwest. Am J Public Health. 2006;96(6):1104–10.

75. Roberts AL, Rosario M, Corliss HL, Koenen KC, Austin SB. Elevated risk of posttraumatic stress in sexual minority youths: mediation by childhood abuse and gender nonconformity. Am J Public Health. 2012;102:1587–93.

76. Kosciw JG, Greytak EA, Bartkiewicz MJ, Boesen MJ, Palmer NA. The 2011 National School Climate Survey: the experiences of lesbian, gay, bi-sexual, and transgender youth in our nation's schools. GLSEN [Internet]. 2011 [cited 30 Dec 2015]. Available from: file:///C:/Users/ashle/Downloads/2011%20National% 20School%20Climate%20Survey%20Full%20Report.pdf.

77. Bird ST, Bogart LM, Delahanty DL. Health-related correlates of perceived discrimination in HIV care. AIDS Patient Care STDs. 2004;18:19–26.

78. Nadal KL, Issa MA, Leon J, Meterko V, Wideman M, Wong Y. Sexual orientation microaggressions: "death by a thousand cuts" for lesbian, gay, and bisexual youth. J LGBT Youth. 2011;8:234–59.

79. Nadal KL, Skolnik A, Wong Y. Interpersonal and systemic microaggressions toward transgender people: implications for counseling. J LGBT Issues Couns. 2012;6:55–82.

80. Nadal KL, Wong Y, Issa M, Meterko V, Leon J, Wideman M. Sexual orientation microaggressions: processes and coping mechanisms for lesbian, gay, and bisexual individuals. J LGBT Issues Couns. 2011;5(1):21–46.

81. Nadal KL. Preventing racial, ethnic, gender, sexual minority, disability, and religious microaggressions: recommendations for promoting positive mental health. Prev Couns Psychol Theory Res Pract Train. 2008;2(1):22–7.

82. Blume AW, Lovato LV, Thyken BN, Denny N. The relationship of microaggressions with alcohol use and anxiety among ethnic minority college students in a historically white institution. Cultur Divers Ethnic Minor Psychol. 2012;18(1):45–54.

83. Wang J, Leu J, Shoda Y. When the seemingly innocuous "stings": racial microaggressions and their emotional consequences. Personal Soc Psychol Bull. 2011;37(12):1666–78.

84. Feinstein BA, Goldfried MR, Davila J. The relationship between experiences of discrimination and mental health among lesbians and gay men: an examination of internalized homonegativity and rejection sensitivity as potential mechanisms. J Consult Clin Psychol. 2012;80(5):917–27.

85. Hatzenbuehler ML. How does sexual minority stigma "get under the skin"? A psychological mediation framework. Psychol Bull. 2009;135:707–30.

86. Earnshaw V, Bogart LM, Dovidio J, Williams D. Stigma and racial/ethnic HIV disparities: moving towards resilience. Am Psychol. 2013;68:225–36.

87. Herek GM, Gillis JR, Cogan JC. Internalized stigma among sexual minority adults: insights from a social psychological perspective. Stigma Health. 2015;1:18–34.

88. Mizock L, Mueser K. Employment, mental health, internalized stigma, and coping with transphobia among transgender individuals. Psychol Sex Orientation Gend Divers. 2014;1 (2):146–58.

89. Vogel D, Bitman R, Hammer J, Wade N. Is stigma internalizes? The longitudinal impact of public stigma on self-stigma. J Couns Psychol. 2013;60(2):311–6.

90. Breslow A, Brewster M, Velez B, Wong S, Geiger E, Soderstrom B. Resilience and collective action: exploring buffers against minority stress for transgender individuals. Psychol Sex Orientation Gend Divers. 2015;2:253–65.

91. Newcomb ME, Mustanski B. Internalized homophobia and internalizing mental health problems: a meta-analytic review. Clin Psychol Rev. 2010;30:1019–29.

92. Meyer I. Minority stress and mental health in gay men. 2nd ed. - New York: Columbia University Press; 2003.

93. Meyer I, Dietrich J, Schwartz S. Lifetime prevalence of mental disorders and suicide attempts in diverse lesbian, gay, and bisexual populations. Am J Public Health. 2007;97:1–4.

94. Alessi EJ. A framework for incorporating minority stress theory into treatment with sexual minority clients. J Gay Lesbian Ment Health. 2013;18(1):47–66.

95. Lazarus RS, Folkman S. Stress, appraisal, and coping. New York: Springer; 1984.

96. DiPlacido J. Minority stress among lesbians, gay men, and bisexuals: a consequence of heterosexism, homophobia, and stigmatization. In: Herek GE, editor. Stigma and sexual orientation: understanding prejudice against lesbians, gay men, and bisexuals. Thousand Oaks: Sage; 1998.

97. Ryan C, Russell S, Huebner D, Diaz R, Sanchez J. Family acceptance in adolescents and the health of LGBT young adults. J Child Adolesc Psychiatr Nurs. 2010;23(4):205–13.

98. Kelleher C. Minority stress and health: implications for lesbian, gay, bisexual, transgender and questioning young people. Couns Psychol Q. 2009;22:373–9.

99. Birkett M, Espelage DL, Koenig B. LGB and questioning students in schools: the moderating effects of homophobic bullying and school climate on negative outcomes. J Youth Adolesc. 2009;38 (7):989–1000.

100. Public Health Agency of Canada. HIV surveillance data (unpublished data). Surveillance and Epidemiology Division, Centre for Communicable Diseases and Infection Control. Public Health Agency of Canada; 2013.

101. Marcellin R, Scheim A, Bauer G, Redman N. Experiences of transphobia among trans Ontarians. Trans PULSE e-Bulletin [Internet]. 2013 [cited 30 Dec 2015];3(2). Available from: http:// www.transpulseproject.ca.

102. Testa R, Jimenez C, Rankin S. Risk and resilience during transgender identity development: the effects of awareness and engagement with other transgender people on affect. J Gay Lesbian Ment Health. 2014;18:31–46.

103. Bockting WO, Miner MH, Swinburne Romine RE, Hamilton A, Coleman E. Stigma, mental health, and resilience in an online sample of the US transgender population. Am J Public Health. 2013;103(5):943–51.

104. Flicker S, Flynn S, Larkin J, Travers R, Guta A, Pole J, et al. Sexpress: the Toronto teen survey report. Toronto: Planned Parenthood Toronto; 2009.

105. Hoffman ND, Freeman K, Swann S. Healthcare preferences of lesbian, gay, bisexual, transgender, and questioning adolescents. J Adolesc Health. 2009;45(3):222–9.

106. Bess JA, Staab SD. The experiences of transgendered persons in psychotherapy: voices and recommendations. J Ment Health Couns. 2009;31(3):264–82.

107. Zucker K, Bradley S. Gender identity and psychosexual disorders. Focus. 2005;3(4):598–617.

108. American Medical Association. Report 9 of the council on science and public health: optimizing care for gay men and lesbians. American Medical Association [Internet]. 2008 [cited 4 Feb 2010]. Available from http://www.ama-assn.org/ama1/pub/ upload/mm/443/csaph9a08-summary.pdf.

109. D'Augelli AR, Hershberger SL, Pilkington NW. Suicidality patterns and sexual orientation-related factors among lesbian, gay, and bisexual youths. Suicide Life Threat Behav. 2002;31 (3):250–65.

110. Allen LB, Glicken AD, Beach RK, Naylor KE. Adolescent health care experiences of gay, lesbian, and bisexual young adults. J Adolesc Health. 1998;23:212–20.

111. Meckler GD, Elliott MN, Kanouse DE, Beals KP, Schuster MA. Nondisclosure of sexual orientation to a physician among a sample of gay, lesbian, and bisexual youth. Arch Pediatr Adolesc Med. 2006;160:1248–54.

112. Craig SL, McInroy LB, McCready LT, Alaggia R. Media: a catalyst for resilience in sexual minority youth. J LGBT Youth. 2015;12(3):254–75.

113. Mustanski B, Newcomb ME, Garofalo R. Mental health of lesbian, gay, and bisexual youth: a developmental resiliency perspective. J Gay Lesbian Soc Serv. 2011;23:204–25.

114. Goldstein S, Brooks R. Why we study resilience? In: Goldstein S, Brooks R, editors. Handbook of resilience in children. New York: Kluwer; 2005.

115. Hall D, Vine C, Gardner S, Molloy C. Resilience. Toronto: Ministry of Children and Youth Services [Internet]. 2010 [cited 1 Oct 2013]. Available from: http://www.reachinginreachingout.com/documents/MCYS%20Resilience%20Report%2011-16-10%20Dissemination.pdf.

116. Rosen D, Neinstein L. Preventive health care for adolescents. In: Neinstein L, Gordon C, Katzman D, Rosen D, Woods E, editors. Handbook of adolescent health care: a practical guide. Philadelphia: Wolters Kluwer Health/Lippincott Williams & Wilkins; 2009.

117. Eisenberg ME, Resnick MD. Suicidality among gay, lesbian and bisexual youth: the role of protective factors. J Adolesc Health. 2006;39(5):662–8.

118. Hatzenbuehler ML. The social environment and suicide attempts in lesbian, gay, and bisexual youth. Pediatrics. 2011;127(5):896–903.

119. Hatzenbuehler ML, McLaughlin KA. Structural stigma and hypothalamic-pituitary-adrenocortical axis reactivity in lesbian, gay, and bisexual young adults. Ann Behav Med. 2014;47(1):39–47.

120. Higa D, Hoppe MJ, Lindhorst T, Mincer S, Beadnell B, Morrison DM, et al. Negative and positive factors associated with the well-being of lesbian, gay, bisexual, transgender, queer, and questioning (LGBTQ) youth. Youth Soc. 2014;46(5):663–87.

121. Williams T, Connolly J, Pepler D, Craig W. Peer victimization, social support, and psychosocial adjustment of sexual minority adolescents. J Youth Adolesc. 2005;34(5):471–82.

122. Simons L, Schrager SM, Clark LF, Belzer M, Olson J. Parental support and mental health among transgender adolescents. J Adolesc Health. 2013;53:791–3.

123. Needham BL, Austin EL. Sexual orientation, parental support, and health during the transition to young adulthood. J Youth Adolesc. 2010;39:1189–98.

124. Berkman LF. The role of social relations in health promotion. Psychosom Med. 1995;57:245–54.

125. Detrie PM, Lease SH. The relation of social support, connectedness, and collective self-esteem to the psychological well-being of lesbian, gay, and bisexual youth. J Homosex. 2008;53(4):173–99.

126. Lee RM, Robbins SB. The relationship between social connectedness and anxiety, self esteem, and social identity. J Couns Psychol. 1998;45:338–45.

127. Snapp SD, Watson RJ, Russell ST, Diaz RM, Ryan C. Social support networks for LGBT young adults: low cost strategies for positive adjustment. Fam Relat. 2015;64(3):420–30.

128. Grossman AH, Kerner MS. Support networks of gay male and lesbian youth. J Gay Lesbian Bisexual Identity. 1998;3:27–46.

129. Cash SJ, Thelwall M, Peck SN, Ferrell JZ, Bridge JA. Adolescent suicide statements on MySpace. Cyberpsychol Behav Soc Netw. 2013;16(3):166–74.

130. Craig SL, McInroy L, McCready L, Di Cesare D, Pettaway L. Connecting without fear: clinical implications of the consumption of information and communication technologies by sexual minority youth and young adults. Clin Soc Work. 2015;43:159–68.

131. Swan M. The quantified self: fundamental disruption in big data science and biological discovery. Big Data. 2013;1(2):85–100.

132. Craig SL, McInroy L. You can form a part of yourself online: the influence of new media on identity development and coming out for LGBTQ youth. J Gay Lesbian Ment Health. 2014;18(1):95–109.

133. Ybarra ML, Mitchell KJ, Palmer NA, Reisner SL. Online social support as a buffer against online and offline peer and sexual victimization among U.S. LGBT and non-LGBT youth. Child Abuse Negl. 2015;39:123–36.

134. Mustanski B, Greene GJ, Ryan D, Whitton SW. Feasibility, acceptability, and initial efficacy of an online sexual health promotion program for LGBT youth: the queer sex Ed intervention. J Sex Res. 2015;52(2):220–30.

135. Collazo A, Austin A, Craig SL. Facilitating transition among transgender clients: components of effective clinical practice. Clin Soc Work. 2013;41(3):1–10.

136. Austin A. There I am: a grounded theory study of young adults navigating a transgender or gender nonconforming identity within a context of oppression and invisibility. Sex Roles (In press).

137. Newman PA, Fantus S. A social ecology of bias-based bullying of sexual and gender minority youth: towards a conceptualization of conversion bullying. J Gay Lesbian Soc Serv. 2015;27:46–63.

138. Horn SS. Contemporary attitudes about sexual orientation. In: Patterson C, D'Augelli A, editors. The handbook for the psychology of sexual orientation. Oxford: Oxford University Press; 2010.

139. Craig SL, Austin A. The AFFIRM Open Pilot Feasibility Study: a brief affirmative cognitive behavioral coping skills group intervention for sexual and gender minority youth. Child Youth Serv (In press).

140. Craig SL. Strengths-first: an empowering case management model for multiethnic sexual minority youth. J Gay Lesbian Soc Serv. 2012;39(3):274–88.

141. Craig SL, McInroy L, Austin A, Smith M, Engle B. Promoting self-efficacy and self-esteem for multiethnic sexual minority youth: an evidence-informed intervention. J Soc Serv Res. 2012;38(5):688–98.

142. Craig SL. Affirmative supportive safe and empowering talk [ASSET]: leveraging the strengths and resiliencies of sexual minority youth in school-based groups. J LGBT Issues Couns. 2013;7:1–15.

143. Craig SL, Austin A, McInroy LB. School based groups to support multiethnic sexual minority youth resiliency: preliminary effectiveness. Child Adolesc Soc Work J. 2014;31(1):87–106.

144. Craig SL, Austin A, Alessi E. Gay affirmative cognitive behavioral therapy for sexual minority youth: a clinical adaptation. Clin Soc Work. 2013;41(3):25–35.

145. Meininger E, Remafedi G. Gay, lesbian, bisexual, and transgender adolescents. In: Neinstein L, Gordon C, Katzman D, Rosen D, Woods E, editors. Handbook of adolescent health care: a practical guide. Philadelphia: Wolters Kluwer Health/Lippincott Williams & Wilkins; 2009.

146. Ehrensaft D. From gender identity disorder to gender identity creativity: true gender self child therapy. J Homosex. 2012;59(3):337–56.

147. Price-Minter S. Supporting transgender children: new legal, social, and medical approaches. J Homosex. 2012;59:422–33.

148. Austin A, Craig SL. Transgender* affirmative cognitive behavioral therapy: clinical considerations and applications. Prof Psychol Res Pract. 2015;46(1):21–9.

149. Frankowski BL. Sexual orientation and adolescents. Pediatrics. 2004;113:1827–32.

150. Rosenthal SL, Lewis LM, Succop PA, Burklow KA. Adolescents' views regarding sexual history taking. Clin Pediatr. 1999;38:227–33.

151. Mizock L, Lewis TK. Trauma in transgender populations: risk, resilience, and clinical care. J Emot Abus. 2008;8:335–54.

152. Saleebey D. The strengths perspective in social work practice: extensions and cautions. Soc Work. 1996;41:296–305.

153. Woods E, Neinstein L. Office visit, interview techniques, and recommendations to parents. In: Neinstein L, Gordon C, Katzman D, Rosen D, Woods E, editors. Handbook of adolescent health care: a practical guide. Philadelphia: Wolters Kluwer Health/Lippincott Williams & Wilkins; 2009.

154. Lebolt J. Gay affirmative psychotherapy: a phenomenological study. Clin Soc Work J. 1999;27:335–70.

155. Langridge D. Gay affirmative therapy: a theoretical framework and defense. J Gay Lesbian Psychother. 2007;11(1/2):27–43.

156. Association of American Medical Colleges. Implementing curricular and institutional climate changes to improve health care for individuals who are LGBT, gender nonconforming, or born with DSD. 2014. Available from: http://offers.aamc.org/lgbt-dsd-health.

157. Craig SL, Doiron C, Dillon F. Cultivating multiethnic professional allies for sexual minority youth: a community-based educational intervention. J Homosex. 2015;62(12):1703–21.

158. Orr A, Baum J. Schools in transition: a guide for supporting transgender students in K-12 schools. 2015. Available from https://www.nea.org/assets/docs/Schools_in_Transition_2015.pdf.

Nathan Grant Smith

Resilience has been defined as successful adaption to adverse circumstances, including recovery from adversity and the ability to sustain well-being while facing adversity [1]. While it may seem reasonable to assume that trauma, discrimination, loss, and other adverse events will result in negative outcomes, resilience in the face of these stressors is commonly observed [1]. Such is the case with lesbian, gay, bisexual, and transgender (LGBT) individuals, who face similar adversities as people in the general population (e.g., adverse childhood experiences, employment insecurity, financial stress) as well as adversities that are more specific or unique to LGBT communities (e.g., anti-LGBT discrimination, coming out) [2, 3].

An important process in adapting resiliently to adversity is coping. In their cognitive theory of stress and coping, Lazarus and Folkman [4] stated that stress results when an environmental challenge exceeds a person's capacity to cope successfully. When an individual encounters such a challenge, they[1] engage in a process of primary cognitive appraisal in which the impact of the challenge on well-being is evaluated. If the encounter is deemed to be threatening, then the individual engages in a secondary appraisal process to identify coping strategies to mitigate the threat to well-being. One or more coping strategies may be selected; these strategies may be emotion focused, aimed at changing the way one feels about the challenge (such as minimizing the importance of the stressor or identifying positive aspects of the stressor), or problem focused, aimed at changing the challenge itself (such as engaging in problem solving or

taking behavioral steps to address the stressor). In general, emotion-focused coping is more adaptive for stressors that are unchangeable, whereas problem-focused coping is more adaptive for stressors that are changeable. A coping strategy is deemed to be adaptive if it reduces the negative impact of an environmental encounter on an individual's well-being (see Fig. 7.1).

Resilience Resulting from Minority Stressors

Stress and coping theory is a useful framework to understand the impact of anti-LGBT stigma and discrimination on the well-being of LGBT adults. Studies comparing LGBT to heterosexual adults have revealed a number of health disparities, including increased risk for depressive and anxiety disorders; behavioral health problems such as tobacco, alcohol, and illicit drug use; suicidal ideation and attempts; non-suicidal self-injury; and access to healthcare [6]. However, the health professions have long noted that there is nothing inherently pathological about identifying as lesbian, gay, bisexual, or transgender. Indeed, homosexuality was declassified as a mental illness by the American Psychiatric Association in 1973. Further, in 1975, the American Psychological Association stated that "homosexuality, per se, implies no impairment in judgment, stability, reliability, or general social and vocational capabilities" [7] (p633). Rather, the heightened risk of poor health outcomes among LGBT populations is attributed to the stress of living in a society that stigmatizes nonheterosexual sexual orientations and gender identities that do not conform to binary and stereotypical notions of the concordance of sex and gender.

The stress of living in a stigmatizing society has been termed *minority stress*. Meyer [8] operationalized minority stress into five separate components: (a) prejudice events, (b) expectations of stigma/rejection, (c) internalized homonegativity (subsequent authors have expanded this component to include internalized binegativity and

---

[1] Note that "they" is used as a singular pronoun to avoid the false dichotomy of "he or she" that reinforces binary notions of sex and gender.

N.G. Smith, PhD (✉)
Department of Psychological, Health, and Learning Sciences, University of Houston, 3657 Cullen Boulevard, Room 491, Houston, TX 77204-5029, USA
e-mail: ngsmith@central.uh.edu

© Springer International Publishing AG 2017
K.L. Eckstrand, J. Potter (eds.), *Trauma, Resilience, and Health Promotion in LGBT Patients*,
DOI 10.1007/978-3-319-54509-7_7

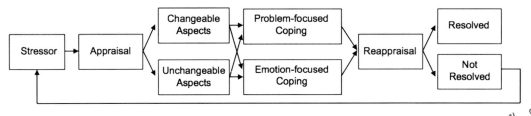

Fig. 7.1 The general stress and coping model (Adapted from Folkman et al. [5] with permission from Springer)

internalized transnegativity for bisexual and transgender persons, respectively), (d) sexual orientation concealment, and (e) ameliorative coping processes. Meyer [2] further noted that minority stress is (a) unique to sexual/gender minorities and thus additive to the stress experienced by all people, (b) chronic, and (c) socially based, meaning that the stress is due to social, institutional, and structural processes rather than due to any factors inherent in the LGBT person experiencing the stress.

While Meyer's [8] minority stress model focuses predominantly on the processes resulting from stigma and the negative outcomes of those processes, the fifth component of his model—compensatory coping, which includes social support and community affiliation—is of particular importance in understanding resilience among LGBT adults. As noted previously, when faced with a stressor, individuals respond by engaging in coping behaviors to mitigate the threat of the stressor; [4] this is also the case with LGBT adults faced with minority stressors. Indeed, Allport [9] noted the resilience of minority group members in engaging in coping strategies to deal with prejudice.

Research on coping in LGBT adults has predominately focused on maladaptive coping processes and the ways in which minority stress activates maladaptive coping (e.g., substance use), in turn increasing negative health outcomes. Indeed, Hatzenbuehler's [10] psychological mediation framework posits that minority stressors (including distal stressors, such as discrimination and violence, and proximal stressors, such as internalized homonegativity) lead to coping, emotion dysregulation, social isolation, and negative cognitive processes. These coping processes, in turn, lead to such outcomes as substance use, depression, and anxiety (see Fig. 7.2). This view of the relations between stress, coping, and outcomes is consistent with Lazarus and Folkman's [4] cognitive theory of stress and coping, which states that maladaptive coping strategies will increase risk for negative outcomes. However, stress and coping theory also states that effective coping strategies are likely to result in resilience. For example, in a qualitative study of 40 gay and lesbian couples, Rostosky et al. [11] found that couples engaged in four types of coping to deal with minority stress. These coping strategies included reframing negative experiences, concealing the relationship to avoid rejection

from others, accessing social support, and affirming the self and the couple. Moreover, the couples viewed these coping strategies as instrumental in allowing them to overcome adversity. However, despite viewing concealment of the relationship as a helpful survival technique, it caused additional stress for couples where differences existed in the level of outness between the partners. In another quantitative study, Lehavot [12] examined almost 1400 lesbian and bisexual women and found that adaptive coping strategies (i.e., active coping, planning, positive reframing, acceptance, humor, religion, and using emotional and instrumental social support) were negatively associated with depression, mental health concerns, and physical health concerns. Similarly, in a sample of Latinx lesbian women and gay men, active coping was negatively associated with depression and positively associated with self-esteem [13].

By engaging in adaptive coping strategies, LGBT adults are able to experience stress-related growth (SRG), a term from positive psychology that explains the occurrence of favorable outcomes following stress [14]. Vaughan and Rodriguez noted that the "link between SRG and psychological wellbeing indicate that SRG may serve as an important pathway by which other strengths develop. In this context, these strengths may go on to serve as protective factors that buffer future experiences of minority stress" [15] (p328).

General Strengths Using a Positive Psychology Framework

With the rise of the positive psychology movement, scholars have recently begun to explore the positive aspects of, or strengths associated with, being LGBT. Positive psychology as a discipline focuses on the strengths of human beings and includes positive individual traits (e.g., forgiveness), positive subjective experiences (e.g., sense of well-being), civic virtues (e.g., altruism), and institutional factors (e.g., workplaces that promote employee growth) that help individuals reach their potential [16]. Vaughan and colleagues [3] recently examined the published literature to identify positive psychology topics explored in LGBT research. The positive psychology themes identified in

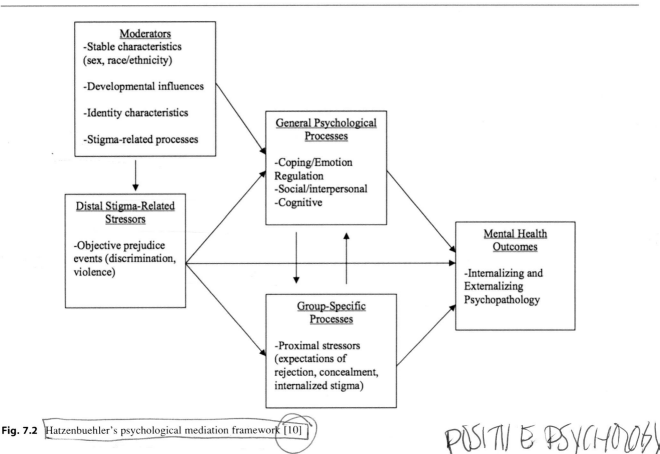

Fig. 7.2 Hatzenbuehler's psychological mediation framework [10]

POSITIVE PSYCHOLOGY (handwritten)

their review included creativity in creating one's identity and in redefining ideas of family; self-acceptance and living honestly, in regard to being authentic both to self and to others; positive affect; love and support in the context of interpersonal relationships; community building and advocacy that is inclusive of a range of marginalized groups (e.g., people of color); connection to community; self-regulation; spirituality; and positive adaptation in the face of adversity. Despite the importance of these topics, the authors found that only one in six LGBT-focused articles included positive psychology themes, pointing to the need for additional research examining strengths in LGBT samples.

Many of these broad positive psychology themes identified in the literature also emerged in the first empirical study to directly ask participants about the positive aspects of being lesbian or gay. Riggle and colleagues [17] asked 553 lesbians and gay men (this study did not examine positive aspects of being bisexual or transgender) to identify the positive aspects of being LG. Only 1% of the sample reported that there were no positive aspects to being LG. Of the remaining 99% who identified positive aspects, their responses fell into three broad categories: disclosure and social support, insights into and empathy for self and others, and freedom from societal definitions. In the disclosure and social support category, positive aspects of being LG included community belongingness, the ability to create families of choice, deeper connections with others, and

being a positive role model. Within the insights into and empathy for self and others domain, participants identified a number of positive aspects of being LG. These included authenticity and honesty with self and others, a deeper sense of self, increased empathy for other people who are oppressed, more cultural sensitivity, and the promotion of social justice and activism. Finally, the freedom from societal definitions theme included ideas such as not being bound by rigid gender role stereotypes, the ability to explore sexuality and ways of being in intimate relationships, and having more egalitarian relationships.

A number of these factors have been identified in qualitative and quantitative research. For example, Russell and Richards [18] found five resilience factors among LGB adults facing anti-LGB stressors: social support, connection with the LGB community, emotional coping, coming out/self-acceptance, and positive reframing. Other strengths identified in the literature include hope and optimism [19], emotional expression [20], and having a positive LGB identity [21]. All of these factors have been shown to be related to positive mental health outcomes among LGB adults. Moreover, while research examining positive psychology constructs specifically in LGBT samples remains scarce, a number of authors (e.g., Hill and Gunderson [22]) have suggested that the strengths predictive of resilience in the general population, such as coping styles and personality traits, should be similarly adaptive among sexual and gender minorities.

Coming Out Growth

As noted in minority stress theory, LGBT individuals have unique stressors. In addition to needing to engage in adaptive coping to successfully overcome these stressors, there is evidence that LGBT-specific stressors can provide opportunities for SRG. Thus, resilience in the face of minority stress may encompass both successful adaptation to adversity and growth as a result of adversity—growth that might not have occurred in the absence of adversity. One such example of LGBT-specific SRG is growth related to coming out. The idea that adopting an LGBT identity and coming out to self and others is adaptive has been discussed in the literature for decades. Indeed, early authors noted that sexual minorities have "our own special, life-affirming gay growth track" [23] (p12). For example, lesbian and bisexual women who completed a measure of SRG regarding the growth they experienced as a result of "coming to terms with [their] sexual identity" (p10) on average scored between 38 (for lesbian women) and 34 (for bisexual women), which approached the maximum for the scale of 45 [24]. Moreover, sexual-orientation-related SRG was positively associated with participants' connectedness to the LGB community and their feelings of generativity (i.e., efforts to promote the next generation). In addition, the original version of the SRG scale was positively associated with optimism, positive affect, and social support in a college sample [14].

Vaughan and Waehler [25] identified five domains of coming out growth in the theoretical and empirical literature: gains in honesty and authenticity, growth in social and personal identity, increases in mental health and well-being, better social and relational functioning, and development of advocacy efforts (see Fig. 7.3). They developed a scale to measure the growth associated with coming out as LG. Their scale included individualistic growth—including gains in mental health, self-acceptance, and social support/relationship satisfaction—and collectivistic growth, including gains in advocating for self and the LG community, community connection, and positive views of the LG community. Both individualistic and collectivistic growth were positively associated with optimism, involvement with the LGBT community, and outness. Moreover, they found a positive relationship between coming out growth and time since beginning the coming out process, where those who had been out longer reported more growth.

The finding that coming out growth increased commensurate with more time elapsed since beginning the coming out process highlights the iterative nature of the coming out process. Coming out to others is a continual process, with each new interpersonal situation (e.g., family/friend interactions, new job) representing a new opportunity to come out; those who have navigated multiple different iterations of coming out may attain the greatest benefits from this process. This explanation is consistent with research indicating that LGB adolescents and young adults evidence greater health disparities than older LGB adults [26, 27]. Thus, LGB adults and those who have had more time to progress through the coming out process may fare better in terms of health outcomes and the growth associated with coming out, although a direct link between the duration of outness and long-term health outcomes has not been studied.

While there is evidence that coming out results in growth, it is important to note that disclosure of a nonheterosexual orientation is not always associated with positive outcomes. While most studies have demonstrated positive associations between outness and health [28], some found no significant relationships [29]. In addition, McGarrity and Huebner [28] found worse physical health outcomes related to outness among gay and bisexual men of lower socioeconomic status (SES). While outness among high SES GB men was associated with fewer physician visits and less perceived stress, levels of outness were associated with more nonprescription drug use, physical symptoms, and perceived stress among low SES GB men. Thus, the benefits of sexual orientation disclosure may not be applicable for those of lower SES, although the degree to which the challenges associated with coming out and disclosure of sexual orientation are related to SRG in lower SES adults is unknown. Moreover, a population-based study of California adults revealed sex differences in the relationship between outness and mental health, with women who were out being less depressed than those who were closeted but men who were out being more depressed than those who were closeted [30]. Thus, it will be important for researchers and care providers to be cognizant of the complex interplay of outness, SRG, resilience, and demographic characteristics such as SES and sex among LGBT adults.

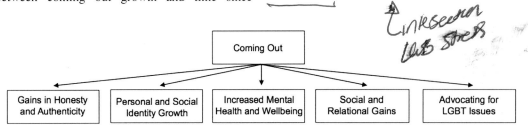

Fig. 7.3 Five broad domains of coming out growth identified in the theoretical and empirical literature by Vaughan and Waehler [25]

Possible explanations for the equivocal findings regarding the adaptiveness of outness include the risk of experiencing discrimination as a result of coming out and subsequent fears of rejection. An early empirical study examining the impact of anti-LGB discrimination on psychological well-being found that individuals who were more out in their workplace were more likely to experience overt or blatant experiences of discrimination [31]. More recent research has examined outness, rejection, and fears of rejection based on sexual orientation. A study of gay men asked participants to indicate whether they had come out to their parents and, if so, how accepting their parents are of their sexual orientation. Participants also completed a measure of gay-related rejection sensitivity by responding to a number of ambiguous hypothetical situations (e.g., not being invited to a party, being seated in a remote part of a restaurant) as to how concerned they were that the situation was a result of their sexual orientation. Those with more rejecting parents had more gay-related rejection sensitivity (i.e., they were more likely to attribute potential rejection to their sexual orientation). Moreover, parental rejection was related to more internalized homonegativity, which mediated the relationship between parental rejection and gay-related rejection sensitivity [32]. Similar findings were observed in a sample of lesbian women and gay men: Experiences of discrimination were related to more LG-related rejection sensitivity and more internalized homonegativity [33]. It appears that experiences of rejection or discrimination may contribute to the development of cognitive distortions and faulty schemas. However, clinicians can work to address these distorted schemas. As the authors of the study focusing on gay men's rejection sensitivity note: "Although gay men's expectations of rejection may not always be inaccurate, rejection-sensitive gay clients may benefit from therapeutic techniques that have proven effective for promoting schema revision, especially if internalized homophobia drives their rejection sensitivity" [32] (p313). Thus, while outness can be resilience promoting, being out also puts one at risk for being rejected or experiencing discrimination, which increases negative feelings about one's sexual orientation and increases the potential for cognitive distortions. Healthcare providers are in a unique position to help sexual minority patients navigate both the risks and rewards of coming out.

Interpersonal Factors Implicated in Resilience

Social support has been studied extensively and shown to be associated with well-being [34]. Research on LGBT adults has explored the role of social support in resilience and well-being via studies examining LGBT individuals' engagement with and connection to the LGBT community, family of origin, and couple/family of choice.

In general, connection to one's community helps to satisfy humans' powerful need to belong and is associated with positive outcomes [35]. LGBT adults who feel connected to an LGBT community are able to compare themselves positively to others in their ingroup, as opposed to comparing themselves negatively to heterosexuals in their outgroup. Positive community connection is believed to be protective against the negative impact of minority stress on health [8]. Frost and Meyer [36] noted that community connection has been linked in a variety of studies to mental health and well-being, increased safer sex practices and decreased sexual risk, and medication adherence and effective coping among HIV-positive individuals. In addition, they found that community connection was positively associated with psychological well-being and negatively associated with internalized homonegativity. Moreover, individuals who were active members of LGBT clubs, organizations, gyms, and/or religious congregations felt more strongly connected to the LGBT community. Connectedness to the transgender community has been shown to be related to less depression and anxiety for transwomen, though a similar relationship was not observed for transmen. However, both transmen and transwomen benefit from general social support, with greater general social support (regardless of the gender identity of the members of the support network) related to less depression and anxiety [37]. For lesbian women, sense of belonging to the lesbian community was a protective factor that reduced the strength of the relationship between body image dissatisfaction and depression [38]. Among gay and bisexual men, engagement in the LGBT community has been conceptualized as a protective factor against HIV risk behaviors. Ramirez-Valles [39], based on a review of the literature, proposed a framework in which LGBT community involvement (a) lessens the impact of poverty, homophobia, and racism on HIV risk behaviors and (b) increases positive peer norms, self-efficacy, and positive self-identity, which all lead to reductions in sexual risk behaviors among GB men.

While engagement with and feeling connected to an LGBT community have been shown to promote resilience in LGBT adults, engagement with and connection to one's family of origin can serve both as a resource and as a source of stress. Whereas LGBT adults can and often do create families of choice [40] made up of supportive individuals who may or may not be biologically related, they cannot choose their families of origin. As such, reactions of family members to the disclosure of an LGBT identity can vary greatly, from distancing of an LGBT person from their family of origin when the reactions are negative, or deepening family cohesion when the reactions are positive [41]. Families that are supportive of their LGBT family members may engage in a number of processes to promote resilience. Oswald [42] categorized these processes into intentionality and redefinition. Intentionality refers to efforts of LGBT persons and their families (of origin and chosen) to engage in strategies that legitimize and support LGBT identities, in the absence of larger societal support for these identities. These intentional behavioral efforts include integrating LGBT and heterosexual family members, providing social support, engaging in the LGBT and ally communities (e.g., PFLAG [Parents, Families, and Friends of Lesbians and Gays] provides resources and education to family members of LGBT individuals), and taking part in supportive rituals (e.g., family members attending pride events or same-sex weddings). Redefinition refers to meaning-making processes that create affirming linguistic and symbolic structures. Such processes include understanding the broader context of heterosexism and transphobia that impact LGBT people's lives, developing and using inclusive language (e.g., family members calling co-mothers by their chosen names, such as one mother being called "mommy" and the other being called "mama"), integrating LGBT identities into other cultural identities, and re-envisioning ideas of what it means to be family.

In addition to supportive families of origin, LGBT adults create families of choice. These include friends, partners, and "gay families." Whereas tight-knit groups of friends become families of choice for a variety of LGBT adults [40], "gay families" or "houses" have emerged in communities of color, predominately among African American and Latino LGBT-identified individuals. Both gay families and houses tend to have family structures that often consist of a gay man or transwoman who is regarded as a role model serving as the parent, with younger gay men and transwomen (and to a lesser degree lesbian women and transmen) as the children. Houses tend to have a performance focus, as is the case in the ballroom community (which was depicted in the 1990 film *Paris Is Burning*), whereas gay families may not have a performance focus [43]. Research has found that houses and gay families serve as important sources of resilience by providing social support, strategies to cope with hetero/cissexism and racism, and tools for safer sex [43, 44].

Creation of families of choice in the LGBT community has redefined the meaning of family in the United States. In addition, rapid political change at the beginning of the twenty-first century has resulted in the increased legitimization of LGBT families. In June 2015, the US Supreme Court ruled in *Obergefell v. Hodges* [45] that all states must recognize marriage between two same-sex individuals, thus allowing for same-sex marriage nationwide. This decision allowed same-sex couples access to federal and state benefits, including employer-sponsored spousal health insurance (*United States v. Windsor* [46] provided some of these benefits, but not necessarily nationwide). Research into the impact of *Obergefell* on same-sex couples is needed to

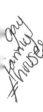

determine if these changes will translate into increased resiliency. However, Perone [47] reviewed the research showing the negative health impacts of denying same-sex couples access to marriage and concluded that *Obergefell* "moves LGBT persons one step closer to better health by affirming marriage equality and thus the dignity of LGBT couples to have equal rights as their opposite-sexed peers in this legal arena" (p197).

Legalization of same-sex marriage and increasing public recognition of LGBT families notwithstanding, Patterson's 2000 review of the literature on same-sex couples and their children "yield[ed] a picture of families thriving, even in the midst of discrimination and oppression. Certainly, [the research] provide[s] no evidence that psychological adjustment among lesbians, gay men, their children, or other family members is impaired in any significant way" [48] (p1064). Indeed, research to date suggests that lesbian and gay couples fare just as well, and in some cases better, than heterosexual couples. A 5-year longitudinal study demonstrated no differences between married heterosexual couples and cohabiting lesbian and gay couples in relationship satisfaction both at initial assessment and over time. In addition, lesbian couples reported more intimacy, autonomy, and equality than heterosexual couples. Gay male couples reported more autonomy than heterosexual couples; levels of intimacy and equality were also greater, though not significantly different. Moreover, lesbian and gay couples were both similar to heterosexual couples in using constructive problem solving to address conflict resolution [49]. Thus, despite additional minority stress and a long history of lack of recognition of their relationships, lesbian and gay families demonstrate resilience.

Individual Difference Factors Implicated in Resilience

A number of individual difference factors that predict resilience in LGBT adults have been explored in the literature. These include, but are not limited to, faith, religion, and spirituality; personality-related factors; and cultural factors. Religious traditions vary in their attitudes toward LGBT persons, with some viewing sexual and gender minorities as abnormal and sinful and others viewing them as normal and/or morally neutral [50, 51]. For example, Unitarian-Universalist, Unity, United Church of Christ, Episcopalian, and Metropolitan Community churches, among others, adopt an affirming view of LGBT issues [52]. As such, faith and religion may be sources of stress or of strength for LGBT adults. When viewed through a resilience lens, faith and religion can offer social support, adaptive coping strategies, and meaning for some LGBT persons. For example, Bowleg et al. [53] found that Black lesbian adults viewed spirituality as a resilience-strengthening factor. Similarly, among Black LGB young adults, for those with high levels of internalized homonegativity, religious faith was associated with more resilience [54]. Among White LGB adults, personal spirituality was positively associated with psychological health. In addition, spirituality mediated the relationship between affirming faith experiences (e.g., feeling welcomed by a religious community, belonging to an LGB-affirming faith community) and psychological well-being. Likewise, affirming faith experiences decreased internalized homonegativity, which was a risk factor for poor psychological health [55]. A qualitative study of transgender female Christian adults revealed a number of positive, as well as negative, experiences with organized religion and spirituality [56]. One participant said, "I go to a very evangelical church ... where I transitioned. I am accepted by the people, and indeed was baptized by immersion there several years ago as my new self" (p27). Other participants discussed the ways in which their faith provided support as they struggled with their gender identity and grew stronger as a result of identifying as transgender. Thus, spirituality and religious engagement, especially engagement with LGBT-affirming religious communities, may be sources of resilience for LGBT adults.

A number of personality-related factors have been examined to explain resilience in LGBT adults. For example, Carter and colleagues [57] found that locus of control moderated the relationship between workplace-based heterosexist discrimination and psychological distress among LGB adults (see Fig. 7.4). For those with a stronger *internal*

locus of control (i.e., the belief that outcomes of one's behavior are determined by internal factors, such as one's own actions), workplace discrimination was not significantly correlated with distress, while for those with a stronger *external* locus of control (i.e., the belief that outcomes of one's behavior are determined by external factors, such as the actions of others), there was a significant and positive relationship between discrimination and distress, such that more discrimination was related to more distress. Thus, it appears that an internal locus of control can buffer the effects of heterosexist discrimination on psychological function among LGB adults. As noted previously, hope, optimism, and emotion regulation have also been examined among LGBT adults. Kwon [20] developed a research-based theoretical model that included emotional openness and hope and optimism (collectively referred to as future orientation) as predictors of psychological health. Specifically, this model posited that emotional openness and future orientation both lead to lower emotional reactivity to anti-LGB prejudice, which in turn lead to better psychological health outcomes. Additional research is needed to fully test Kwon's model; however, existing data support a role for future orientation in explaining individual variation in LGB resilience.

Finally, the impact of cultural factors on LGBT resilience has also been investigated. Moradi et al. [58] noted that in both theoretical and empirical literature, LGB people of color have been conceptualized as having both more risk and more resilience than White LGB people. The assumption is that communities of color are more heterosexist and, as a result, LGB persons of color are exposed to more

Fig. 7.4 The moderating role of locus of control in the relationship between workplace-based prejudice events and psychological distress among LGB adults, as presented in Carter et al. [57]

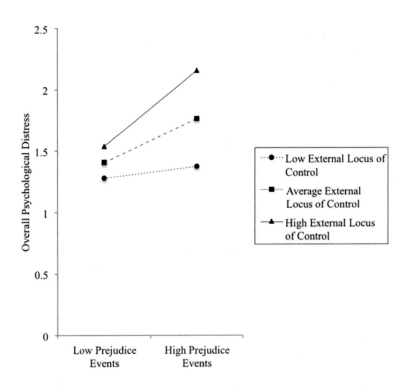

heterosexism, thus placing them at greater risk. In addition, LGB individuals of color are assumed to have greater resilience because of strong faith traditions in communities of color, increased skill in coping with racism translating into skill in coping with heterosexism, and greater flexibility in terms of outness and disclosure. To test these assumptions, Moradi and colleagues directly assessed whether LGB persons of color had more risk and resilience than White LGB persons. There were no group differences between participants of color and White participants on perceived heterosexist stigma, internalized homonegativity, or level of comfort with sexual orientation disclosure; however, White participants were more out than participants of color. The authors suggested that concealment of sexual orientation may be a "reasonable self-protective strategy in the face of widespread heterosexist stigma" (p413) that may be reflective of role flexibility. In addition, the relationship between perceived heterosexist stigma and internalized homonegativity was nonsignificant for persons of color but was significant and positive for White persons. Thus, participants of color appear to be fairly equal in terms of risk, but do show some evidence of heightened resilience in response to heterosexist stigma. Similar results were found in a sample of racially diverse young (18–25) lesbian and bisexual women: there were no racial differences in sexual-orientation-based victimization, depression, anxiety, or heavy drinking [59].

While these studies suggest that there are more similarities than differences between LGB adults of color and White LGB adults in terms of risk and resilience, qualitative studies have revealed specific resilience factors in various LGB racial communities. For example, Sung and colleagues [60] examined resilience factors in Asian American lesbian and bisexual women. Their qualitative results identified a number of coping strategies participants used to deal with challenges associated with being Asian American and lesbian/bisexual (i.e., having multiple minority identities and experiencing heterosexism), including engaging in activism and seeking social support. Participants also identified a number of positive aspects to being Asian American lesbian/bisexual women, such as belonging to multiple (Asian American, LGBT, Asian American lesbian/bisexual female) communities, as well as using Asian cultural values as sources of strength and increased empathy for others. Increased empathy with minority status was also seen in a sample of White gay and bisexual men, who reported more racial empathy toward people of color and more positive racial attitudes than White heterosexual men; moreover, experiences of heterosexist discrimination led to increased empathy, which in turn led to more positive racial attitudes [61]. Similar to findings among Asian American lesbian/bisexual women, a qualitative study of Black lesbians revealed several resilience themes including

confronting oppression, engaging in social support, finding strength in the Black community, and using internal strengths such as humor and spirituality [53].

Resilience Against Suicidality

One outcome of minority stress is an increased risk for suicidal ideation and behavior. Indeed, in a systematic review of the literature, King and colleagues [62] found that the 12-month prevalence of suicide attempts was 2.5 times greater among LGB persons than among heterosexuals. Likewise, lifetime suicidal ideation was twice as common among LGB individuals compared to heterosexuals. A convenience sample of LGB adults in New York City found that 8.7% of LGB adults aged 18–29, 5.9% of LGB adults aged 30–44, and 15.6% of LGB adults aged 45–59 had made a serious suicide attempt [63]. A population-based study in California found that bisexual women were almost six times as likely as heterosexual women to have attempted suicide; bisexual men were almost three times as likely as heterosexual men to have attempted suicide [64]. Rates of suicidality are even more alarming among transgender adults, with studies reporting suicide attempt rates between 23 and 32% [65–67]. In addition, a recent national survey of 6450 transgender adults found a lifetime suicide attempt rate of 41% [68].

In the face of these high rates of suicidal ideation and attempts, it is heartening that protective factors against suicidality have been identified. These factors include social support [69], cognitive reappraisal of suicidal thoughts (i.e., the ability to regulate suicidal thoughts and not act on them) [70], problem solving/coping [69], and identifying reasons for living (i.e., responsibility to others) [71], among others. Most research examining suicide protective factors in LGB samples has focused on youth, described in detail in Chap. 6. While research on suicide resilience in LGB adults is lacking, recent research has explored suicide resilience among transgender adults. In a quantitative study, Moody and Smith [72] found that social support from family, emotional stability, and concern related to one's children (i.e., concern for the effect one's death would have on one's children) were all negatively associated with risk for suicidal behavior in a sample of Canadian transgender adults. Though social support from family was protective against suicidal behavior, the authors found that the amount of perceived social support from family was significantly less than the amount of perceived social support from friends. Thus, interventions aimed at fostering support and acceptance among family members of transgender adults may be lifesaving.

Social support was also an important suicide protective factor in a qualitative study of Canadian transgender adults, in which participants who had experienced suicidal ideation were asked why they had not acted on those thoughts [73]. The authors analyzed participants' answers and grouped their responses into five broad categories: (a) social support, (b) transition-related factors, (c) individual difference factors, (d) reasons for living, and (e) gender identity-related factors. Social support from friends and family, as well as from mental health and community service workers, was viewed by transgender adults as protective. For those participants who wished to transition, disclosing one's gender identity, hope of being able to transition, and actually transitioning were all seen as protective. Next, a number of individual difference factors were protective against suicidal behavior, including coping and problem solving, optimism, and the capacity to withstand suicidal ideation without acting upon it. Reasons for living included feelings of responsibility to others, including children; religious, spiritual, or personal objections to suicide; fear of suicide; desire to keep living; and wanting to be a positive role model to other transgender persons. Finally, a number of gender identity-related factors emerged as protective. Realizing oneself to be transgender eased the pain and confusion related to questioning one's gender identity, thereby reducing suicidality. Establishing a stable sense of one's transgender identity, gaining self-acceptance of one's identity, and having the opportunity to live authentically were also protective against suicide. In regard to self-acceptance, participants discussed a process of moving from distress and discomfort to feeling comfortable with themselves. Participants reported feelings of distress prior to identifying as transgender; however, once they began to express their gender identity and identify themselves as transgender, they were able to better accept themselves for who they are. Subsequently, their feelings of distress decreased. Taken together, these results suggest numerous ways to reduce suicide risk among transgender adults (e.g., improve access to transition-related care and encourage patients to seek social connection and identify reasons for living). More research is needed to continue to identify suicide protective factors in both transgender and LGB adults.

Emerging Data

As discussed in Chap. 4, emerging data examining stress biomarkers, such as cortisol, show promise for the exploration of resilience among LGB adults. Cortisol is the stress hormone produced as a result of hypothalamic-pituitary-adrenal (HPA) axis activation in response to stress. Cortisol production in response to an acute stressor mobilizes the body for "fight or flight," but continued exposure to stress and the resulting HPA axis activation cause wear and tear on the body, known as allostatic load. Researchers in Montreal,

QC, Canada [74], found that gay and bisexual men had lower cortisol concentrations than heterosexual men in response to a laboratory-induced stressor (i.e., a mock job interview and engaging in mental arithmetic in front of a one-way mirror). While it is unclear whether this blunted cortisol response is adaptive or maladaptive, the same researchers found that gay and bisexual men had lower allostatic load and less depression than heterosexual men [75]. In addition, in a US-based sample of young LGB adults, those who had grown up in more LGB-accepting environments showed a less blunted acute cortisol response to a laboratory-induced stressor than those who had grown up in more stigmatizing environments [76]. While more research is needed to fully explore the clinical implications of cortisol responses on stress reactivity and resilience in LGBT adults, these emerging data suggest that resilience may be evident in biological markers of stress.

Emerging data regarding LGB-affirmative treatment approaches have shown promise for integrating resilience-fostering strategies into clinical treatment. Pachankis and colleagues [77] developed a cognitive-behavioral therapy for young adult gay and bisexual men that focused on providing participants with skills to manage the impact of minority stress on cognitive, affective, and behavioral processes (e.g., development of emotion regulation skills, assertive communication skills, and cognitive restructuring skills). A total of 63 participants were randomized to the treatment or to a waitlist control group. Results indicated that those in the treatment group had reduced depression, alcohol use problems, sexual compulsivity, and condomless sex. My colleagues and I [78] developed a similar intervention focused on helping young adult gay and bisexual men develop effective coping strategies for dealing with minority stress. We presented three case studies that each demonstrated reductions in condomless sex at 3-month follow-up. In addition, we found reductions in alcohol use, number of sex partners, loneliness, and internalized homonegativity, combined with increases in self-esteem [79]. These new affirmative treatment models offer specific guidelines for promoting resilience in gay and bisexual men. Additional affirmative interventions with LGBT clients have been discussed in the literature, but few studies have actually examined the efficacy of specific treatment approaches. For a recent overview of the state of LGB-affirmative psychotherapy, see Johnson's [80] 2012 review of existing meta-analyses and systematic reviews.

Resilience Promotion in Patient/Provider Relationships

Because of experiences or fears of discrimination by healthcare workers, some LGBT patients are concerned about receiving poor care and thus may not disclose their sexual orientation or gender identity to providers [81]. However, like all patients, LGBT individuals want and deserve competent and effective healthcare. For example, a study of lesbian women found that participants wanted, but did not always receive, healthcare that is comprehensive, person centered, free from discrimination, and integrative of their lesbian identities [82]. Moreover, when patients are provided with this type of healthcare, they are more likely to be open about their sexual orientation and gender identity with healthcare providers and to engage more actively in seeking and utilizing healthcare. A study of Canadian lesbian adults found that women who were more open about their sexual orientation were more likely to disclose to their healthcare providers, which in turn was related to greater healthcare utilization. In addition, those who were more comfortable with their healthcare providers were more likely to seek routine preventive care [83]. In order to promote resilience in LGBT adult patients, healthcare providers must be knowledgeable about LGBT issues and create a welcoming healthcare environment. Indeed, establishing an accepting and supportive provider-patient relationship can provide the cornerstone for the development of additional social connections in the future, and the guidance of a knowledgeable provider can help direct patients toward community supports and affirmative coping practices.

A number of professional organizations have developed guidelines or standards for working effectively with LGBT patients; provider knowledge and healthcare environment are central to these guidelines. For example, the American Psychological Association has published guidelines for psychological practice with both LGB [84] and transgender [85] patients. Though focused on psychologists, these guidelines are applicable to a variety of healthcare providers as they provide a frame of reference and basic information for working with LGBT patients. Similarly, the Association of American Medical Colleges (AAMC) Advisory Committee on Sexual Orientation, Gender Identity, and Sex Development developed competencies that all physicians should be able to demonstrate when working with LGBT patients [86]. The guidelines direct healthcare providers to be knowledgeable about the issues facing LGBT patients, including issues of stigma, family and partner issues, workplace issues, cultural diversity, and unique issues facing bisexual and transgender patients. The guidelines also discuss the important role that provider attitudes and knowledge have in the care they provide to LGBT patients. Provider bias and lack of knowledge can negatively impact the care they provide and subsequent patient outcome.

The Gay, Lesbian, Bisexual and Transgender Health Access Project [87] produced standards for the provision of healthcare services to LGBT patients. The standards include administrative and service delivery components, including personnel, patient rights, intake and assessment, service planning and delivery, confidentiality, and community outreach and health promotion. The standards focus on the knowledge base of providers and agency staff, nondiscriminatory treatment of patients and agency employees, and culturally appropriate intake and assessment procedures, as well as other foci including methods of health promotion and outreach.

GLMA: Health Professionals Advancing LGBT Equality [88] published guidelines for care of LGBT patients, which include suggestions for creating a welcoming environment for LGBT patients, ways to make paperwork and patient-provider interactions more inclusive, staff training suggestions, and specific considerations when working with lesbian and bisexual women and when working with gay and bisexual men. Suggestions for creating a more welcoming climate include having visible displays of LGBT-inclusive materials in offices, such as brochures about LGBT health, posters that include LGBT people, and nondiscrimination statements that include sexual orientation and gender identity; avoiding using heterosexist language in intake forms or in in-person assessments, such as using gender-neutral language such as "partner" rather than "husband/wife"; avoiding asking transgender persons unnecessary questions; mirroring patients' language; avoiding making assumptions; and having at least one gender-inclusive restroom that is not labeled as "men" or "women." The guidelines also provide some basic information about health issues facing LGBT persons, such as minority stress issues; tobacco, alcohol, and drug use; safer sex and sexually transmitted infections; and violence. Finally, the guidelines contain specific recommendations for working with sexual minority women, such as pap screening, and sexual minority men, such as hepatitis immunization.

Summary

LGBT adults show remarkable resilience in the face of societally based adversity. Sources of resilience include effective coping strategies; focusing on positive aspects of being LGBT; growth resulting from stress; support from family, community, and partners; and individual strengths. Healthcare providers wishing to help promote the resilience of their LGBT adult patients need to be knowledgeable about the issues facing their patients and to create a welcoming environment in which to see their patients. LGBT-affirmative healthcare practice can help to promote resilience in sexual and gender minority patients and facilitate better healthcare utilization and health-promoting behaviors.

While LGBT adults have the capacity for resilience, focusing solely on individual resilience ignores the important role that policies and institutions have in reducing the stigma and discrimination faced by people with diverse sexual orientations and gender identities. If LGBT people lived in a more affirming social context, they would not need to expend as many resources on developing and maintaining their resilience. Thus, healthcare providers are encouraged to foster the resilience of their LGBT patients while simultaneously working to accomplish structural changes to alleviate the pathogenic social environment that causes health disparities in the first place [89]. As Meyer [8] (p691) noted in laying out his minority stress theory:

> As researchers are urged to represent the minority person as a resilient actor rather than a victim of oppression, they are at risk of shifting their view of prejudice, seeing it as a subjective stressor—an adversity to cope with and overcome—rather than as an objective evil to be abolished.

Given their important role in society at large, healthcare providers are well situated to advocate for LGBT patients and to work to abolish the evils LGBT people face.

Case Scenario

Wanda is a 40-year-old Black female who presents for her yearly physical. During initial discussion, she reveals that she has been feeling more stress than usual at work and as a result has been drinking alcohol and smoking cigarettes more often (Fig. 7.5). She perceives that alcohol and tobacco use are relaxing and help her to cope with the stress of her job. She is concerned about her weight and knows that the alcohol is contributing to her weight gain, but also notes that the cigarettes help to decrease her appetite. When you inquire about the stress at work, she states that coworkers have been "targeting" her and describes a colleague who has been cold to her and gives her "funny looks" ever since Wanda mentioned her girlfriend of several years. She was initially

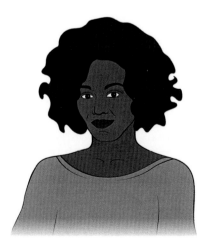

Fig. 7.5 Wanda is a 40-year-old Black female who presents for her yearly physical

hesitant to come out at work given the prior negative reaction of her mother to her identifying as a same-gender-loving woman, but wanted to participate in office discussions regarding families and children. In addition, she complains of low energy and often not wanting to get out of bed.

Discussion Questions

1. What adaptive and maladaptive coping strategies are more frequently observed among LGBT adults in response to discrimination and rejection?
2. How does minority stress impact the mental and physical health of LGBT adults? How does this vary by race, ethnicity, and religion?
3. What interpersonal and individual resilience strategies support improved health among LGBT adults?
4. How do affirmative treatments help to foster resilience development in LGBT adults?
5. What strategies can health professionals utilize to promote resilience and positive health outcomes among LGBT adults?

Summary Practice Points

- Maladaptive coping strategies in response to interpersonal rejection and/or discrimination observed among LGBT adults include behaviors (such as tobacco, alcohol, and/or substance use, higher-risk sexual practices, self-injury, or suicide attempts) or thought processes including suicidal ideation, rumination, or internalization of rejection.
- Anti-LGBT stigma and rejection are associated with depression, anxiety, and physical health sequelae of maladaptive behaviors including STIs, hepatitis, certain cancers, and chronic obstructive pulmonary disease.
- Bias and discrimination can affect LGBT adults across the life span; for example, 38% of LGB and 78% of transgender adults report LGBT-related workplace discrimination.
- Adaptive coping and resilience-enhancing strategies used by LGBT adults include engaging family and/or chosen social support networks, cognitive reappraisal of rejection or suicidal thoughts, strengthening self-acceptance, positioning an internal locus of control, and forward thinking.
- Health professionals can accept and affirm the experiences of LGBT adults, explore and strengthen adaptive coping strategies with patients, and openly discuss treatment options for addressing maladaptive coping strategies that individuals are motivated to change.

Resources

1. Resources from the Gay and Lesbian Medical Association at http://www.glma.org/index.cfm?fuseaction= Page.viewPage&pageId=534.
2. Gay and Lesbian Medical Association. Guidelines for care of lesbian, gay, bisexual and transgender patients. San Francisco, CA: Gay and Lesbian Medical Association; 2006. Available from: http://glma.org/_data/n_0001/ resources/live/GLMA%20guidelines%202006%20FINAL. pdf.
3. LGBT resources from the American Medical Association at http://www.ama-assn.org/ama/pub/about-ama/our-peo ple/member-groups-sections/glbt-advisory-committee/ glbt-resources.page.
4. LGBT resources from the American Psychological Association at http://www.apa.org/pi/lgbt/.

References

1. Zautra AJ, Hall JS, Murray KE. Resilience: a new definition of health for people and communities. HandbAdult Resilience. 2010;1:3–34.
2. Meyer IH. Prejudice and discrimination as social stressors. In: The health of sexual minorities. Boston: Springer; 2007. p. 242–67.
3. Vaughan MD, Miles J, Parent MC, Lee HS, Tilghman JD, Prokhorets S. A content analysis of LGBT-themed positive psychology articles. Psychol Sex Orientation Gend Divers. 2014;1 (4):313–24.
4. Lazarus RS, Folkman S. Stress, appraisal, and coping. New York: Springer; 1984.
5. Folkman S, Chesney M, McKusick L, Ironson G, Johnson D, Coates T. Translating coping theory into an intervention. In: Eckenrode J, editor. The social context of coping. New York: Plenum Press; 1991. p. 239–60.
6. Institute of Medicine. The health of lesbian, gay, bisexual, and transgender people: building a foundation for better understanding. Washington, DC: National Academies Press; 2011.
7. Conger JJ. Proceedings of the American Psychological Association, incorporated, for the year 1974: minutes of the annual meeting of the Council of Representatives. Am Psychol. 1975;30:620–51.
8. Meyer IH. Prejudice, social stress, and mental health in lesbian, gay, and bisexual populations: conceptual issues and research evidence. Psychol Bull. 2003;129(5):674–97.
9. Allport GW. The nature of prejudice. Reading: Addison- Wesley; 1954.
10. Hatzenbuehler ML. How does sexual minority stigma "get under the skin"? A psychological mediation framework. Psychol Bull. 2009;135(5):707–30.
11. Rostosky SS, Riggle ED, Gray BE, Hatton RL. Minority stress experiences in committed same-sex couple relationships. Prof Psychol Res Pract. 2007;38:392–400.
12. Lehavot K. Coping strategies and health in a national sample of sexual minority women. Am J Orthopsychiatry. 2012;82 (4):494–504.
13. Zea MC, Reisen CA, Poppen PJ. Psychological well-being among Latino lesbians and gay men. Cultur Divers Ethnic Minor Psychol. 1999;5(4):371–9.

14. Park CL, Cohen LH, Murch RL. Assessment and prediction of stress-related growth. J Pers. 1996;64:71–106.
15. Vaughan MD, Rodriguez EM. LGBT strengths: incorporating positive psychology into theory, research, training, and practice. Psychol Sex Orientation Gend Divers. 2014;1(4):325–34.
16. Seligman MEP, Csikszentmihalyi M. Positive psychology: an introduction. Am Psychol. 2000;55(1):5–14.
17. Riggle ED, Whitman JS, Olson A, Rostosky SS, Strong S. The positive aspects of being a lesbian or gay man. Prof Psychol Res Pract. 2008;39:210–7.
18. Russell GM, Richards JA. Stressor and resilience factors for lesbians, gay men, and bisexuals confronting antigay politics. Am J Community Psychol. 2003;31(3–4):313–28.
19. Kwon P, Hugelshofer DS. The protective role of hope for lesbian, gay, and bisexual individuals facing a hostile workplace climate. J Gay Lesbian Ment Health. 2010;14(1):3–18.
20. Kwon P. Resilience in lesbian, gay, and bisexual individuals. Personal Soc Psychol Rev. 2013;17(4):371–83.
21. Riggle ED, Mohr JJ, Rostosky SS, Fingerhut AW, Balsam KF. A multifactor lesbian, gay, and bisexual positive identity measure (LGB-PIM). Psychol Sex Orientation Gend Divers. 2014;1 (4):398–411.
22. Hill CA, Gunderson CJ. Resilience of lesbian, gay, and bisexual individuals in relation to social environment, personal characteristics, and emotion regulation strategies. Psychol Sex Orientation Gend Divers. 2015;2(3):232–52.
23. Berzon B. Positively gay. Millbrae: Celestial Arts; 1979.
24. Bonet L, Wells BE, Parsons JT. A positive look at a difficult time: a strength based examination of coming out for lesbian and bisexual women. J LBGT Health Res. 2007;3(1):7–14.
25. Vaughan MD, Waehler CA. Coming out growth: conceptualizing and measuring stress-related growth associated with coming out to others as a sexual minority. J Adult Dev. 2010;17(2):94–109.
26. Bränström R, Hatzenbuehler ML, Pachankis JE. Sexual orientation disparities in physical health: age and gender effects in a population-based study. Soc Psychiatry Psychiatr Epidemiol. 2016;51(2):289–301.
27. Thomeer MB. Sexual minority status and self-rated health: the importance of socioeconomic status, age, and sex. Am J Public Health. 2013;103(5):881–8.
28. McGarrity LA, Huebner DM. Is being out about sexual orientation uniformly healthy? The moderating role of socioeconomic status in a prospective study of gay and bisexual men. Ann Behav Med. 2014;47(1):28–38.
29. McGregor BA, Carver CS, Antoni MH, Weiss S, Yount SE, Ironson G. Distress and internalized homophobia among lesbian women treated for early stage breast cancer. Psychol Women Q. 2001;25(1):1–9.
30. Pachankis JE, Cochran SD, Mays VM. The mental health of sexual minority adults in and out of the closet: a population-based study. J Consult Clin Psychol. 2015;83(5):890–901.
31. Waldo CR. Working in a majority context: a structural model of heterosexism as minority stress in the workplace. J Couns Psychol. 1999;46(2):218–32.
32. Pachankis JE, Goldfried MR, Ramrattan ME. Extension of the rejection sensitivity construct to the interpersonal functioning of gay men. J Consult Clin Psychol. 2008;76(2):306–17.
33. Feinstein BA, Goldfried MR, Davila J. The relationship between experiences of discrimination and mental health among lesbians and gay men: an examination of internalized homonegativity and rejection sensitivity as potential mechanisms. J Consult Clin Psychol. 2012;80(5):917–27.
34. Cohen S, Wills TA. Stress, social support, and the buffering hypothesis. Psychol Bull. 1985;98(2):310–57.
35. Baumeister RF, Leary MR. The need to belong: desire for interpersonal attachments as a fundamental human motivation. Psychol Bull. 1995;117(3):497–529.

36. Frost DM, Meyer IH. Measuring community connectedness among diverse sexual minority populations. J Sex Res. 2012;49(1):36–49.

37. Pflum SR, Testa RJ, Balsam KF, Goldblum PB, Bongar B. Social support, trans community connectedness, and mental health symptoms among transgender and gender nonconforming adults. Psychol Sex Orientation Gend Divers. 2015;2(3):281–6.

38. Hanley S, McLaren S. Sense of belonging to layers of lesbian community weakens the link between body image dissatisfaction and depressive symptoms. Psychol Women Q. 2015;39(1):85–94.

39. Ramirez-Valles J. The protective effects of community involvement for HIV risk behavior: a conceptual framework. Health Educ Res. 2002;17(4):389–403.

40. Weston K. Families we choose: Lesbians, gays, kinship. New York: Columbia University Press; 1991.

41. Patterson CJ. Lesbian and gay family issues in the context of changing legal and social policy environments. In: Bieschke KJ, Perez RM, DeBord KA, editors. Handbook of counseling and psychotherapy with lesbian, gay, bisexual, and transgender clients. 2nd ed. Washington, DC: American Psychological Association; 2007. p. 359–77.

42. Oswald RF. Resilience within the family networks of lesbians and gay men: intentionality and redefinition. J Marriage Fam. 2002;64(2):374–83.

43. Levitt HM, Horne SG, Puckett J, Sweeney KK, Hampton ML. Gay families: challenging racial and sexual/gender minority stressors through social support. J GLBT Fam Stud. 2015;11(2):173–202.

44. Arnold EA, Bailey MM. Constructing home and family: how the ballroom community supports African American GLBTQ youth in the face of HIV/AIDS. J Gay Lesbian Soc Serv. 2009;21(2–3):171–88.

45. Obergefell v. Hodges (2015).

46. United States v. Windsor (2013).

47. Perone AK. Health implications of the Supreme Court's Obergefell vs. Hodges marriage equality decision. LGBT Health. 2015;2:196–9.

48. Patterson CJ. Family relationships of lesbians and gay men. J Marriage Fam. 2000;62(4):1052–69.

49. Kurdek LA. Relationship outcomes and their predictors: longitudinal evidence from heterosexual married, gay cohabiting, and lesbian cohabiting couples. J Marriage Fam. 1998;60:553–68.

50. Ontario consultants on religious tolerance. n.d. Available from: http://www.religioustolerance.org.

51. Porter KE, Ronneberg CR, Witten TM. Religious affiliation and successful aging among transgender older adults: findings from the trans MetLife survey. J Religion Spirituality Aging. 2013;25(2):112–38.

52. Schuck KD, Liddle BJ. Religious conflicts experienced by lesbian, gay, and bisexual individuals. J Gay Lesbian Psychother. 2001;5(2):63–82.

53. Bowleg L, Huang J, Brooks K, Black A, Burkholder G. Triple jeopardy and beyond: multiple minority stress and resilience among black lesbians. J Lesbian Stud. 2003;7(4):87–108.

54. Walker JNJ, Longmire-Avital B. The impact of religious faith and internalized homonegativity on resiliency for black lesbian, gay, and bisexual emerging adults. Dev Psychol. 2013;49(9):1723–31.

55. Lease SH, Horne SG, Noffsinger-Frazier N. Affirming faith experiences and psychological health for caucasian lesbian, gay, and bisexual individuals. J Couns Psychol. 2005;52(3):378–88.

56. Yarhouse MA, Carrs TL. MTF transgender Christians' experiences: a qualitative study. J LGBT Issues Couns. 2012;6(1):18–33.

57. Carter LW, Mollen D, Smith NG. Locus of control, minority stress, and psychological distress among lesbian, gay, and bisexual individuals. J Couns Psychol. 2014;61:169–75.

58. Moradi B, Wiseman MC, DeBlaere C, Goodman MB, Sarkees A, Brewster ME, et al. LGB of color and white individuals' perceptions of heterosexist stigma, internalized homophobia, and outness: comparisons of levels and links. Couns Psychol. 2010;38(3):397–424.

59. Balsam KF, Molina Y, Blayney JA, Dillworth T, Zimmerman L, Kaysen D. Racial/ethnic differences in identity and mental health outcomes among young sexual minority women. Cultur Divers Ethnic Minor Psychol. 2015;21(3):380–90.

60. Sung MR, Szymanski DM, Henrichs-Beck C. Challenges, coping, and benefits of being an Asian American lesbian or bisexual woman. Psychol Sex Orientation Gend Divers. 2015;2(1):52–64.

61. Kleiman S, Spanierman LB, Smith NG. Translating oppression: understanding how sexual minority status is associated with white men's racial attitudes. Psychol Men Masculinity. 2015;16:404–15.

62. King M, Semlyen J, Tai SS, Killaspy H, Osborn D, Popelyuk D, et al. A systematic review of mental disorder, suicide, and deliberate self harm in lesbian, gay and bisexual people. BMC Psychiatry. 2008;8:70.

63. Meyer IH, Dietrich J, Schwartz S. Lifetime prevalence of mental disorders and suicide attempts in diverse lesbian, gay, and bisexual populations. Am J Public Health. 2008;98(6):1004–6.

64. Blosnich JR, Nasuti LJ, Mays VM, Cochran SD. Suicidality and sexual orientation: characteristics of symptom severity, disclosure, and timing across the life course. Am J Orthopsychiatry. 2016;86(1):69–78.

65. Mathy RM. Transgender identity and suicidality in a nonclinical sample: sexual orientation, psychiatric history, and compulsive behaviors. J Psychol Hum Sex. 2002;14:47–65.

66. Nuttbrock L, Hwahng S, Bockting W, Rosenblum A, Mason M, Macri M, et al. Psychiatric impact of gender-related abuse across the life course of male-to-female transgender persons. J Sex Res. 2010;47:12–23.

67. Clements-Nolle K, Marx R, Katz M. Attempted suicide among transgender persons: the influence of gender-based discrimination and victimization. J Homosex. 2006;51:53–69.

68. Grant JM, Mottet LA, Tanis J, Harrison J, Herman JL, Keisling M. Injustice at every turn: a report of the National Transgender Discrimination Survey. Washington, DC: National Center for Trans- gender Equality and National Gay and Lesbian Task Force; 2011.

69. Johnson J, Wood AM, Gooding P, Taylor PJ, Tarrier N. Resilience to suicidality: the buffering hypothesis. Clin Psychol Rev. 2011;31:563–91.

70. Osman A, Gutierrez PM, Muehlenkamp JJ, Dix-Richardson F, Barrios FX, Kopper BA. Suicide resilience inventory-25: development and preliminary psychometric properties. Psychol Rep. 2004;94:1349–60.

71. Linehan MM, Goodstein JL, Nielsen SL, Chiles JA. Reasons for staying alive when you are thinking of killing yourself: the reasons for living inventory. J Consult Clin Psychol. 1983;51:276–86.

72. Moody C, Smith NG. Suicide protective factors among trans adults. Arch Sex Behav. 2013;42:739–52.

73. Moody C, Fuks N, Pelaez S, Smith NG. "Without this, I would for sure already be dead": a qualitative inquiry regarding suicide protective factors among trans adults. Psychol Sex Orientation Gend Divers. 2015;2:266–80.

74. Juster R-P, Hatzenbuehler ML, Mendrek A, Pfaus JG, Smith NG, Johnson PJ, et al. Sexual orientation modulates endocrine stress reactivity. Biol Psychiatry. 2015;77(7):668–76.

75. Juster R-P, Smith NG, Ouellet É, Sindi S, Lupien SJ. Sexual orientation and disclosure in relation to psychiatric symptoms, diurnal cortisol, and allostatic load. Psychosom Med. 2013;75(2):103–16.

76. Hatzenbuehler ML, McLaughlin KA. Structural stigma and hypothalamic–pituitary–adrenocortical axis reactivity in lesbian, gay, and bisexual young adults. Ann Behav Med. 2014;47(1):39–47.

77. Pachankis JE, Hatzenbuehler ML, Rendina HJ, Safren SA, Parsons JT. LGB-affirmative cognitive-behavioral therapy for young adult

gay and bisexual men: a randomized controlled trial of a transdiagnostic minority stress approach. J Consult Clin Psychol. 2015;83:875–89.

78. Smith NG, Hart TA, Moody C, Willis AC, Andersen MF, Blais M, et al. Project PRIDE: a cognitive-behavioral group intervention to reduce HIV risk behaviors among HIV-negative young gay and bisexual men. Cogn Behav Pract. 2016;23:398–411.

79. Moody C, Smith NG, Hart T, Willis AC, Stratton NL, Blais M, et al. Project PRIDE (Promoting Resilience In Discriminatory Environments): results of a pilot test of an HIV-prevention intervention for gay and bisexual men. Counseling Psychology Conference; Atlanta, 2014.

80. Johnson SD. Gay affirmative psychotherapy with lesbian, gay, and bisexual individuals: implications for contemporary psychotherapy research. Am J Orthopsychiatry. 2012;82(4):516–22.

81. Eliason MJ, Schope R. Original research: does "don't ask don't tell" apply to health care? Lesbian, gay, and bisexual people's disclosure to health care providers. J Gay Lesbian Med Assoc. 2001;5 (4):125–34.

82. Seaver MR, Freund KM, Wright LM, Tjia J, Frayne SM. Healthcare preferences among lesbians: a focus group analysis. J Womens Health. 2008;17(2):215–25.

83. Bergeron S, Senn CY. Health care utilization in a sample of Canadian lesbian women: predictors of risk and resilience. Women Health. 2003;37(3):19–35.

84. American Psychological Association. Guidelines for psychological practice with lesbian, gay, and bisexual clients. Am Psychol. 2012;67(1):10–42.

85. American Psychological Association. Guidelines for psychological practice with transgender and gender nonconforming people. Am Psychol. 2015;70(9):832–64.

86. Hollenbach A, Eckstrand KL, Dreger AD. Implementing curricular and institutional climate changes to improve health care for individuals who are LGBT, gender nonconforming, or born with DSD: a resource for medical educators. Washington, DC: Association of American Medical Colleges; 2014. Available from: http://www.aamc.org/lgbtdsd.

87. Gay, Lesbian, Bisexual and Transgender Health Access Project. Community standards of practice for the provision of quality health care services to lesbian, gay, bisexual, and transgender clients. Boston: Gay, Lesbian, Bisexual and Transgender Health Access Project. Available from: http://www.glbthealth.org/CommunityStandardsofPractice.htm.

88. Gay and Lesbian Medical Association. Guidelines for care of lesbian, gay, bisexual and transgender patients. San Francisco: Gay and Lesbian Medical Association; 2006. Available from: http://glma.org/_data/n_0001/resources/live/GLMAguidelines 2006 FINAL.pdf.

89. Meyer IH. Resilience in the study of minority stress and health of sexual and gender minorities. Psychol Sex Orientation Gend Divers. 2015;2(3):209–13.

Older Adults

Charles P. Hoy-Ellis

According to the US Census Bureau, the number of Americans aged 50 and older will exceed 134 million by 2030 and 172 million by 2060 [1]. Although lesbian, gay, bisexual, and transgender (LGBT) older adults are an increasingly visible segment of the aging US population, accurate assessments of their true numbers are exceedingly difficult to come by. According to a 2012 Gallup poll, 2.6% of Americans aged 50 to 64 years and 1.9% of those aged 65 and older self-identify as LGBT, compared to 3.4% of the overall adult population [2]. This is probably a conservative underestimate. Many older adults who engage in same-sex behavior or report same-sex attraction may not endorse a lesbian, gay, or bisexual identity; gender nonconforming older adults may not identify as transgender, although others (e.g., researchers, healthcare providers) might characterize them as such. Historical trauma and continued discrimination are among the factors that contribute to older adults being less likely than younger adults to self-identify as LGBT. Cohorts are also shaped by generational influences that change over time.

Some research reported in this publication was supported in part by grants from the National Institute on Aging of the National Institutes of Health under Award Numbers R01AG026526 and 2R01AG026526-03A1 (Fredriksen-Goldsen, PI). The content is solely the responsibility of the authors and does not necessarily represent the official views of the National Institutes of Health, National Institute of Aging, or the University of Utah.

Correspondence regarding this article should be addressed to Charles P. Hoy-Ellis, College of Social Work, University of Utah. 395 South 1500 East, #311 Salt Lake City, UT 84112. Email: Charles.Hoy-Ellis@socwk.utah.edu

C.P. Hoy-Ellis, MSW, PhD, LICSW (✉)
College of Social Work, The University of Utah, 395 South 1500 East, Salt Lake City, UT 84112, USA
e-mail: Charles.Hoy-Ellis@socwk.utah.edu

There are three cohorts of LGBT older adults living today: those born between 1901 and 1924 (Greatest Generation), 1925 and 1945 (Silent Generation), and 1946 and 1964 (Baby Boom Generation) [3]. The Greatest Generation came of age in the years preceding World War II and is lauded as the heroic generation that fought "the greatest war." Members of the Silent Generation were just coming of age during the waning years of World War II and are typically unacknowledged as a discrete cohort (i.e., silent), eclipsed by both the Greatest and post-World War II Baby Boom generations. World War II is a unifying theme that connects these cohorts, yet the political, cultural, and social contexts within which this momentous event was situated and the consequent fallout that ensued challenged the lived experiences and generational identities of these cohorts in differing ways (see Table 8.1 for an overview of historical events according to cohort and chronological age). An awareness of the common and unique lived histories of today's LGBT older adults is crucial to understanding how different generational cohorts collectively and individually conceptualize and approach healthcare today. These histories lead to complexities and nuances in perceptions and behaviors that often play out in dramatic, sometimes seemingly counterintuitive ways. For example, results from the Caring and Aging with Pride Project (CAP), a national, community-based sample of 2,650 self-identified LGBT adults aged 50 to 95 years old, found that 40% of transgender older adults feared accessing mainstream healthcare services, in contrast to only 13% of their nontransgender, lesbian, gay, and bisexual (LGB) peers [13]. On the other hand, LGBT Baby Boomers in this study were significantly *more* likely to fear accessing mainstream healthcare services than their older counterparts of the Greatest and Silent Generations [13].

© Springer International Publishing AG 2017

K.L. Eckstrand, J. Potter (eds.), *Trauma, Resilience, and Health Promotion in LGBT Patients*,
DOI 10.1007/978-3-319-54509-7_8

Table 8.1 LGBT midlife and older adults and historic events by cohort [3]

Historical event	Year of event	Greatest Generation (born 1901–1924)	Silent Generation (born 1925–1945)	Baby Boom Generation (born 1946–1964)
		Cohort ages in years when experienced		
Emergence of medical discourse of "sexual inversion" as illness [4]	~1860s			
First known use of term "homosexual" in English language [5]	1892			
First of Greatest Generation cohort (born 1901–1924)	1901	0		
First of Silent Generation cohort (born 1925–1945)	1925	1–24	0	
Great Depression begins	1929	5–28	0–4	
World War II begins	1939	15–38	0–14	
World War II ends	1945	21–44	0–20	
First of Baby Boom Generation cohort (born 1946–1964)	1946	22–45	1–21	0
Lavender Scare, a witch-hunt against homosexuals begins [6]	1950	26–49	5–25	0–4
Homosexuality designated as mental illness in *DSM-I* [6]	1952	28–51	7–27	0–6
Mandated firing of federal and civilian homosexual employees [6]	1953	29–52	8–28	0–7
McCarthy hearings broadcast on television [7]	1954	30–53	9–29	0–8
Illinois becomes first state to decriminalize sodomy [8]	1962	38–61	17–37	0–16
Civil Rights Act	1964	40–63	19–39	0–18
Stonewall riots [8]	1969	45–68	24–44	5–23
Homosexuality as pathology removed from *DSM-II-R* [4]	1973	49–72	28–48	9–27
Gender identity differentiated from homosexuality in *DSM-III* [4]	1980	56–79	35–55	16–34
159 cases reported of what would come to be known as HIV/AIDS [10]	1981	57–80	36–56	17–35
Total US AIDS cases reported: 733,374; died: 429,825 [10]	1989	65–88	44–64	25–43
"Don't Ask, Don't Tell" military policy enacted [9]	1994	70–93	49–69	30–48
1st protease inhibitors approved; HIV/AIDS soon becomes chronic [10]	1995	71–94	50–70	31–49
Defense of Marriage Act (DOMA) enacted [9]	1996	72–95	51–71	32–50
US Supreme Court rules sodomy laws unconstitutional [9]	2003	79–102	58–78	39–57
Massachusetts first state to legalize same-sex marriage [4]	2004	80–103	59–79	40–58
First Baby Boomers turn 65 years old "Don't Ask, Don't Tell" military policy ends [9]	2011	87–110	66–86	47–65
Supreme Court strikes down Section III of DOMA [11] Gender identity disorder becomes gender dysphoria in *DSM-5* [40]	2013	89–112	68–88	49–67
Supreme Court rules bans on same-sex marriage unconstitutional; full marriage equality state and federal [12]	2015	91–114	70–90	51–69

Reprinted from Fredriksen-Goldsen and Hoy-Ellis [3] with permission from Baywood Publishing Company

Understanding the Context and Impact of Trauma

Cultural, political, and social contexts are constituent forces of dominant discourses that foster discrimination, victimization, and marginalization; these contexts are also shaped by the very discourses they create [14]. Primary constituents of discourse include both language and practice; dominant discourses are "an institutionalized way of talking that regulates and reinforces action and thereby exerts power"

[15]. Central to this conceptualization are language (i.e., "way of talking") and power. Dominant discourses are situated within particular historical moments that profoundly influence public spheres and private domains of lived experience, which may vary significantly by cohort. The socially constructed self is constituted by language and sustained through discourse [16]. *Heterosexism* is a dominant discourse that has constructed heterosexuality as "normal and natural" and same-sex desires and gender-variant expressions deviant and abnormal. During the early and mid-twentieth century, medical, legal, and military

institutions produced language that defined nonheterosexuality as "sickness and perversion" and recast unnatural behaviors into aberrant identities. The social and psychological consequences for many LGBT people were devastating and traumatic.

During the waning years of WWII and the beginnings of the McCarthy Era, the dominant discourse around homosexuality underwent a subtle but important shift from behavior to identity. Although Western medical and legal characterizations of "sexual inversion" (i.e., homosexuality, gender-variant expression/identity) can be traced back to the mid- to late nineteenth century [4], homosexuality was formally described as a "sociopathic personality disturbance" by the American Psychiatric Association (APA) in the first edition of the *Diagnostic and Statistical Manual of Mental Disorders (DSM)* in 1952 [17]. It was not until 1973 that the APA voted to remove homosexuality as a mental disorder per se [17]; gender identity was not differentiated from sexual orientation until 1980 in the *DSM-III* [18]. Prior to this time, LGBT people were considered mentally ill by definition and were subjected to involuntary institutionalization and "curative" invasive medical treatments, including but not limited to electroshock therapy, castration, and lobotomy [4]. Legal and political discourses characterized same-sex desire and gender variance as "perversion."

Beginning in the late 1940s and extending into the 1950s, persecution against LGBT people was fueled in large part by an offshoot of the Red Scare fear of a communist takeover – the Lavender Scare [6] – that cast LGBT people as either sympathetic to communism or vulnerable to blackmail by communists. LGBT individuals were barred from military and federal employment [19], and the Veterans Administration ruled that service members discharged for "homosexual acts or tendencies" were ineligible for GI-related employment services and educational benefits [6]. A keystone of both the Red and Lavender Scares were the McCarthy Hearings of the 1950s, now commonly characterized as "witch trials" [6], because they reinvoked the hysteria that surrounded the Salem witch trials in the late 1600s. These hearings coincided with the birth of and widespread access among Americans to television [20]. For the first time, "sexual perversion" [6] (i.e., homosexuality) became an open and vociferous topic of discussion in living rooms, neighborhoods, and newspapers across the USA. In response to this series of events, LGBT people congregated increasingly in what came to be known by the mainstream as "notorious" venues—gathering places that on the one hand provided opportunities for community-building and connection, while at the same time increasing the vulnerability of community members to institutional victimization and discrimination [21].

Bars and nightclubs that served as safe havens for LGBT people were routinely raided by police, while newspapers routinely published the names of those apprehended and arrested on "moral charges," which typically led to being fired from jobs and finding new employment more difficult to secure [19]. In June of 1969, LGBT patrons of the Stonewall Inn in New York City fought back against a typical routine police raid, sparking the Stonewall Riots; an historical event that is now memorialized annually by Pride celebrations around the world. Although a handful of groups had quietly begun organizing to reframe medical, legal, and social perspectives of nonheterosexuality and gender variance in a more positive light in the 1950s, it was Stonewall that marked the birth of the modern and very public gay rights movement that flowered during the 1970s. This movement focused on gay and lesbian individuals, largely omitting bisexual and transgender individuals. Countering the hitherto dominant discourse of sickness and perversion, this movement spawned a resistance discourse of "pride and liberation." However, two momentous events would all too quickly create yet another dominant discourse portraying LGBT people as sick and perverse, albeit in a somewhat different light.

In reaction to advancing civil rights for gay and lesbian-identified people during the latter part of the 1970s, political and religious conservatives began to coalesce under the banner of a "moral majority," promulgating an amalgam of putative Christian and American values [9]. Nearly simultaneously in the early 1980s, what would eventually become known as the acquired immuno-deficiency syndrome (AIDS) pandemic in America began to surface. An emergent dominant discourse reformulated AIDS as *disease*, in juxtaposition to the historic sickness of psychiatric *disorder*, and subsequent death the result of divine retribution for purported *sin*, in contrast to previous characterizations of LGBT people as *perverse*. Gay and bisexual men in particular were disproportionately impacted by initial characterizations of AIDS as the "gay plague," and numerous medical care providers refused to treat those who were infected [22]. Politicians publicly debated legislation that would mandate that gay and bisexual men be quarantined *en masse* in order to curtail the spread of AIDS in the USA [4]. The majority argument in the 1986 Supreme Court ruling *Bowers v. Hardwick* upheld the right of states to criminalize same-sex behavior; this opinion was couched primarily in terms of morality – Judco-Christian values – [8] and influenced by public and private fear of the spread of AIDS [4]. Actions and responses of medical, political, legal, and religious institutions have been significant contributors to heterosexist dominant discourses that have marginalized LGBT older adults.

Sources of External Trauma

The impact of ongoing, day-to-day stigmatization experienced by members of marginalized social groups has been described as *insidious trauma* [23, 24]. Political, legislative, and social discrimination continue to deprive LGBT older adults of important resources, one of the hallmarks of stigma. For example, despite national recognition of marriage equality, discrimination in employment and public accommodations based on sexual orientation and gender identity is still legal in at least half of the states [25]. Such institutionalized discrimination has a major impact on the economic security of older LGBT adults. The majority of economic resources in the USA flow from employment [26]. Direct benefits accrue income through wages and benefits, such as insurance and pension plans, which can have profound consequences when LGBT individuals can arbitrarily and legally be fired or denied promotions. Indirectly, 90% of older Americans receive retirement benefits through Social Security, which are directly based on earlier individual and/or spousal employment histories [27]. As a result of ongoing discrimination, LGBT older adults typically accrue lower lifetime earnings and have less access to pension plans and employer-sponsored health insurance [28]. In addition, spousal benefits only recently became available to LGBT older adults when the US Supreme Court ruled in favor of full marriage quality in June of 2015 [12]; older individuals who had partners who died before same-sex marriage was legalized will never receive spousal benefits. It is no wonder then that there are disparities in poverty rates upon turning 65 years old, with poverty rates for married lesbian and gay male couples rising to 9.1% and 4.9%, respectively, compared to a poverty rate for heterosexual married couples of 4.6% [28].

The effects of anti-LGBT legislation on economic security are in many ways easier to discern than the psychological risk. Nonetheless, the deleterious effects of discriminatory anti-LGBT legislation on mental health have been established by prospective, longitudinal, state-level population-based studies [29, 30]. Regardless of outcome, the political rhetoric and public debate associated with attempts to legislate LGBT lives is such that the heated debates over LGBT topics including same-sex marriage, access to gender affirming care, etc. that occur during election season can be a subtle reminder of ongoing insidious trauma [31]. Arguably more subtle yet inarguably as traumatic are findings from the General Social Survey (GSS) linked with the National Death Index (NDI). Compared to their counterparts living in communities with low levels of bias against sexual minorities, LGB adults living in in communities with high levels of such bias have significantly higher rates of premature mortality and cardiovascular disease [32], which is strongly associated with chronic stress [33].

Sources of Internal Trauma

In addition to discriminatory conditions and events external to the individual, Meyer's minority stress model describes expectations of rejection, concealment of minority identity, and *internalized heterosexism*, a term used to explain the internalization of stigmatized attitudes toward nonheterosexual identities and gender variance, which then become internal stressors in the lives of lesbian, gay, bisexual [34], and transgender people [35]. Expectations of rejection are understandable, as they are rooted in historic heterosexist discourses that fostered a social atmosphere wherein biological family members, particularly children and parents, as well as friends, neighbors, and employers actually did reject today's older LGBT adults. Seeking to protect themselves from possible rejection and being targeted for discrimination, some LGBT older adults continue to conceal their identities, which may increase their risk for chronic stress-related disease and depression [36]. Internalized heterosexism and cisgenderism are insidious minority stressors [34], contributing to a devalued sense of self and concomitant shame [37], the long-term effects of which can negatively impact mental, physical, and social well-being [34, 38]. Hate crimes motivated by sexual orientation and gender identity are an assault on one's personhood; the resulting trauma is more likely than non-biased victimization to result in significant psychological disruption, including posttraumatic stress disorder (PTSD) and other mood and anxiety disorders [39]. Although not meeting *DSM-5* Criteria A of "exposure to actual or threatened death, serious injury, or sexual violence..." [40, p. 271], past-year experiences of heterosexist rejection and harassment were found to be associated with PTSD symptoms in an Internet sample of 247 lesbians who were on average 41 years old ($SD = 11$) [24]. Such experiences occur all too frequently: in the national, community-based CAP survey, 81% of LGBT adults aged 50 and older reported at least one experience of discrimination or victimization (e.g., physical assault, verbal threats, being hassled or ignored by police) in their lifetimes; 64% indicated three or more such experiences [13]. Data from this same study suggest that both internalized stigma and lifetime experiences of discrimination and victimization are associated with depression and disability among LGB [41] and transgender older adults [42].

Pooled data from the Washington State Behavioral Risk Factor Surveillance System (BRFSS) of nearly 100,000 adults aged 50 and older found that compared to heterosexuals aged 50 and older, LGB older adults are at significantly greater risk for both excessive drinking and smoking [43]. The risk for transgender older adults is likely to be at least as great [42]. While clearly a major health concern, these disparities in health aversive behaviors can be understood as a synergistic effect resulting from a confluence and interactions of trauma-response and other social, historical, cultural, economic, political, and psychological factors. As we previously discussed, overt social and political hostility, coupled with de facto legal discrimination and victimization by police, led to bars and nightclubs becoming underground safe havens for LGBT people during the middle decades of the twentieth century [19]. Alcohol – in addition to a space to socialize – was and continues to be the primary product of such establishments; while tobacco use in such venues has become increasingly challenged in recent years, smoking was also part and parcel of social life in the past. Coupled with ready access to these substances, both smoking and drinking are common behavioral responses used to cope with general stress [44], which is compounded by the layering minority stressors observed among LGBT people [34]. Furthermore, LGBT communities have been recognized as a niche market by purveyors of alcohol [45] and tobacco [46], leading to targeted marketing of LGBT communities and sponsorship of events, such as annual Pride celebrations.

LGBT older adults are also at increased risk for elder abuse, neglect, and consequent trauma. Domestic elder abuse refers to intentional mistreatment of a vulnerable older adult by someone in a trusting relationship, such as a friend, family member, partner, and/or caregiver [47]. Definitions of elder abuse and neglect vary by state but are commonly categorized as (a) physical abuse – threatening to or causing physical harm; (b) emotional abuse – verbally or non-verbally causing psychological distress and emotional pain; (c) sexual abuse – being coerced in any manner to participate in or witness any form of nonconsensual sexual activity; (d) exploitation – the misappropriation or misuse of financial assets; (e) neglect – failing to provide for basic needs or failing to protect a vulnerable older adult from abuse or neglect by someone else; and (f) abandonment – being deserted by an individual who has custodial care [47]. A national probability sample of Americans aged 60 and older found that previously experiencing traumatic events increases the risk of elder abuse and neglect [48]. In a New York State sample of 3,500 LGBT adults aged 55 and older, between 8% and 9% had been abused, neglected, blackmailed, or otherwise financially exploited by caregivers due to their sexual orientation or gender identity [49]. Five percent of a community sample of 616 LGBT adults aged 60 and older in a San Francisco reported being abused [50]. The majority of LGBT elder abuse victims do not report their experiences, many because of an understandable lack of trust in authorities [51]. Nearly a quarter (23%) of LGBT CAP participants reported that they had been threatened with being outed [13], which may increase their vulnerability to abuse and neglect.

LGBT older adults also continue to be impacted by historical trauma stemming from the US AIDS pandemic of the 1980s and early 1990s. A number of researchers have characterized that epochal experience as being akin to a natural disaster, with death on vast scale, and destruction of social and community fabric [4]. Individuals initially responded with shock, but as the death toll from AIDS continued to mount into the tens of thousands, their emotional response gave way to a sense of numbness and depletion. Coexistent with this individual trauma was the collective trauma of loss of community, which led community members to question their sense of the LGBT community as a part of a meaningful and coherent world [4]. To date, more than 650,000 Americans have died from AIDS, a majority of them gay and bisexual men [52], an entire generation lost. Many older gay and bisexual continue to experience "survivor's guilt," another form of ongoing trauma.

Although providers' attitudes toward sexual and gender minorities have become increasingly positive in recent decades, prior experiences of trauma remain a significant contributor to LGBT older adults' fear of accessing and utilizing healthcare and related services. A literature review of 66 studies found that discrimination seriously and negatively impacts LGBT older adults' access to healthcare, the quality of care received, and utilization of healthcare, housing, and social services [53]. Many LGBT older adults are fearful of accessing other community support systems, such as senior centers, assisted living facilities, and skilled nursing facilities [54]. In addition to expectations of discrimination from both staff and other consumers in such facilities, many LGBT older adults fear institutional abuse and neglect from staff, and isolation from other service users. Experiences of stigma and fear may create significant barriers to accessing healthcare, and provider bias may influence the quality of care [55].

Transgender older adults share many of the same challenges as nontransgender LGB older adults; they also have unique experiences. Many have faced closets within closets – concealing their gender identities in both dominant and lesbian and gay male cultures due to transphobia (more accurately the gendered aspect of heterosexist discourses) in both. This stems in part from the reality that gender identity was not widely differentiated from sexual orientation until the 1980s. With no preexistent public language from which to constitute "nonnormative" gender identities, some older transgender and gender nonconforming individuals are only now constructing congruent and authentic selves. Emergent themes from a small ($n = 22$) qualitative study that examined the experiences of individuals who did not seriously contemplate or start gender transition until they were 50 or older provide compelling insights. Having lived a significant portion of their lives within the deeply entrenched enforcement of "traditional" gender expressions and expectations, participants described this period as "time-served" [56]. In a recent qualitative study, a major theme highlighting the process of finally embracing one's gender and expressing one's true self at an older age was highlighted by Fabbre (2015) as: "fraught with emotional anguish and anger, which took a toll on … mental health … [but resulted in] the sheer peace of accepting oneself and feeling comfortable in one's own skin" (p. 149). Emotions of shame and anger were balanced with great fortitude and a sense of joy and liberation for most participants [56].

Among other reasons, transgender individuals may choose to delay disclosing their gender identity and transitioning because of family concerns. It is extremely common for children who learn that a parent is transgender to experience grief at the loss of either a "mother" or a "father" [57]. Although most of these children eventually reconcile to the change in parental role and expression of gender identity, many do not, choosing rather to treat the transgender parent as truly dead [57]. This may explain why 40% of children of transgender adults aged 55 and older in the National Transgender Discrimination Survey (NTDS) have no communication whatsoever with the transgender parent [58]. Transgender older adults experience a similar conundrum when considering accessing healthcare. Disclosure of gender identity and choosing to pursue transition may provide psychological relief [35] and increase appropriate care planning [59]; however, it can also make one a more visible target for discrimination [34].

In the national, community-based CAP survey, transgender participants had significantly higher rates of being denied or provided inferior healthcare (40%) than nontransgender LGB participants (11%), even after controlling for age, income, and education [13]. In an ongoing needs assessment of LGBT older adults (64–88 years old) utilizing the LGBT Elders Needs Assessment Scale, 42% of 1,100 respondents to date report being treated in an aversive manner in the healthcare system [60]. One CAP participant stated, "I was advised by my primary care doctor (at my HMO) to not get tested there, but rather do it anonymously, because he knew they were discriminating" (57, S42). Discrimination in healthcare settings leads many LGBT older adults to put off or even do without needed healthcare [61]. Fearing discrimination, many do not disclose their sexual orientation or gender identity to their primary care provider [62]. In a recent survey conducted by Harris Polling on behalf of SAGE (Services and Advocacy for GLBT Elders), 36% of 1,857 LGBT adults aged 45 to 75 years old had not disclosed their sexual orientation to their primary care physician; 44% believed that disclosing their sexual orientation or gender identity to staff in healthcare settings would be detrimental to their relationships with these providers [63]. In addition to suboptimal healthcare, nondisclosure may also contribute to poor mental health outcomes, in part by exacerbating internalized heterosexism [36].

Supporting Resilience When Working with LGBT Older Adults

In the face of such adversity, LGBT older adults demonstrate amazing resilience. The interaction of background characteristics and numerous risk and protective factors can either support competent engagement of resources or undermine adaptation and resilience among older adults in the general population. These include mobility, physical activity, self-reliance, not abusing substances, social support, and positive self-identity [64, 65]. Drawing on Resilience Theory [66], Fredriksen-Goldsen and colleagues [41, 42] conceptualized a resilience framework that highlights the ways in which these factors also apply to resilience among LGBT older adults, although resources that support resilience development in this population may be more difficult to access. For example, physical activity promotes mental and physical health and is protective against mobility loss [67]; however, programs that target physical activity among older adults are often provided through community aging programs such as senior centers that may be unsafe for LGBT older adults. Historically, bars and nightclubs provided safe havens where LGBT people could congregate; however, such venues also provided ready access to alcohol, tobacco, and other substance use. Adding insult to injury, programs designed to reduce substance misuse among older adults typically do not target LGBT elders, while companies that produce and distribute alcohol have disproportionately targeted LGBT communities [45]. Similarly, LGBT agencies and programs that promote health are typically geared toward younger LGBT people. Understanding how these dynamic forces interact with multiple psychological and social characteristics is instrumental in supporting resilience when working with LGBT older adults.

Exposure to pervasive marginalization, discrimination, and trauma may also provide opportunities for development of heightened resilience. For example, in a sample of 141 transgender adults aged 61 plus in the online *Trans Metropolitan Life Survey*, 71% indicated that they had "aged successfully" [68]. The MetLife Survey of 1,201 LGBT Baby Boomers aged 45–64 found that while half of respondents indicated that being LGBT made aging more challenging, most (about 75%) reported that it made them better prepared for aging [69]. The idea that successfully navigating a lifetime of heterosexist discrimination and victimization could better prepare LGBT people for the vicissitudes of aging through *crisis competence* was first put forth in the latter part of the twentieth century [70, 71]. The gay character Arnold in the 1988 movie *Torch Song Trilogy* is emblematic of the notion of crisis competence in the context of a lifetime of marginalization when he announces: "There's one more thing you better understand. I have taught myself to sew, cook, fix plumbing, build furniture – I can even pat myself on the back when necessary – all so I don't have to ask anyone for anything. There's nothing I need from anyone except for love and respect and anyone who can't give me those two things has no place in my life" [72].

Cultivating crisis competence may be challenging for some LGBT older adults, considering the overwhelmingly negative dominant discourses of LGBT sickness, perversion, and sin that permeated so much of the American landscape when they were growing up, coming of age and forming their identities. Conversely, because LGBT older adults' identities as sexual and gender minorities were typically constructed and integrated in such a hostile social climate, such adversity may actually promote resilience and positive identity – in the words of Nietzsche "that which does not destroy, strengthens." The experience of trauma can shatter one's expectations of the world as predictable and orderly. The process of reconstructing that world, making sense of the incomprehensible, can contribute to resilience through *posttraumatic growth*, providing a new appreciation of internal strengths and interpersonal relationships [73]. In her explication of *positive marginality*, Unger [74] argues that minority individuals can reappraise their experiences of marginalization as meaningful influences that provide impetus for recasting previously stigmatized attributes (e.g., sexual orientation, gender identity) as essential aspects of a valued, agentic, resilient self. The reappraisal of discrimination and victimization as a "challenge" rather than a "threat" engages responses that support resilience rather than hopelessness and helplessness [75]. This process can also be bolstered by personal spirituality, one of the *resilience repertoires* articulated by transgender older adults as being key to positive aging [68]. Beyond individual level factors – the exercise of agency, creation of meaning from adversity, and increasing self-acceptance – caring interpersonal relationships and social and political action are additional repertoires that support resilience [68].

In tandem with broader community and social exclusion, many LGBT older adults have been rejected by their biological families; they are less likely than heterosexual older adults to have children of their own. *Families-of-choice*, also characterized by Maupin as "logical kin" in juxtaposition to "biological kin," [76] are typically composed of friends, neighbors, and often former partners. The majority of LGBT older adults indicate that they have such families [69], which they describe in terms of "trust, shared values, acceptance, compatibility, and care" [77]. In addition to being foundational to the caring interpersonal relationships of LGBT older adults, these families can provide an anchor for positive identities that support resilience. Unfortunately, members of families-of-choice are generally not accorded automatic legal standing [78], which may be a barrier to LGBT older adults' ability to "age in place."

Overwhelmingly, regardless of sexual orientation or gender identity, most older adults would prefer to age in or close to their communities (i.e., "place") and their formal and informal supports [60]. Research also provides evidence that moving from community living to institutional living typically results in *life expectancy compression*, significantly reducing remaining life expectancy [79]. LGBT older adults are less likely to have children, an important resource for aging in place. Nearly 31% of LGBT older adults in the CAP study reported annual household incomes at or below 200% of the Federal Poverty Level [13], further restricting access to important community support. Fearing discrimination makes it less likely that they will access mainstream community-based supports, such as senior centers and the social health-promoting programming they offer. In an ouroboros-type fashion, this can contribute to social isolation that is associated with increased risk for premature morbidity and consequent institutionalization. With the exception of very few states, the Family Medical Leave Act (FMLA) does not recognize or provide protections to such families-of-choice. However, the National Family Caregiver Support Program (NFCSP) has extended its definition of family constitutions beyond legally related family members to include "other caregivers" [80]. Armed with this knowledge, providers can assist LGBT older adults and their families-of-choice in accessing programs funded under the NFCSP to support aging in place.

The tempestuous years of the height of the AIDS pandemic in the USA offers not only posttraumatic growth but also positive marginality, reflective of the incredible resilience of LGBT older adults. In the face of overt hostility and discrimination at the hands of governmental and healthcare institutions, today's LGBT older adults were in the vanguard of political action responding to the "violence, ignorance, and stigma with which they were confronted by educating themselves and others" [77]. The models and programs they created to care for their dying loved ones and their communities have been recreated and implemented across the globe [77]. By recognizing and acknowledging these profound contributions when working with LGBT older adults, providers can further reinforce resilience.

Health Promotion

The cornerstones of competency are awareness, attitudes, knowledge, and skills, which are necessary to promote equitable access to healthcare for LGBT older adults and communities. Implicit biases of healthcare providers can have a major impact on quality of care; in fact past exposure to such biases may even drive an LGBT individual's decision as to whether to seek future care at all [62]. Healthcare providers can and must play an active role in addressing elder abuse and neglect as mandatory reporters. If the danger to an older adult is immediate and serious, call 911 or your local police. If the situation is not imminently hazardous, the Administration on Aging and the National Center on Elder Abuse operate a State Resources website that provides easy access to reporting agencies, laws, and other resources (http://ncea.aoa.gov/Stop_Abuse/Get_Help/State/index.aspx). Most violence recovery programs (VRPs) in LGBT communities do not specifically target older adults. However, the programs that do exist, such as Fenway Health Center's VRP (http://fenwayhealth.org/care/behavioral-health/vrp/), provide services that encompass the multiple forms of violence that LGBT people experience, from intimate partner violence to hate crimes. An overview of this program is covered in an archived webinar that addresses particular issues in same-sex intimate relationships, including healthcare access, sponsored by the National LGBT Health Education Center at the Fenway Institute [52]. While explicit bias on the part of healthcare providers has diminished in recent decades, implicit bias continues to impact the health and healthcare of LGBT older adults. A nonprobability international sample ($n = 247, 030$) of healthcare and associated workers' implicit and explicit attitudes regarding sexual orientation found that heterosexual providers across the board had an implicit bias in favor of heterosexuality [81]. Interestingly, heterosexual nurses had the highest levels of such bias [81], an important consideration as they generally have more contact with those seeking healthcare services. Because of their long history of discrimination and marginalization, LGBT older adults are likely to be acutely aware of implicit bias on the part of healthcare providers. Such bias may impede open communication and could potentially influence treatment recommendations [81], further contributing to health disparities among LGBT older adults [62, 81]. Utilizing Hays ADDRESSING (*a*ge, *d*evelopment/*d*isability, *r*eligion, *e*thnicity/race, *s*ocial status, *s*exual orientation, *i*ndigenous heritage, *n*ationality, *g*ender/gender identity-expression/sex) framework [82], healthcare providers can increase their awareness by understanding how power dynamics inherent in implicit bias can impact interactions with LGBT older adults. This framework calls for individuals to explore how their own and their clients' various social identities locate and modulate interpersonal communications and professional decision-making.

Fredriksen-Goldsen and colleagues' health equity promotion model [83] can be invaluable in aiding healthcare providers to expand their knowledge, facilitating resilience among older LGBT adults (see Fig. 8.1). This model situates LGBT health and well-being within a lifecourse perspective, recognizes the potential and actual negative impact of social structures and institutions, and the central roles of agency and resilience on health outcomes. This framework "highlights (a) heterogeneity and intersectionality within LGBT communities; (b) the influence of structural and environmental contexts; and (c) both health-promoting and adverse pathways that encompass behavioral, social, psychological, and biological processes" [83].

Healthcare providers can also foster resilience among LGBT older adults through the development and utilization of specific competencies and strategies. These skills and knowledge offer a guide for best practice [84]. Some of these have already been discussed, such as incorporating the ADDRESSING framework to increase awareness of implicit biases and how these biases inform all decision-making processes, including ethical dilemmas. The ADDRESSING framework can also be applied on a systems level to raise awareness of the ways that services, programs, and agencies may unwittingly contribute to ongoing marginalization. It is important to become cognizant of the ways in which historical and current social contexts, including discriminatory policies and laws, deleteriously and differentially have impacted and continue to affect the development, life transitions, and health and well-being of LGBT older adults [84], as this information is crucial to a thorough biopsychosocial assessment. Effective and sensitive treatment planning is only possible when one recognizes the heterogeneity of LGBT subgroups (i.e., unique experiences of people who are bisexual and transgender) and considers the impact of intersectionality (i.e., different life experiences that result from exposure to multiple intersecting identities in addition to sexual orientation and gender identities). Providers should explore with clients the language they favor and use this language to demonstrate respect and understanding [84]. For example, as a result of historic discourses, older lesbians may consider themselves to be "gay", while older gay men may prefer the term "homosexual." Similarly, although often well-meaning, the term "sexual preference" as opposed to "sexual orientation" or "sexual identity" implies choice, which is rarely the case. The American Psychological Association's (APA) *Publication Manual* (6th edition) offers additional guidance on appropriate terminology [85].

Healthcare professionals also have unique opportunities to empower LGBT older adults, their families, and their informal caregivers in negotiating the fragmented aging, health, and social services systems. At the same time, healthcare systems have an unparalleled opportunity to "defragment" themselves by applying innovative strategies to promote health equity. Fenway Health – a Federally Qualified Health Center in Boston, Massachusetts – provides a ready example. While a central tenet of Fenway Health's mission focuses on promoting the well-being of LGBT people, the health center is inclusive of all members of its geographic community, rather than the larger community being inclusive of LGBT people. Fenway Health has been a pioneer in providing wrap-around, intergenerational health

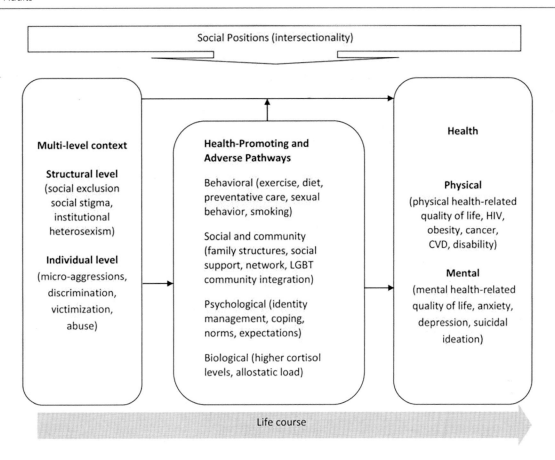

Fig. 8.1 Health equity promotion model [83]

services (e.g., mental, physical, dental, social) through a network of locations with dedicated programming that recognizes LGBT diversity. Offering a single gateway portal (http://fenwayhealth.org/care/) transforms a fragmented maze into an integrated web. In addition, Fenway Health now houses the LGBT Aging Project (http://fenwayhealth.org/the-fenway-institute/lgbt-aging-project/), a nonprofit organization dedicated to ensuring that LGBT older adults in Massachusetts have equal access to the life-prolonging benefits, protections, services, and institutions that their heterosexual neighbors take for granted. Additional training and other resources that can help social service agencies develop the capacity to provide competent care to LGBT elders can be found at the National Resource Center on LGBT Aging (https://www.lgbtagingcenter.org/).

The LGBT community itself can be an invaluable resource to address social isolation among LGBT older adults. For example, the Seniors Preparing for Rainbow Years (SPRY) program at the Montrose Center in Houston, Texas (http://www.montrosecenter.org/hub/services/spry/) offers communal lunches and drop-in space three times a week for LGBT adults aged 60 and older. Older LGBT adults also volunteer to engage other LGBT older adults; provision of peer counseling and "friendly visits" decreases

social isolation *and* the need for more formal clinical services. Funding for services and programs specific to LGBT older adults can be a perceived barrier in both mainstream and LGBT agencies. In addition to actively engaging members of the LGBT community to identify solutions, organizations that seek to promote the health and well-being of LGBT communities through institutional philanthropy, such as Funders for LGBT Issues (https://www.lgbtfunders.org/), can provide valuable consultation.

Healthcare providers and programs have an unparalleled opportunity to promote health equity among older LGBT adults, families, and communities. The first step in this transformation is to recognize and acknowledge the roles that governmental and healthcare institutions and societal norms have historically played in inflicting and perpetuating trauma on these populations. The second step is to understand how historical traumas continue to affect individual patients' motivations and actions. The third step is to support individual change toward happier/healthier lives using evidence-based practice. As important is to use our individual and collective knowledge and experience to continue to advocate for structural/systemic changes to better meet the needs of older LGBT adults. This historically marginalized and invisible population is inarguably resilient, yet significant health disparities and barriers to healthcare access remain. Education, awareness, knowledge, and skill are essential to culturally competent practice and to further promote resilience and the health and well-being of LGBT older adults.

Case Study

Jiao, an 86-year-old Asian American woman, is referred to your facility by Adult Protective Services (APS) for suspected neglect (Fig. 8.2). She reports that she lives alone and has two adult children that she claims visit her once a month, and she has been divorced for 40 years. Upon further questioning about her situation, she states that she keeps to herself, doesn't leave the house often or speak to her neighbors, and in a very hushed tone mentions "... Abbie... passed on many years now but can't talk about that..." She is alert and oriented to the conversation and able to participate in brief cognitive testing. A MOCA exam was performed with a score of 27/30, and she has no family history of dementia. She has no personal history of schizophrenia or substance use. Prior to retirement at the age of 65, she worked as an administrative assistant for 40 years. She is very quiet, makes poor eye contact when discussing "Abbie," and appears despondent. You are concerned about safety, health, and mental health issues.

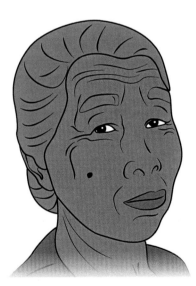

Fig. 8.2 Jiao, an 86-year-old Asian American woman, is referred to your facility by Adult Protective Services for suspected neglect

Discussion Questions

- What are your initial assumptions?
- What ADDRESSING factors might be influencing those assumptions?
- How might you explore those assumptions as part of a biopsychosocial assessment?
- How would you assess for possible mood and anxiety disorders? Suicidality? Loneliness versus depression?
- What other questions would you ask as part of the assessment process?
- What resilience factors can you identify?
- Discuss how you might think about accessing resources in this case.

Summary Practice Points

1. Older LGBT adults have unique lived experiences and generations influences that shape their understanding of their sexual orientation identity and gender identity (e.g. older adults may not use an LGBT identity).
2. Older LGBT adults may be more likely to have been rejected by both their parents and their children, and rely on families of choice for support.
3. Mobility, physical activity, self-reliance, substance non-use, social support, and positive self-identity are associated with resilience and positive coping among older LGBT adults.
4. The ADDRESSING framework can be helpful when considering how implicit bias and power dynamics affect older LGBT adults, and provide a better understanding of how to engage in respectful clinical communication.
5. Numerous social support services are available for older LGBT adults including Services and Advocacy for LGBT Elders (SAGE), the LGBT Aging Project, and Aging with Pride.

References

1. U.S. Census Bureau. 2014 National population projections: summary tables. Table 9. Projections of the population by age and sex for the United States: 2015 to 2060: U.S. Census Bureau; 2015. Available from: https://www.census.gov/population/projections/data/national/2014/summarytables.html.
2. Gates GJ, Newport F. Special report: 3.4% of U.S. adults identify as LGBT. Inaugural Gallup findings based on more than 120,000 interviews. Princeton: Gallup Polls; 2012. Available from: http://

www.gallup.com/poll/158066/special-report-adults-identify-lgbt.
aspx

3. Fredriksen-Goldsen IK, Hoy-Ellis CP. LGBT older adults emerging from the shadows: health disparities and risks and resources. In: Wilmoth J, Silverstein M, editors. The hierarchy of social support revisited. New York: Baywood Publishing Company, Inc.; (in press).

4. Institute of Medicine. The health of lesbian, gay, bisexual, and transgender people: building a foundation for better understanding. Washington, DC: The National Academies Press; 2011.

5. Penhallurick RJ. Studying the English language. 2nd ed. Basingstoke/New York: Palgrave MacMillan; 2010. xv, 358 pp.

6. Canaday M. The straight state: sexuality and citizenship in twentieth-century America. Princeton: Princeton University Press; 2009. xiv, 277 pp.

7. Johnson DK. The lavender scare: the Cold War persecution of gays and lesbians in the federal government. Chicago: University of Chicago Press; 2004. xii, 277 pp.

8. Carpenter D. Flagrant conduct: the story of Lawrence v. Texas. 1st ed. New York: W.W. Norton; 2012. xv, 345 p, 8 p. of plates p.

9. Carpenter D. Flagrant conduct: The story of Lawrence v. Texas. 1st ed. New York: W.W. Norton; 2012.

10. AVERT. History of HIV & AIDS overview Brighton, UK; 2015. Available from: http://www.avert.org/professionals/history-hiv-aids/overview.

11. Supreme LA. Court bolsters gay marriage with two major rulings. New York; 26 June 2013. Available from: http://www.nytimes.com/2013/06/27/us/politics/supreme-court-gay-marriage.html?page wanted=all&_r=0.

12. Obergefell v. Hodges. No. 14-556, slip op. at 22 (U.S. June 26, 2015) ("The Court now holds that same-sex couples may exercise the fundamental right to marry."). Available at: https://www.supremecourt.gov/opinions/14pdf/14-556_3204.pdf

13. Fredriksen-Goldsen KI, Kim H-J, Emlet CA, Muraco A, Erosheva EA, Hoy-Ellis CP, et al. The aging and health report: disparities and resilience among lesbian, gay, bisexual, and transgender older adults. Seattle: Institute for Multigenerational Health; 2011.

14. Foucault M. The history of sexuality. 1st American ed. New York: Pantheon Books; 1978.

15. van Dijk TA. Critical discourse studies: a sociocognitive approach. In: Wodak R, Meyer M, editors. Methods of critical discourse analysis. 2nd ed. Los Angeles: Sage; 2009. p. 62–86.

16. Foucault M. The care of the self. 1st Vintage Books ed. New York: Vintage Books; 1988.

17. Silverstein C. The implications of removing homosexuality from the DSM as a mental disorder. Arch Sex Behav. 2009;38(2):161–3.

18. Koh J. The history of the concept of gender identity disorder. Seishin Shinkeigaku Zasshi. 2012;114(6):673–80.

19. D'Emilio J. Sexual politics, sexual communities: the making of a homosexual minority in the United States, 1940–1970. Chicago: University of Chicago Press; 1983.

20. Archive, of American Television. TV history Los Angeles academy of television arts & sciences foundation; 2013. Available from: http://www.emmytvlegends.org/resources/tv-history.

21. Berube A. Coming out under fire: the history of gay men and women in World War II. New York: Free Press; 1990.

22. Curran JW, Jaffe HW, (CDC) CfDCaP. AIDS: the early years and CDC's response. MMWR Surveill Summ. 2011;60 Suppl 4:64–9.

23. Root PM. Reconstructing the impact of trauma on personality. In: Brown LS, Ballou M, editors. Personality and psychopathology: feminist reappraisals. New York: Guilford; 1992. p. 229–65.

24. Szymanski DM, Balsam KF. Insidious trauma: examining the relationship between heterosexism and lesbians' PTSD symptoms. Traumatology. 2011;17(2):4–13.

25. Human Rights Campaign. Why the equality act? Washington, DC: Human Rights Campaign; 2015. Available from: http://www.hrc.org//resources/entry/why-the-equality-act

26. Esping-Anderson G. De-commodification in social policy. The three worlds of welfare capitalism. Cambridge: Polity Press; 1990. p. 35–54.

27. Social Security Administration. Social security basic facts. Washington, DC: Social Security Administration; 2015. Available from: http://www.ssa.gov/pressoffice/basicfact.htm.

28. Fitzgerald E. No golden years at the end of the rainbow: how a lifetime of discrimination compounds economic and health disparities for LGBT older adults. Washington, DC: National Gay and Lesbian Task Force; 2013.

29. Hatzenbuehler ML, Keyes KM, Hasin DS. State-level policies and psychiatric morbidity in lesbian, gay, and bisexual populations. Am J Public Health. 2009;99(12):2275–81.

30. Rostosky SS, Riggle EDB, Horne SG, Miller AD. Marriage amendments and psychological distress in lesbian, gay, and bisexual (LGB) adults. J Couns Psychol. 2009;56(1):56–66.

31. Russell GM, Bohan JS, McCarroll MC, Smith NG. Trauma, recovery, and community: perspectives on the long-term impact of anti-LGBT politics. Traumatology. 2011;17(2):14–23.

32. Hatzenbuehler ML, Bellatorre A, Lee Y, Finch BK, Muennig P, Fiscella K. Structural stigma and all-cause mortality in sexual minority populations. Soc Sci Med. 2014;103:33–41.

33. Chobanian AV, Bakris GL, Black HR, Cushman WC, Green LA, Izzo JL, et al. The seventh report of the joint National Committee on prevention, detection, evaluation, and treatment of high blood pressure: the JNC 7 report. JAMA. 2003;289(19):2560–72.

34. Meyer IH. Prejudice, social stress, and mental health in lesbian, gay, and bisexual populations: conceptual issues and research evidence. Psychol Bull. 2003;129(5):674–97.

35. Hendricks ML, Testa RJ. A conceptual framework for clinical work with transgender and gender noncomforming clients: an adaptation of the minority stress model. Profess Psychol Res Pract. 2012;43 (5):460–7.

36. Hoy-Ellis CP. Concealing concealment: the mediating role of internalized heterosexism in psychological distress among lesbian, gay, and bisexual older adults. J Homosex. 2015;63(4):487–506.

37. Hammack PL, Cohler BJ. Narrative, identity, and the politics of exclusion: social change and the gay and lesbian life course. Sex Res Soc Policy. 2011;8:162–82.

38. Kertzner RM, Meyer IH, Frost DM, Stirratt MJ. Social and psychological well-being in lesbians, gay men, and bisexuals: the effects of race, gender, age, and sexual identity. Am J Orthopsychiatry. 2009;79(4):500–10.

39. Herek GM, Gillis JR, Cogan JC. Psychological sequelae of hate-crime victimization among lesbian, gay, and bisexual adults. J Consult Clin Psychol. 1999;67(6):945–51.

40. American Psychiatric Association. Diagnostic and statistical manual of mental disorders: DSM-5. 5th ed. Arlington: American Psychiatric Publishing; 2013.

41. Fredriksen-Goldsen KI, Emlet CA, Kim H-J, Muraco A, Erosheva EA, Goldsen J, et al. The physical and mental health of lesbian, gay male, and bisexual (LGB) older adults: the role of key health indicators and risk and protective factors. Gerontologist. 2013;53 (4):664–75.

42. Fredriksen-Goldsen KI, Cook-Daniels L, Kim H-J, Erosheva EA, Emlet CA, Hoy-Ellis CP, et al. Physical and mental health of transgender older adults: an at-risk and underserved population. Gerontologist. 2013;54(3):488–500.

43. Fredriksen-Goldsen KI, Kim H-J, Barkan SE, Muraco A, Hoy-Ellis CP. Health disparities among lesbian, gay male and bisexual older

adults: results from a population-based study. Am J Public Health. 2013;103(10):1802–9.

44. Zucker AN, Landry LJ. Embodied discrimination: the relation of sexism and distress to women's drinking and smoking behaviors. Sex Roles. 2007;56(3/4):193–203.

45. Absolut ES. Celebrates its 30 years of marketing to gay consumers. New York Times [Internet]. 2011; (Business Day Media & Advertising). Available from: http://www.nytimes.com/2011/10/27/business/media/absolut-heralds-its-marketing-to-gay-consumers.html?_r=0.

46. Blosnich J, Lee JG, Horn K. A systematic review of the aetiology of tobacco disparities for sexual minorities. Tob Control. 2013;22:66–73.

47. National Center on Elder Abuse. Elder abuse FAQs. 2011. Updated 19 July 11. Available from: http://www.ncea.aoa.gov/faq/index.aspx.

48. Acierno R, Hernandez MA, Amstadter AB, Resnick HS, Steve K, Muzzy W, et al. Prevalence and correlates of emotional, physical, sexual, and financial abuse and potential neglect in the United States: the National Elder Mistreatment Study. Am J Public Health. 2010;100(2):292–7.

49. Frazer S. LGBT health and human services needs in New York State. Albany: Empire State Pride Agenda Foundation; 2009.

50. Fredriksen-Goldsen KI, Kim H-J, Hoy-Ellis CP, Goldsen J, Jensen D, Adelman M, et al. Addressing the needs of LGBT older adults in San Francisco: recommendations for the future. Seattle: Institute for Multigenerational Health; 2013.

51. Cook-Daniels L. Lesbian, gay male, bisexual and transgendered elders: elder abuse and neglect issues. J Elder Abuse Negl. 1997;9(2):35–49.

52. and CfDC, Prevention. HIV in the United States: at a glance. Atlanta: Centers for Disease Control and Prevention; 2015. Available from: http://www.cdc.gov/hiv/statistics/overview/ataglance.html

53. Addis S, Davies M, Greene G, Macbride-Stewart S, Shepherd M. The health, social care and housing needs of lesbian, gay, bisexual and transgender older people: a review of the literature. Health Soc Care Community. 2009;17(6):647–58.

54. National Senior Citizens Law Center. LGBT older adults in long-term care facilities: stories from the field. 2011. Available from: http://www.lgbtlongtermcare.org/authors/.

55. Nyblade L, Stangl A, Weiss E, Ashburn K. Combating HIV stigma in health care settings: what works? J Int AIDS Soc. 2009;12:15.

56. Fabbre VD. Gender transitions in later life: a queer perspective on successful aging. The Gerontologist. 2015;55(1):144–53.

57. Cook-Daniels L. Transgender elders and significant others, friends, family and allies (SOFFAs): a primer for service providers and advocates. Milwaukee: Transgender Aging Network; 2007.

58. Witten T. End of life, chronic illness, and trans-identities. J Soc Work End Life Palliat Care. 2014;10:1–26.

59. American Medical Association. Removing financial barriers to care for transgender patients, House of delegates. Washington, DC: American Medical Association; 2008. p. 4.

60. Orel NA. Investigating the needs and concerns of lesbian, gay, bisexual, and transgender older adults: the use of qualitative and quantitative methodology. J Homosex. 2014;61(1):53–78.

61. Krehely J. How to close the LGBT health disparities gap. Washington, DC: Center for American Progress; 2009.

62. Foglia MB, Fredriksen-Goldsen KI. Health disparities among LGBT older adults and the role of nonconscious bias. Garrison: The Hastings Center; 2014. Contract No.: no. 5

63. LGBT SSaAf, Elders. Out & visible: the experiences and attitudes of lesbian, gay, bisexual and transgender older adults, ages 45–75. New York: SAGE; 2014.

64. Hildon Z, Montgomery SM, Blane D, Wiggins RD, Netuveli G. Examining resilience of quality of life in the face of health-related and psychosocial adversity at older ages: what is "right" about the way we age? Gerontologist. 2010;50(1):36–47.

65. Netuveli G, Wiggins RD, Montgomery SM, Hildon Z, Blane D. Mental health and resilience at older ages: bouncing back after adversity in the British Household Panel Survey. J Epidemiol Community Health. 2008;62(11):987–91.

66. Yates TM, Masten AS. Fostering the future: resilience theory and the practice of positive psychology. In: Linley PA, Joseph S, editors. Positive psychology in practice. Hoboken: Wiley; 2004. p. 521–39.

67. Centers for Disease Control and Prevention. Physical activity for everyone: older adults 2011. Available from: http://www.cdc.gov/physicalactivity/everyone/guidelines/olderadults.html.

68. McFadden SH, Frankowski S, Flick H, Witten TM. Resilience and multiple stigmatized identities: lessons from transgender persons' reflections on aging. In: Sinnott JD, editor. Positive psychology. New York: Springer; 2013. p. 247–67.

69. Metlife Mature Market Institute. American society on aging. Still out, still aging: the Metlife study of lesbian, gay, bisexual, and transgender baby boomers. New York: Metlife Mature Market Institute and American Society on Aging; 2010.

70. Friend RA. Older lesbian and gay people: a theory of successful aging. J Homosex. 1991;20(3):99–118.

71. Kimmel DC. Adult development and aging: a gay perspective. J Soc Issues. 1978;34(3):113–30.

72. Bogart P. Torch song trilogy. United States: New Line Cinema; 1988.

73. Tedeschi RG, Calhoun LG. Posttraumatic growth: conceptual foundations and empirical evidence. Psychol Inq. 2004;15(1):1–18.

74. Unger RK. Outsiders inside: Positive marginality and social change. J Soc Issues. 2000;56(1):163–79.

75. Lazarus RS, Folkman S. Stress, appraisal, and coping. New York: Springer Publishing Company; 1984.

76. de Vries B, Croghan C. LGBT aging: the contributions of community-based research. J Homosex. 2014;61:1–20.

77. de Vries B. Stigma and LGBT aging: negative and positive marginality. In: Orel NA, Fruhauf CA, editors. The lives of LGBT older adults: understanding challenges and resilience. Washington, DC: American Psychological Association; 2015. p. 55–71.

78. Knauer NJ. Navigating a post-windsor world: the promise and limits of marriage equality (August 28, 2014). Available at SSRN: https://ssrn.com/abstract=2448296.

79. House JS, Lantz PM, Herd P. Continuity and change in the social stratification of aging and health over the life course: evidence from a nationally representative longitudinal study from 1986 to 2001/2002 (Americans' changing lives study). J Gerontol Series B-Psychol Sci Social Sci. 2005;60B(Special Issue II):15–26.

80. American, Aging So. What's different about LGBT informal caregiving? San Francisco: American Society on Aging; 2016. Available from: http://www.asaging.org/blog/whats-different-about-lgbt-informal-caregiving

81. Sabin JA, Riskind RG, Nosek BA. Health care providers' implicit and explicit attitudes toward lesbian women and gay men. Am J Public Health. 2015;105(9):1831–41.

82. Hays AP. Addressing cultural complexities in practice: a framework for clinicians and counselors. Washington, DC: American Psychological Association; 2001.

83. Fredriksen-Goldsen KI, Simoni JM, Kim H-J, Lehavot K, Walters KL, Yang J, et al. The health equity promotion model: reconceptualization of lesbian, gay, bisexual, and transgender (LGBT) health disparities. Am J Orthopsychiatry. 2014;84(6):653–83.

84. Fredriksen-Goldsen KI, Hoy-Ellis CP, Goldsen J, Emlet CA, Hooyman NR. Creating a vision for the future: key competencies and strategies for culturally competent practice with lesbian, gay, bisexual, and transgender (LGBT) older adults in the health and human services. J Gerontol Soc Work. 2014;57:80–107.

85. American Psychological Association. Publication manual of the American Psychological Association. 6th ed. Washington, DC: American Psychological Association; 2010.

86. American Psychological Association. Practice guidelines for LGB clients: guidelines for psychological practice with lesbian, gay, and bisexual clients. Washington, DC: American Psychological Association; 2011. Available from: http://www.apa.org/pi/lgbt/resources/guidelines.aspx.

87. Knochel KA, Croghan CF, Moone RP, Quam JK. Training, geography, and provision of aging services to lesbian, gay, bisexual, and transgender older adults. J Gerontol Soc Work. 2012;55(5):426–43.

88. Orel NA, Fruhauf CA. The lives of LGBT older adults: understanding challenges and resilience. 1st ed. Washington, D.C: American Psychological Association; 2015.

Transgender and Gender Nonconforming Individuals

Asa E. Radix, Laura Erickson-Schroth, and Laura A. Jacobs

Introduction

Gender identity refers to one's internal sense of gender. Transgender individuals are those whose gender identities do not align with their assigned sex at birth. Included in this umbrella term are people with binary identities, e.g., who were assigned female at birth and identify as male, as well as individuals who identify outside the gender binary of either male or female and who may use nontraditional terms to describe themselves, such as genderqueer, androgynous, bigender, and two-spirited gender [1]. Transgender individuals are also diverse in sexual orientation and may identify as heterosexual, bisexual, lesbian/gay, or pansexual. Data on transgender individuals are not routinely collected or reported in US surveys; however, the prevalence of gender nonconformity in the population may be as high as 0.5% [2].

Gender dysphoria is a term used to describe distress that is caused by a discrepancy between gender identity and sex assigned at birth. Not all transgender people will experience distress, and some may only experience distress at a particular point in their lives. The use of the term may be seen as pathologizing by some and also facilitates access to gender-affirming treatment and changes to gender markers, e.g., on identification cards and birth certificates [3]. Transgender persons who wish to have their physical appearance congruent with their current gender identity may seek out medical interventions such as hormone therapy and/or surgeries, a process called medical/surgical transition [4, 5].

Health Outcomes for Transgender People

Over the last two decades, an increasing number of peer-reviewed publications have addressed the health and well-being of transgender individuals; however, the literature is still limited and predominantly focuses on specific areas, such as the diagnosis of gender dysphoria and its treatment, mental health disorders, and communicable diseases such as HIV, which affects transgender women disproportionately [6]. A recent Institute of Medicine Report underscored the need for more research to be done on all aspects of transgender health [7].

Despite greater visibility, transgender individuals continue to experience high rates of stigma and discrimination manifested by macro- and microaggressions on many levels. Transgender persons may experience external (enacted) stigma as a result of their gender nonconformity, including outright violence, verbal harassment, bullying, denial of health-care services, and discrimination in public accommodations [8–16]. Enacted stigma does not affect transgender and gender nonconforming people equally. Studies have shown higher rates of discrimination against those who are gender nonconforming or "visibly trans" [8, 16]. Transgender people who "pass" or "blend" (i.e., do not appear to be transgender) may avoid overt discrimination; however, they may experience heightened anxiety instead due to fear of disclosure [17]. Expectations of discrimination, even when not actualized, can result in adverse health outcomes as a result of nondisclosure of gender identity and avoidance of health care due to fear of discrimination [8, 12].

Microaggressions are verbal and nonverbal messages that send often unintended yet nevertheless demeaning messages that may impact self-esteem negatively. Examples include

A.E. Radix, MD, MPH (✉)
Director of Research and Education at Callen-Lorde Community Health Center, Assistant Clinical Professor of Medicine at New York University, 356 West 18th Street, New York, NY 10011, USA
e-mail: aradix@callen-lorde.org

L. Erickson-Schroth, MD, MA
Mount Sinai Beth Israel, Hetrick Martin Institute, 461 Central Park West #2A, New York, NY 10025, USA
e-mail: Erickson.schroth@gmail.com

L.A. Jacobs, LCSW-R
239 North Broadway, Sleepy Hollow, New York, NY 10591, USA
e-mail: Laura@LauraAJacobs.com

© Springer International Publishing AG 2017
K.L. Eckstrand, J. Potter (eds.), *Trauma, Resilience, and Health Promotion in LGBT Patients*,
DOI 10.1007/978-3-319-54509-7_9

exoticization of transgender people, endorsing the gender binary, and reinforcing stereotypes, e.g., that all transgender people want to undergo gender-affirming surgeries [18]. Microaggressions, enacted and felt stigma, and internalized transphobia can all contribute to adverse psychosocial and physical health outcomes, including high rates of HIV and other sexually transmitted infections, substance use, depression, anxiety, suicidal thoughts and actions, avoidance of health care, poverty, homelessness, and incarceration [6, 8, 10, 15, 19–22]. Barriers to routine and emergent care can have dire consequences. For example, transgender people may opt to access hormones outside of medical settings or undertake gender-affirming procedures such as silicone and soft tissue filler injections, leading to serious medical complications [17, 23, 24]. It is therefore critical to frame stigma and health outcomes, including quality of life, within a minority stress model so as to aid in the development of targeted strategies for building resilience (Chap. 4, Fig. 4.2).

Studies of Resilience in Transgender Populations

Given the high levels of discrimination and violence experienced by transgender people and the mental health outcomes that can result from these traumatic experiences, a number of researchers have begun to focus on resilience within transgender communities. Instead of asking which risk factors lead to poor coping, they are attempting to determine which protective factors help transgender people to thrive despite difficult situations (Fig. 9.1).

In general, studies of resilience in transgender people have been small and qualitative, though some larger quantitative studies include measures related to resilience. Defining resilience as an outcome has been one of the most difficult tasks for researchers. Some have used resilience scales already developed for the general population [25], while others have attempted to create resilience scales specific to transgender people [26]. Most studies have not used resilience scales, instead focusing on factors that differentiate those trans people who have "good outcomes" (i.e., high self-esteem, good quality of life) from those who have "poor outcomes" (i.e., depression, anxiety).

Examining factors that contribute to resilience is not the only way researchers have approached the study of transgender resilience. Some studies have also examined strategies employed by transgender people that allow them to be resilient, including seeking out LGBT peers for social support [25]. Notably limited are studies of interventions to promote resilience, although it can be argued that transition-related health interventions such as hormones and surgeries are resilience-building; certainly, studies have supported the fact that initiation of gender-affirming care reduces

gender dysphoria and improves psychological functioning [27, 28]. While every day across the country transgender people engage in activities such as attending support groups and doing advocacy work, these activities have rarely been studied formally as resilience-promoting interventions.

Two factors that have been established as contributing to resilience among transgender individuals are family and social support [8, 15, 25, 29–31]. Family support has been correlated with less distress among transgender people [15], while social support has been linked to lower levels of anxiety and depression [29]. Moreover, support from friends and family is associated with a decrease in suicidal behavior [31].

It has been somewhat difficult to tease out the types of social support that are most influential. Increased size of the transgender community has been shown to correlate with decreased distress, and transgender peer support moderates the relationship between stigma and mental distress [15]; however, it is not known whether support from transgender peers is a crucial ingredient or if general social support might be sufficient. Very little is known about how helpful it is for transgender people to have connections with LGBT communities where most of the members are not transgender. For some people this may be very rewarding. One study showed that having frequent contact with LGBT peers was associated with higher scores on a resilience scale [25]. However, LGB communities can sometimes be subtly or even outwardly discriminatory toward transgender people, so how composition of and contact with LGBT support networks impact resilience remains unclear.

There are certain demographic characteristics that appear to influence resilience in transgender communities. Several studies have shown that younger age is correlated with greater psychological distress among transgender people [25], while older age is associated with resilience, specifically with regard to the impact of gender-related abuse [15, 22]. It may be that transgender people learn resilience strategies over the course of their lifetimes; however, it may also be that those who are not as resilient do not live as long.

Those transgender people who are employed and/or have higher incomes or levels of education appear to show lower levels of depression and higher resilience scores [15, 25, 29, 30]. These correlations may not represent causation, as it is possible that those who are more resilient or less depressed are able to finish college, achieve employment, and make good incomes more frequently than others. While employment may correlate with resilience, the work environment can be difficult to navigate for a transgender person. In fact, one study demonstrated that employed transgender people face higher levels of stigma than nonemployed transgender people [32]; in another study, 90% of transgender people reported experiencing harassment, mistreatment, or discrimination on the job or taking actions to avoid it [8].

Fig. 9.1 Factors contributing to
the resilience of transgender
individuals

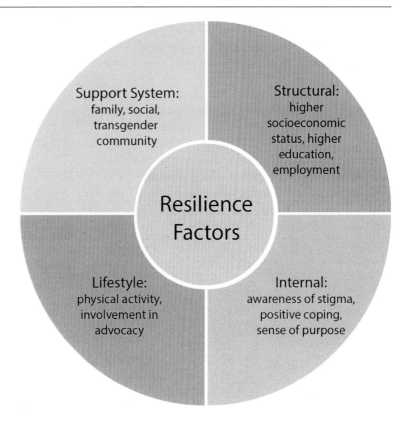

This information underscores the need to enact anti-discrimination legislation in employment and public accommodations for transgender and gender nonconforming individuals. Similarly, in schools, providing trans-affirming environments free of violence and bullying may help to improve graduation rates of transgender students.

In general, it appears that like other people, transgender people benefit from having full lives. This includes receiving family and social support, succeeding in school, and being employed. However, it also depends on other facets of life. Transgender people who have reasons for living, such as children, have fewer suicidal behaviors [31]. Trans men who are sexually satisfied are less likely to be depressed [30]. In a study of 141 older trans individuals, successful aging included caring relationships; engaging in an active, healthy lifestyle; and nurturing their spiritual selves [33].

Research has begun to reveal some of the strategies that transgender people use to remain resilient in difficult circumstances. Many of the studies of resilience strategies are small and qualitative, but a number of topics have emerged that are worthy of further investigation. Importantly, transgender people may need to utilize different coping styles at different points during the transition process [34]. One theme that frequently emerges from trans resilience studies is the potential benefit of increased awareness of stigma [35–38]. In one study of trans people of color,

participants highlighted the importance of recognizing and negotiating gender and racial/ethnic oppression [37]. Another study found that awareness of stigma protects self-esteem in the face of blatant, but not more subtle discrimination [38]. Being involved in advocacy also appears to be a common resilience strategy for transgender people [33, 35, 37, 39]. It is likely that awareness of stigma and involvement in advocacy allow transgender people to see their oppression as a societal issue that affects them as a class of people, rather than as individuals fighting the world on their own.

Despite the increasing number of studies of transgender resilience factors and strategies, there has been little formal research into interventions that promote resilience among transgender people. One reason for this may be that community organizations and health-care centers that engage in activities likely to build resilience are less focused on producing research than results for individual people; however, there is growing consensus that research into resilience-building interventions is an important next step [40–43]. Two peer-led interventions (Life Skills and Girlfriends) show early promise in reducing participants' sexual risk behaviors by increasing participant's use of condoms and reducing the number of their sex partners [44, 45]. These interventions, which address transgender stigma and empowerment and feature skills building exercises and

HIV education, are now being formally studied in clinical trials. Transition-related health care can also be considered a resilience-building intervention for transgender people. While few large-scale prospective studies have been performed, evidence to date demonstrates that desired hormone treatments and surgeries correlate with improved quality of life and mental health outcomes among transgender people [46–49].

Recently published research has highlighted the importance of structural interventions in reducing adverse health outcomes among transgender people. In one study, veterans who live in states that have employment nondiscrimination protection were shown to have lower rates of mood disorders and self-directed violence [50]. Similarly, in 12 city jails in New York implementation of a staff training regarding the needs of transgender detainees was associated with a significant reduction in complaints related to medical care, including access to hormones and medical staff sensitivity [51].

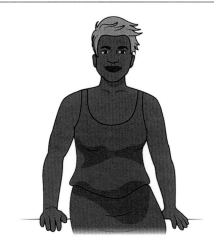

Fig. 9.2 Natasha is a 34-year-old, African-American, transgender female presenting for the first time to an LGBT community health clinic

Summary

Microaggressions, enacted and felt stigma, and internalized transphobia contribute to increased mental health issues among transgender populations, including depression, anxiety, suicidal thoughts and actions, substance use, and engagement in other risk behaviors. Resilience factors among transgender persons include family and social support, employment, recognition of stigma and involvement in advocacy. Structural interventions that improve health and well-being include access to gender-affirming care, including medical transition care, and legal protections. More research needs to be done to study effective individual-, interpersonal-, and community-level interventions for building resilience. Clinicians play an important role by providing culturally competent care in environments that are bias-free, facilitating access to hormonal therapy, providing appropriate referrals for transition care if needed, and linking their clients to community resources, such as support groups and legal assistance.

Case Scenario

Natasha is a 34-year-old, African-American, transgender female presenting for the first time to an LGBT community health clinic to initiate hormones (Fig. 9.2). During the health interview, Natasha discloses that she is an officer in the US Army. She was born in South Carolina, where she completed high school. During college she was a member of the Reserve Officers' Training Corps, and since graduation she has remained on active duty. Natasha is married to

a woman, Sherylyn, and has a 6-year-old son. Her father, a lieutenant in the military, died in an accident when she was 13, but her mother and two sisters are alive and well. Four years ago Natasha started psychotherapy for depression and gradually came to embrace her identity as a transgender woman; however, when she shared this revelation at home, Sherylyn initially was angry and distant. Natasha states that she knew from a young age that that she "was different," but gender nonconformity was not accepted in her conservative family. As the only son, she was expected to follow in her father's footsteps; to this day, no one else in her family knows that she is transgender, and she believes they would not accept her as a transwoman. Natasha is very concerned that she will not be accepted if anyone finds out that she is transgender. She wants to start hormones, but at a low dose so that the physical changes will be less noticeable.

Discussion Questions

1. What strategies can health professionals use when trying to promote health and well-being among transgender clients?
2. How should providers assess support systems for transgender clients who present for hormonal care?
3. What are some examples of enacted stigma experienced by transgender people, and how might this differ for those serving in the military?
4. How does access to transition health services, including hormones and surgeries, impact the health of transgender people?
5. What community resources are available to support transgender people who serve in the military?

Summary Practice Points

1. Medical and mental health providers need to build practice settings that affirm the identity of transgender persons and provide culturally competent and appropriate care. They should be knowledgeable about terminology and ensure that transgender clients are treated respectfully, which includes using requested names and pronouns. Providers should be aware of issues that impact access to care, such as stigma and discrimination, and understand available options for medical and surgical transition.

2. Transgender people who have family and community support appear to have improved mental health outcomes. Providers should therefore be aware of available community resources, support groups, and organizations that can assist with transgender identity development and sense of community belonging [15, 52].

3. Since access to gender-affirming health care and hormone therapy improves psychological health outcomes, [47] providers should stay up to date with the medical options available for medical transition and be able to assist clients with appropriate medical and mental health referrals.

4. There are possibly more than 150,000 transgender people serving in the military. Repeal of "Don't ask, don't tell" allowed gay, lesbian and bisexual service members to serve openly since 2010 however transgender individuals did not receive similar protections until 2016 [53, 54]. The threat of discharge caused many military personnel to hide their transgender identity or delay transition until they left active duty. Transgender veterans experience increased rates of mood disorders, including depression and suicidality, compared with cis-gender persons. Providers should ask about their clients' support network, including family and peers, and be knowledgeable about support resources for active and retired service members.

Resources

SPART*A is a membership organization of LGBT people who currently serve or have served in the military: http://www.spartapride.org/

OutServe-Servicemembers Legal Defense Network (SLDN) represents the US lesbian, gay, bisexual, and transgender (LGBT) community worldwide and provides free and direct legal assistance to service members and veterans: https://www.outserve-sldn.org/

The Transgender American Veterans Association (TAVA) is a nonprofit organization that works with other concerned gay, lesbian, bisexual, and transgender (GLBT) organizations to ensure that transgender veterans will receive appropriate care for their medical conditions with the Veterans Health: http://transveteran.org/

GLAAD Transgender Resources available at http://www.glaad.org/transgender/resources includes general information and resources, health-care and legal resources, and resources for transgender people in crisis.

Transgender Health Learning Center at the UCSF Center of Excellence for Transgender Health available at http://transhealth.ucsf.edu/trans?page=lib-00-00 provides courses for medical and mental health providers on caring for transgender clients, adaptations of interventions for transgender people, and information on incorporating gender identity into data collection.

References

1. Kuper LE, Nussbaum R, Mustanski B. Exploring the diversity of gender and sexual orientation identities in an online sample of transgender individuals. J Sex Res. 2012;49(2–3):244–54.
2. Conron KJ, Scott G, Stowell GS, Landers SJ. Transgender health in Massachusetts: results from a household probability sample of adults. Am J Public Health. 2012;102(1):118–22.
3. Knudson G. Process toward consensus on recommendations for revision of the diagnoses of gender identity disorders by the world professional association for transgender health. Int J Transgend. 2010;12(2):54–9.
4. Hembree WC, Cohen-Kettenis P, Delemarre-van de Waal HA, Gooren LJ, Meyer 3rd WJ, Spack NP, et al. Endocrine treatment of transsexual persons: an endocrine society clinical practice guideline. J Clin Endocrinol Metab. 2009;94(9):3132–54.
5. Coleman E, Bockting W, Botzer M, Cohen-Kettenis P, DeCuypere G, Feldman J, et al. Standards of care for the health of transsexual, transgender, and gender-nonconforming people, version 7. Int J Transgend. 2011;13:165.
6. Herbst JH, Jacobs ED, Finlayson TJ, McKleroy VS, Neumann MS, Crepaz N, et al. Estimating HIV prevalence and risk behaviors of transgender persons in the United States: a systematic review. AIDS Behav. 2008;12(1):1–17.
7. IOM (Institute of Medicine). The health of lesbian, gay, bisexual, and transgender people: building a foundation for better understanding. Washington, DC: The National Academies Press; 2011.
8. Grant JM, Mottet LA, Tanis J. National transgender discrimination survey report on health and health care. Washington, DC: National Center for Transgender Equality and the National Gay and Lesbian Task Force; 2010.
9. Nuttbrock L, Bockting W, Rosenblum A, Hwahng S, Mason M, Macri M, et al. Gender abuse and major depression among transgender women: a prospective study of vulnerability and resilience. Am J Public Health. 2014;104(11):2191–8.
10. Garofalo R, Deleon J, Osmer E, Doll M, Harper GW. Overlooked, misunderstood and at-risk: exploring the lives and HIV risk of ethnic minority male-to-female transgender youth. J Adolesc Health. 2006;38(3):230–6.
11. Garofalo R, Osmer E, Sullivan C, Doll M, Harper G. Environmental, psychosocial, and individual correlates of HIV risk in ethnic minority male-to-female transgender youth. J HIV AIDS Prev Child Youth. 2007;7(2):89–104.

12. Lombardi EL, Wilchins RA, Priesing D, Malouf D. Gender violence: transgender experiences with violence and discrimination. J Homosex. 2001;42(1):89–101.

13. Kenagy GP. Transgender health: findings from two needs assessment studies in Philadelphia. Health Soc Work. 2005;30(1):19–26.

14. Reisner SL, Greytak EA, Parsons JT, Ybarra ML. Gender minority social stress in adolescence: disparities in adolescent bullying and substance use by gender identity. J Sex Res. 2015;52(3):243–56.

15. Bockting WO, Miner MH, Swinburne Romine RE, Hamilton A, Coleman E. Stigma, mental health, and resilience in an online sample of the US transgender population. Am J Public Health. 2013;103(5):943–51.

16. Reisner SL, Hughto JM, Dunham EE, Heflin KJ, Begenyi JB, Coffey-Esquivel J, et al. Legal protections in public accommodations settings: a critical public health issue for transgender and gender-nonconforming people. Milbank Q. 2015;93 (3):484–515.

17. Sevelius JM. Gender affirmation: a framework for conceptualizing risk behavior among transgender women of color. Sex Roles. 2013;68(11–12):675–89.

18. Nadal KL, Skolnik A, Wong Y. Interpersonal and systemic Microaggressions toward transgender people: implications for counseling. J LGBT Issues Couns. 2012;6(1):55–82.

19. Goldblum P. The relationship between gender-based victimization and suicide attempts in transgender people. Prof Psychol Res Pr. 2012;43(5):468–75.

20. Nemoto T, Sausa LA, Operario D, Keatley J. Need for HIV/AIDS education and intervention for MTF transgenders: responding to the challenge. J Homosex. 2006;51(1):183–202.

21. Nuttbrock L, Hwahng S, Bockting W, Rosenblum A, Mason M, Macri M, et al. Psychiatric impact of gender-related abuse across the life course of male-to-female transgender persons. J Sex Res. 2010;47(1):12–23.

22. Nuttbrock L, Bockting W, Rosenblum A, Hwahng S, Mason M, Macri M, et al. Gender abuse and major depression among transgender women: a prospective study of vulnerability and resilience. Am J Public Health. 2013;104:2191–8.

23. Bradford J, Reisner SL, Honnold JA, Xavier J. Experiences of transgender-related discrimination and implications for health: results from the Virginia transgender health initiative study. Am J Public Health. 2013;103(10):1820–9.

24. Xavier JH, Honnold JA, Bradford, JB. The health, health-related needs, and lifecourse experiences of transgender Virginians. 2007. Available at: http://www.vdh.virginia.gov/epidemiology/diseaseprevention/documents/pdf/THISFINALREPORTVol1.pdf.

25. Bariola E, Lyons A, Leonard W, Pitts M, Badcock P, Couch M. Demographic and psychosocial factors associated with psychological distress and resilience among transgender individuals. Am J Public Health. 2015;105(10):2108–16.

26. Testa RJ, Habarth J, Peta J, Balsam K, Bockting W. Development of the gender minority stress and resilience measure. Psychol Sex Orientat Gend Divers. 2015;2(1):65–77.

27. de Vries AL, McGuire JK, Steensma TD, Wagenaar EC, Doreleijers TA, Cohen-Kettenis PT. Young adult psychological outcome after puberty suppression and gender reassignment. Pediatrics. 2014;134(4):696–704.

28. Keo-Meier CL, Herman LI, Reisner SL, Pardo ST, Sharp C, Babcock JC. Testosterone treatment and MMPI-2 improvement in transgender men: a prospective controlled study. J Consult Clin Psychol. 2015;83(1):143–56.

29. Budge SL, Adelson JL, Howard KA. Anxiety and depression in transgender individuals: the roles of transition status, loss, social support, and coping. J Consult Clin Psychol. 2013;81(3):545–57.

30. Rotondi NK, Bauer GR, Travers R, Travers A, Scanlon K, Kaay M. Depression in male-to-female transgender Ontarians: results from the trans PULSE project. Can J Commun Ment Health. 2011;30(2):113–33.

31. Moody C, Smith NG. Suicide protective factors among trans adults. Arch Sex Behav. 2013;42(5):739–52.

32. Mizock L, Mueser KT. Employment, mental health, internalized stigma, and coping with transphobia among transgender individuals. Psychol Sex Orientat Gend Divers. 2014;1(2):146–58.

33. McFadden SH. Resilience and multiple stigmatized identities: lessons from transgender persons' reflections on aging. New York: Springer; 2013. p. 247–267.

34. Budge SL. Transgender emotional and coping processes: facilitative and avoidant coping throughout gender transitioning. Couns Psychol. 2013;41(4):601–47.

35. Reisner SL, Gamarel KE, Dunham E, Hopwood R, Hwahng S. Female-to-male transmasculine adult health: a mixed-methods community-based needs assessment. J Am Psychiatr Nurses Assoc. 2013;19(5):293–303.

36. Singh AA, Hays DG, Watson LS. Strength in the face of adversity: resilience strategies of transgender individuals. J Couns Dev. 2011;89(1):20–7.

37. Singh AA, McKleroy VS. "Just getting out of bed is a revolutionary act": the resilience of transgender people of color who have survived traumatic life events. Traumatology. 2011;17(2):34–44.

38. Kosenko K, Rintamaki L, Raney S, Maness K. Transgender patient perceptions of stigma in health care contexts. Med Care. 2013;51 (9):819–22.

39. Pinto RM, Melendez RM, Spector AY. Male-to-female transgender individuals building social support and capital from within a gender-focused network. J Gay Lesbian Soc Serv. 2008;20 (3):203–20.

40. Herrick AL, Lim SH, Wei C, Smith H, Guadamuz T, Friedman MS, et al. Resilience as an untapped resource in behavioral intervention design for gay men. AIDS Behav. 2011;15(Suppl 1):S25–9.

41. McElroy JA, Wintemberg JJ, Cronk NJ, Everett KD. The association of resilience, perceived stress and predictors of depressive symptoms in sexual and gender minority youths and adults. Psychol Sex. 2016;7(2):116–30.

42. Heck NC. The potential to promote resilience: piloting a minority stress-informed, GSA-based, mental health promotion program for LGBTQ youth. Psychol Sex Orientat Gend Divers. 2015;2 (3):225–31.

43. Harper GW, Riplinger AJ, Neubauer LC, Murphy AG, Velcoff J, Bangi AK. Ecological factors influencing HIV sexual risk and resilience among young people in rural Kenya: implications for prevention. Health Educ Res. 2014;29(1):131–46.

44. Garofalo R, Johnson AK, Kuhns LM, Cotten C, Joseph H, Margolis A. Life skills: evaluation of a theory-driven behavioral HIV prevention intervention for young transgender women. J Urban Health. 2012;89(3):419–31.

45. Taylor RD, Bimbi DS, Joseph HA, Margolis AD, Parsons JT. Girlfriends: evaluation of an HIV-risk reduction intervention for adult transgender women. AIDS Educ Prev. 2011;23 (5):469–78.

46. Ainsworth TA, Spiegel JH. Quality of life of individuals with and without facial feminization surgery or gender reassignment surgery. Qual Life Res. 2010;19(7):1019–24.

47. White Hughto JM, Reisner SL. A systematic review of the effects of hormone therapy on psychological functioning and quality of life in transgender individuals. Trans Health. 2016;1(1):21–31.

48. Murad MH, Elamin MB, Garcia MZ, Mullan RJ, Murad A, Erwin PJ, et al. Hormonal therapy and sex reassignment: a systematic review and meta-analysis of quality of life and psychosocial outcomes. Clin Endocrinol. 2010;72(2):214–31.

49. Rotondi NK, Bauer GR, Scanlon K, Kaay M, Travers R, Travers A. Prevalence of and risk and protective factors for depression in female-to-male transgender Ontarians: trans PULSE project. Can J Commun Ment Health. 2011;30(2):135–55.

50. Blosnich JR, Marsiglio MC, Gao S, Gordon AJ, Shipherd JC, Kauth M, Brown GR, Fine MJ. Mental health of transgender Veterans in

US states with and without discrimination and hate crime legal protection. Am J Public Health. 2016;106(3):534–40.

51. Jaffer M, Ayad J, Tungol JG, MacDonald R, Dickey N, Venters H. Improving Transgender Healthcare in the New York City Correctional System. LGBT Health. 2016;3:116–21.

52. Barr SM, Budge SL, Adelson JL. Transgender community belongingness as a mediator between strength of transgender identity and well-being. J Couns Psychol. 2016;63(1):87–97.

53. Goldbach JT, Castro CA. Lesbian, gay, bisexual, and transgender (LGBT) service members: life after don't ask, don't tell. Curr Psychiatry Rep. 2016;18(6):56.

54. U.S. Department of Defense. Transgender service in the U.S. Military: an implementation handbook. September 30, 2016. Washington, D.C. Available at: https://www.defense.gov/Portals/1/features/2016/0616_policy/DoDTGHandbook_093016.pdf?ver=2016-09-30-160933-837

Understanding Trauma and Supporting Resilience with LGBT People of Color

Anneliese A. Singh

This chapter describes common experiences of trauma and the development of resilience among LGBT people of color, and how they influence individual health, healthcare, and treatment outcomes. "People of color" is a term used more recently in the United States (USA) to refer to people who are members of racial/ethnic minority communities (e.g., African American, Asian American/Pacific Islander, Latina/Latino American, Native American/First Nations, multiracial) and emphasizes shared experiences of racism among these communities [1]. When working with LGBT (lesbian, gay, bisexual, transgender) people of color, healthcare providers should be mindful of the multiple minority identities that intersect with one another. For instance, LGBT people of color experience high rates of health disparities, including trauma, due to the intersection of racism, heterosexism, anti-transgender bias, and other systems of oppression such as classism and ableism. In this chapter, several frameworks are used to contextualize trauma and resilience experiences of LGBT people of color so that healthcare providers can use these approaches to effectively serve and support LGBT people of color.

Conceptual Frameworks with LGBT People of Color

There are several conceptual frameworks healthcare providers can use to guide their service provision with LGBT people of color. First, *structural competency* is a foundational theory that can help providers acknowledge the realities of discrimination and health inequities related

A.A. Singh, PhD (✉)
Department of Counseling and Human Development Services,
The University of Georgia, 402 Aderhold, Athens,
GA 30602-7124, USA

75 Wiltshire Drive, Avondale Estates, GA 30002, USA
e-mail: asingh@uga.edu

to systemic injustices [2], LGBT people of color can experience. Mertzi and Hansen [3] called for the field of medical education to attend to five areas of structural competency training. The first competency entails understanding that structures have an influence on the provider-patient relationship, while the second competency includes having accurate language to describe and acknowledge these structures. The third competency area comprises revising and describing patient conceptualizations using the language of structural competency theory, and the fourth competency invites the provider to become an observer and identify potential interventions from a structural perspective. Lastly, there is a focus on developing structural humility as a healthcare provider interacting with patients. Structural competency theory also has a strong focus on empowerment interventions [2, 3]. Applying these five core areas to work with LGBT people of color, providers seek to understand and identify how their identities and issues of power and privilege influence the relationship between patient and provider; in doing so, they use terms that reflect these power differentials (e.g., racism, societal inequities). Also, structural competency theory applied to work with LGBT people of color demands that patient formulations take into account these systemic forces, while continually developing humility related to learning and understanding these oppressive forces.

Intersectionality theory is another foundational theory healthcare providers should be aware of when working with LGBT people of color. This theory posits that individuals and communities are affected by intersections of privilege and oppression identities and experiences. Many times, these identities and experiences are complex and demand focused attention on the specific intersection influencing an individual. For example, as a transgender South Asian man moves through a social and medical transition, he can move from a socialized identity related to oppression (assigned female at birth) to a gender identity with assigned privilege (man). Yet, this entire process of

© Springer International Publishing AG 2017
K.L. Eckstrand, J. Potter (eds.), *Trauma, Resilience, and Health Promotion in LGBT Patients*,
DOI 10.1007/978-3-319-54509-7_10

identity development as a transgender person can be influenced by the intersections of his gender identity with his race/ethnicity and/or other identities. These intersections can be sites of multiplicative stress and negative health outcomes (e.g., racism and heterosexism), but also may be sites of additive resilience if this transgender man has access to job stability, financial resources, and support from family and friends. To add to the complexity of these intersections, LGBT people of color may experience both oppression and resilience to oppression simultaneously, such as this same South Asian transgender man experiencing disability as he moves into older adulthood while "passing" more for his identified gender and "fitting in" more with his South Asian male community.

In addition to structural competency and intersectionality theories, there are constructs describing processes LGBT people of color may experience that healthcare providers should be able to address when working with this group. When LGBT people of color experience societal marginalization, this oppression can be internalized [4, 5] in the form of internalized racism, internalized homonegativity, internalized transnegativity, and/or internalized binegativity, among others. This internalized stigma can result in LGBT people of color having stereotyped and negative belief systems about themselves and others within their community. For instance, a bisexual genderqueer Latino may experience internalized racism and believe negative societal messages about Latino people ("I will not go to a Latino/a doctor"). Again, these intersections of internalized stigma can provide sites of multiple, and potentially chronic, minority stress.

Trauma Prevalence Among LGBT People of Color

LGBT people of color experience a disproportionate burden of health disparities and trauma compared to other sexual and gender minority populations. Large surveys have found that LGBT people of color, particularly African American trans women, experience higher than average rates of poverty, housing discrimination, mental health challenges [6], and violence victimization [7]. In addition to these social class and mental health stressors, LGBT people of color may use substances and be vulnerable to HIV infection as a result of experiencing many sources of discrimination [8]. Discrete experiences of discrimination may be additive and have a multiplicative impact on the trauma load of an LGBT person of color; at the same time, certain combinations of identities may be sources of strength for LGBT people of color and may actually be supportive in times of stress [9].

The trauma load of LGBT people of color is also affected by intergenerational trauma. Systemic practices such as forced immigration imposed by slavery on people of African descent, removal of Native American/First Nations or Latina/Latino heritage from their lands, and stereotyping Asian/Pacific Islander communities as perpetually "foreign" have created legacy burdens for people in these communities. The history of colonization in the USA also served to erase the existence of a nonbinary gender construct (i.e., "two spirit") that was considered sacred within Native American/First Nations communities [10]. Understanding intergenerational trauma and the effects of colonization and structural racism in the USA can be helpful in providing culturally responsive care to LGBT people of color. For instance, many communities of color have developed culturally specific sources of strength and coping that they may access during times of stress and discrimination [11].

To understand why LGBT people of color have such high rates of trauma, it is helpful to examine both systemic/structural experiences of discrimination as well as everyday lived experiences of stigma and discrimination, such as microaggressions. Microaggressions are often unconscious, embedded sources of stigma within society. When LGBT people of color access healthcare, these microaggressions can be additive and chronic in nature as they are vulnerable to both racism and heterosexism. A Latina queer woman may have a doctoral degree, but providers may make assumptions about both her level of education and that she has a husband as a partner. LGBT people of color often find themselves straddling a cultural divide between their experiences of race/ethnicity and their experiences related to being LGBT [12]. For instance, an African American transgender man may feel he needs to conceal his sexual orientation within his family or his workplace. Yet, he may also live in a geographic area where the LGBT community is predominantly white. Therefore, he may simultaneously experience racism within the surrounding LGBT community as well as homophobia in the workplace.

It is important to exercise caution and not make assumptions that communities of color are more heterosexist than white communities, as there are conflicting perspectives regarding this assertion [12, 13]. Nevertheless, providers will frequently run into this type of thinking, even among LGBT people of color themselves. An alternative view posits that high levels of heterosexism in some communities of color are embedded in racism [14]. Families of color exposed to extensive and insidious racism are often quite conscious that having another minority identity will further set them apart and increase the likelihood of additional experiences of oppression. For instance, in studies of African American lesbians disclosing their sexual orientation identity to their mothers, lesbian participants described their mothers having a "don't ask, don't tell" policy, where they accepted their daughter's sexual orientation, but were concerned about what future discrimination they might face [13, 14]. It is important to consider, however, that some data suggest that conflicts in a person's allegiance to either sexual orientation or racial/ethnic identity are most likely to exist when allegiances to both identities are strong [15].

Terms Used by LGBT People of Color Communities

LGBT people of color use a variety of terms to describe their sexual orientation and gender identities. For example, some lesbian-identified women, especially African American women, may use words such as "stud" to describe their sexual orientation (i.e., identification as women with a masculine gender expression). Other communities of color may self-describe as "same gender loving" and transgender people of color may use "masculine of center" to describe themselves [16]. In addition, LGBT people of color whose second language is English may use native terms to describe themselves, such as the "mahu" of Hawaii [10]. It is important to ask permission from the patient before using these terms, as some of these words were previously epithets with negative connotations (such as "queer") that were later reclaimed and embraced by LGBT communities of color. Further, as these terms may have different meanings to different individuals, it is important to understand how each individual relates to the chosen term.

Coming Out to Others

When working with LGBT patients of color, providers will notice a wide range of self-disclosure with respect to sexual orientation and gender identity. In addition to Miller's "don't ask, don't tell" research [13, 14] with African American lesbian women, recent research with Latino/Latina LGBT people explores the construct of "tacitness." Tacitness refers to a lack of explicit disclosure of sexual orientation by LGBT Latino/Latinas to their families due to the desire to maintain strong family ties, yet also encompasses an implicit understanding that these families have about their loved one's sexual orientation [17, 18]. With these considerations in mind, healthcare providers should be careful in how they assess sexual orientation and gender identity with LGBT people of color when family members are present, and should assess the extent to which they are open about their identities to others in their lives. Some LGBT people of color may not "pass" according to societally restrictive gender norms, so healthcare providers should be sure to refrain from assuming what the sexual orientation and gender identities are for these patients [19].

Access to Services

Lack of access to healthcare providers compounds the harmful effects of trauma on the wellbeing of LGBT people of color. For example, while not all transgender women of color want gender-related care, such as gender affirmation surgeries, access to private insurance to cover these medical procedures is rare, due in large part to the high rates of employment and housing discrimination experienced by this population. Transgender women of color may engage in survival sex work in order to support themselves, yet feel hesitant or distrustful of healthcare providers due to prior negative experiences in care, and therefore avoid accessing publicly funded medical services (e.g., mobile HIV testing). In addition, for LGBT people of color who have access to mental health counseling through community centers, there may not be counselors who are trained in working with significant and multiple levels of racial/ethnic and gender trauma (e.g., lack of coverage of Eye Movement Desensitization and Reprocessing Therapy).

LGBT People of Color and Religious/Spiritual Beliefs

For some LGBT people of color, religious and spiritual practices are important sources of coping and healing. Therefore, assessing the extent to which a person endorses such belief systems is important, as well as exploring how spiritual practices may influence how, when, and why they choose to access health care. At the same time, there are also LGBT people of color who have been ostracized or rejected from their religious/spiritual home communities, so their previous source of coping may have become instead a source of pain and/or trauma [11, 20]. In addition, it is important not to assume that all LGBT people of color are religious/spiritual, as there are those who may be atheist, agnostic, or actively questioning their faith traditions. In order to understand the influence of religious/spiritual practices on health and wellbeing, providers should ask LGBT people of color what role faith plays in their lives, whether it is associated with connection or isolation, and to what extent they feel "torn" between their religious/spiritual and their LGBT identities and communities. LGBT people of color may have experienced discrimination within the religious/spiritual communities in which they were raised, and may have difficulty finding or adjusting to new religious/spiritual homes. A Korean American transgender man may have been raised within a Christian church, but when he discloses his gender identity may not feel safe worshiping with a community where he grew up; whereas, when he attends a new LGBT-affirmative church, he may experience racism or feel like he does not "fit in" with this new faith community.

Individual and Collective Resilience of LGBT People of Color

While it is true that LGBT people of color can experience multiple levels and types of oppression and discrimination in society, it is important that healthcare providers be aware of the individual and community resilience that LGBT people of color often experience. Resilience refers to the everyday strategies and processes that LGBT people of color use to address adversity in their lives. Although resilience typically encompasses the buffers, supports, and protective factors an individual may utilize to cope with difficult life experiences, healthcare providers should also consider the protective effect of connection to a resilient community [11, 19, 21].

Adaptive Resilience and Coping Strategies

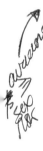

Resilience and coping among LGBT communities have thus far been examined predominantly via a white and Western lens [11] so the literature with respect to LGBT people of color is still nascent. In a study of gay men of color, researchers found that the stress of racism was associated with being more likely to engage in unprotected anal intercourse; however, participants with an avoidant coping style were most likely to manifest sexual risk behaviors. Avoidance coping refers to strategies where people attempt to deal with their difficulties by distancing themselves; however, some studies of people of color have suggested that avoidance coping actually increases rather than decreases stress levels [22, 23]. At the same time, research has found that problem-focused coping strategies – those that entail proactively addressing a stressor or seeking to change a stressor – are helpful for people of color dealing with racism [23]; studies that specifically address the needs of LGBT people of color are needed. In the meantime, healthcare providers are encouraged to explore a variety of coping strategies that LGBT people of color can use to cope with repetitive experiences of racism and LGBT discrimination, with special attention to whether these coping strategies increase or decrease stress.

Collective and Community Resilience

In tandem with exploring individual coping and resilience, healthcare providers should also assess the extent to which LGBT people of color are connected with community sources of resilience. Research with transgender youth and adults of color suggests that these sources of community resilience may include strong connections to not only trans communities of color, but trans activist communities of color who can help them access needed financial and legal resources, in addition to providing mentoring [11, 19]. Similarly, studies of transfeminine African American women have suggested that these communities, despite experiencing exceptionally high levels of societal marginalization, are able to develop close trust networks that are characterized by overt demonstrations of intimacy and affection. Examples entail the use of affectionate language or feelings of immediate emotional intimacy with fellow transfeminine African American women although just meeting for the first time [9]. Scholars have encouraged healthcare providers to work with these trust networks, as opposed to outside of them, as these networks can rapidly gather community members around a need or topic [9, 19]. Specifically, it is critical to work with key constituents and stakeholders within trust networks to develop successful healthcare interventions.

Supporting LGBT People of Color as a Healthcare Provider

There are multiple ways that healthcare providers can increase their ability to provide competent care for LGBT patients of color. First and foremost, healthcare providers must examine their personal experiences of privilege and oppression related to their own race/ethnicity, sexual orientation, gender identity, gender expression, social class, and other identities. This self-examination should include exploration of the messages that one has (or has not) learned from family members, media, medical school, and other sources of potentially stereotyped information. Healthcare providers should explore how racial privilege, class and education privilege, US citizen privilege, and other privileges may obscure their ability to perceive and accurately identify the health concerns of their LGBT patients of color. For example, a white, straight, male healthcare provider working with a Native American bisexual male patient should be sensitive to the power differentials that exist between them in terms of racial/ethnic and sexual orientation identities, rather than being oblivious about how white and straight privilege influences the patient-provider relationship and creating barriers to care.

In addition, healthcare providers can set an explicit intention to periodically assess where their strengths and weaknesses rest. For instance, a black, cisgender provider may lack information about the common health concerns of Latina lesbian women. Seeking professional development to address these growing edges is vital in order to be able to offer competent care to LGBT people of color. These learning experiences must be informed by awareness of the trauma LGBT people of color experience, and also address how to be an affirmative healthcare provider to LGBT people of color who have multiple experiences of both trauma and resilience. Refraining from making assumptions (e.g., all LGBT people of color have a religious or spiritual tradition), while also understanding common concerns of LGBT people of color (e.g., disclosure of gender and sexual orientation identities, conflicts of allegiance) should be intentionally woven into everyday interactions with members of this group.

In doing so, trauma-informed healthcare must also address individual and community resilience, in order to leverage the strengths LGBT people of color may have to address difficulties in their lives and risk factors for negative health outcomes. Specifically exploring patient strengths and community connections and providing resources when these community connections are low are foundational in terms of cultural competence with this group. This exploration can occur during intake session, but also can be an ongoing discussion with patients during the course of treatment.

Because of the extensive societal discrimination LGBT people of color experience and the very real impacts on relationships and health behaviors [24], healthcare providers should develop strong advocacy skills working on systemic change work in their healthcare settings. Partnering with diverse community groups and LGBT people of color networks to design trainings and ongoing professional development is important to assure that LGBT people of color are well served in healthcare settings. Healthcare providers can also utilize information obtained by analyzing individual interactions to inform needed systems interventions. For instance, if healthcare providers are continuously seeing that staff are using incorrect pronouns with transgender people – or inaccurately assessing trauma histories due to internalized racism or transnegativity – they can work to address these issues on a more systemic level in their settings.

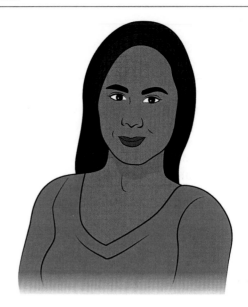

Fig. 10.1 Lynetta is a 33-year old, Hispanic woman who presents in your community clinic

job, Lynetta has had to move back in with her family. The family home is in a rural area, and she has been disconnected from her larger LGBT community. When she is not looking for employment, Lynetta spends a good deal of time at home with her extended family babysitting for her niece and taking care of other projects around the home. Before Lynetta lost her job, she ended a 10-year relationship with a woman and became depressed. She began going to her family's church, but the pastor began preaching anti-LGBT sentiments and she felt that these sentiments were directed at her so she stopped attending. Her family knows about her sexual orientation and gender expression; however, no one in the family talks about it openly. When Lynetta was first coming out, she was sexually assaulted by a cisgender man outside of an LGBT bar. She never told anyone about the experience, and she wondered at the time if it was punishment from God. Lynetta also experienced significant emotional and physical abuse in her last relationship; however, she does not want to disclose this to her family due to their anti-LGBT views. As Lynetta has grown more isolated from her LGBT community after losing her job, she has begun to feel more depressed and anxious and has started having more migraines. During your interview, Lynetta is distant, often staring out of the window for lengths of time before responding to questions.

Clinical Scenario

You are a faculty member at a university that focuses on rural and community healthcare. Lynetta is a 33-year-old Hispanic woman who presents in your community clinic (Fig. 10.1). She was fired from her job six months ago, and she has had difficulty getting in a new job. Since losing her

Discussion Questions

1. As a faculty member, how can you teach your students how to explore their own social locations and experiences of both privilege and oppression?

2. What are the multiple identities of race/ethnicity, sexual orientation, gender identity, gender expression, social class, and other social locations and experiences of both privilege and oppression that you would want your students to reflect on in service provision with Lynetta?

3. What are the trauma and resilience considerations you would want your students to explore with Lynetta when meeting with her?

4. If Lynetta's family were present with her, how would you explore this with your students in order to address potential conflicts in allegiance?

5. How will you explore the healthcare provider's role of advocacy in working with Lynetta?

Summary Practice Points

- LGBT people of color experience multiple levels of oppression in society, from racism and heterosexism to classism, among others.
- LGBT people of color develop resilience and strengths-based coping in response to these multiple levels of oppression.
- Healthcare providers can improve the quality of care for LGBT people of color by using affirmative LGBT language, attending to multiple identities and experiences they have, and understanding.
- Healthcare providers need to develop strong advocacy skills to ensure their LGBT people of color patients receive affirmative care.

References to Support Case

1. FORGE. *Transgender Sexual Violence Survivors: A Self-Help Guide to Healing and Understanding*. September 2015. Available at http://forge-forward.org/2015/09/trans-sa-survivors-self-help-guide/

2. Substance Abuse and Mental Health Services Administration. Trauma-Informed Approach and Trauma-Specific Interventions. Available at http://www.samhsa.gov/nctic/trauma-interventions.

3. American Academy of Family Physicians. AAFP Reprint No. 289D. Recommended Curriculum Guidelines for Family Medicine Residents: Lesbian, Gay, Bisexual, Transgender Health, 2015. Available at: http://www.aafp.org/dam/AAFP/documents/medical_education_residency/program_directors/Reprint289D_LGBT.pdf

4. University of California, San Francisco. LGBT Resource Center. Available at: https://lgbt.ucsf.edu/lgbt-education-and-training. The site includes links to articles, publications, and online trainings.

5. The Fenway Institute. The National LGBT Health Education Center On-Demand Webinars. Available at: http://www.lgbthealtheducation.org/training/on-demand-webinars/

References

1. Vidal-Ortiz S. People of color. In: Shaeffer RT, editor. Encyclopedia of race, ethnicity, and society. Thousand Oaks: Sage; 2008. p. 1037–8.

2. Alisha A, Sichel CE. Structural competency as a framework for training in counseling psychology. Couns Psychol. 2014;42 (7):901–18.

3. Mertzi JM, Hansen H. Structural competency: theorizing a new medical engagement with stigma and inequality. Soc Sci Med. 2014;103:126–33.

3. Balsam KF, Molina Y, Beadnell B, Simoni J, Walters K. Measuring multiple minority stress: the LGBT people of color microaggressions scale. Cult Divers Ethn Minor Psychol. 2011;17 (20):163–74.

4. Chang SC, Singh AA. Affirming psychological practice with transgender and gender nonconforming people of color. Psychol Sex Orientat Gend Divers. 2016;3(2).140–7.

5. Drazdowski TK, Perrin PB, Trujillo M, Sutter M, Benotsch EG, Snipes DJ. Structural equation modeling of the effects of racism, LGBTQ discrimination, and internalized oppression on illicit drug use in LGBTQ people of color. Drug Alcohol Depend. 2016;159:255–62.

6. Grant JM, Mottet LA, Tanis J, Harrison J, Herman JL, Kiesling M. Injustice at every turn: a report of the national transgender discrimination survey. Washington, DC: National Center for Transgender Equality & National Gay and Lesbian Task Force. Available at http://endtransdiscrimination.org/PDFs/NTDS_Report.pdf.

7. National Coalition of Anti-Violence Programs. Hate violence against lesbian, gay, bisexual, transgender, queer, and HIV-affected communities in the United States in 2011: a report from the National Coalition of Anti-Violence Programs. New York: National Coalition of Anti-Violence Programs; 2011.

8. Han C, George A, Boylan R, Gregorich SE, Choi KH. Stress and coping with racism and their role in sexual risk for HIV infection among African American, Asian/Pacific Islander and Latino men who have sex with men. Arch Sex Behav 2015;44(2):411–20. Fussell S. Are Black people more homophobic than White people? 2013, 19 May. Available at http://www.thefeministwire.com/2013/05/are-black-people-more-homophobic-than-white-people/.

9. Hwahng SJ, Nuttbrock L. Adolescent gender-related abuse, androphilia, and HIV risk among transfeminine people of color in New York City. J Homosex. 2014;61(5):691–713.

10. Matzner A. O au no keia: voices from Hawai'I's mahu and transgender communities. In: Ferber AL, Holcomb K, Wentling T, editors. Sex, gender, and sexuality: the new basics: an anthology. 2nd ed. New York: Oxford University Press. p. 109–17.

11. Singh AA, McKleroy VS. "Just getting out of bed is a revolutionary act": the resilience of transgender people of color who have survived traumatic life events. Traumatology. 2011;17(2):34–44.

12. Lewis GB. Black-white differences in attitudes toward homosexuality and gay rights. Public Opin Q. 2003;67(1):59–79.

13. Miller SJ. African-American lesbian identity management and identity development in the context of family and community. J Homosex. 2011;58(4):547–63.

14. Miller SJ. Reframing the power of lesbian daughters' relationships with mothers through black feminist thought. J Gay Lesb Soc Serv. 2009;21(2–3):206–18.

15. Sarno EL, Mohr JJ, Jackson SD, Fassinger RE. When identities collide: conflicts in allegiances among LGB people of color. Cult Divers Ethn Minor Psychol. 2015;21(4):550–9.

16. Brown Boi Project. Freeing ourselves: a guide to health and self love for brown bois. 2011. Available at https://brownboiproject.nationbuilder.com/health_guide.

17. Salcedo J. Deconstructing the outreach experience: renegotiating queer and Latino masculinities in the distribution of safe sex materials. J Gay Lesb Soc Serv. 2009;21(2–3):151–70.

18. Ulises Decena C. Tacit subjects: belonging and same-sex desire among Dominican immigrant men. Raleigh: Duke University Press; 2011.

19. Singh AA, Hwhang SJ, Chang SC, White B. Affirmative counseling with trans/gender-variant people of color. In: Singh AA, Dickey LM, editors. Trans-affirmative counseling and psychological practice. Washington, DC: American Psychological Association; 2017.

20. Everett B, MacFarlane DA, Reynolds VA, Anderson HD. Not on our backs: supporting counsellors in navigating the ethics of multiple relationships within queer, two Spirit, and/or trans communities. Can J Couns Psychother. 2013;47(1):14–28.

21. Singh AA. Transgender youth of color and resilience: negotiating oppression, finding support. Sex Roles J Res. 2012;68(11–12):690–702.

22. Han C, George A, Boylan R, Gregorich SE, Choi KH. Stress and coping with racism and their role in sexual risk for HIV infection among African American, Asian/Pacific Islander and Latino men who have sex with men. Arch Sex Behav. 2015;44(2):411–20.

23. West LM, Donovan RA, Roemer L. Coping with racism: what works and doesn't work for black women. J Black Psychol. 2010;36:331–49.

24. Kattari SK, Walls NE, Whitfield DL, Langenderfer-Magruder L. Racial and ethnic differences in experiences of discrimination in accessing health services among transgender people in the United States. Int J Transgenderism. 2015;16(2):68–79.

LGBT Forced Migrants

Rebecca Hopkinson and Eva S. Keatley

Forced Migrants

Terms and Definitions

Forced migration is used to describe the process by which people flee their home countries due to coercion [1]. Such coercion includes threats to life and livelihood as a result of war, persecution, and natural or environmental disasters. Individuals who are forced to migrate under these circumstances are often referred to as refugees, asylees, or asylum seekers. Terminology used to describe immigrant populations can vary. Words such as "illegal alien" or "illegal immigrant" are still commonly used by the US agencies but have "othering" connotations: preferred terms include "newcomers" or "undocumented persons." It is important to note that the distinction between forced and voluntary migration may not always be clear-cut; most people migrate as a result of various push and pull factors. For example, a person may flee persecution while also seeking better economic opportunities in a developed country. Understanding both factors, and the resultant impact on an individual's life, can be important in providing optimal, culturally responsive care.

Seeking Immigration Status in the USA

There are many reasons why individuals may seek to enter another nation. The impetus may be to find more opportunities or to avoid harm in their home countries. Each country has a unique refugee and asylee immigration process. To be eligible for refugee or asylee status in the USA, an individual must be "unable or unwilling to return to their country because of persecution or a well-founded fear of persecution on account of race, religion, nationality, membership in a particular social group, or political opinion" [2]. To obtain US refugee status, a person must apply while outside the American borders, whereas for asylee status, one must apply while in the USA or at a port of entry. In 2013, the USA admitted almost 70,000 refugees and 25,000 asylees [2]. Refugees generally receive greater support than asylees when entering the country, as they are provided with government assistance and connected to organizations that aid in resettlement (e.g., the International Rescue Committee). In contrast, individuals who apply for asylum generally enter the country under temporary visas or as undocumented immigrants. In the USA, undocumented immigrants must seek asylum within 1 year of entering the country (INA §208(a) [2] (B)). Because many forced migrants are not aware of the 1-year deadline, it is important for all providers to assess immigration status and inform their clients about the asylum process.

While applying for asylum is a way to obtain legal status, it is hardly guaranteed. For example, according to the Department of Justice Executive Office for Immigration Review, in the fiscal year 2015, 45,770 applications for asylum were received. Only 8246 were granted and 8833 were denied; thus, only 18% of applications that year were successful. The remainder that were not directly granted or denied include those withdrawn, abandoned, or "other." Thus, many choose to remain undocumented rather than risk deportation, and it is not uncommon to apply defensively (i.e., requesting asylum as a defense against deportation). In 2015, 42,391 of the total applications were defensive. An asylum seeker is much more likely to gain asylee status if applying affirmatively (i.e., application for asylee status once within 1 year of entering the USA); for

R. Hopkinson, MD (✉)
Department of Psychiatry and Behavioral Medicine, University of Washington, M/S OA.5.154 PO Box 5371, Seattle, WA 98145-5005, USA
e-mail: Rebecca.Hopkinson@seattlechildrens.org

E.S. Keatley, MA
Department of Psychology, University of Windsor, 401 Sunset Avenue, Windsor, ON N9B 3P4, Canada
e-mail: Keatley@uwindsor.ca

© Springer International Publishing AG 2017
K.L. Eckstrand, J. Potter (eds.), *Trauma, Resilience, and Health Promotion in LGBT Patients*,
DOI 10.1007/978-3-319-54509-7_11

Table 11.1 Organizations that provide legal services for forced migrants

Name	Location	Population served	Website
Immigration Equality	National	LGBT and HIV+ immigrants	http://www.immigrationequality.org/
Human Rights First	New York City, Washington D.C., Houston, Tx	All asylum-seekers	http://www.humanrightsfirst.org/
Immigration Law Help, of Immigration Advocates Network	National	List of advocacy organizations, searchable by area	http://www.immigrationlawhelp.org/
International Refugee Rights Initiative	International	List of asylum legal organizations, including law school clinics	http://www.refugeelegalaidinformation.org/united-states-america-pro-bono-directory
US Justice Department	National	List of lawyers providing pro-bono services by state	https://www.justice.gov/eoir/list-pro-bono-legal-service-providers-map

example, the affirmative grant rate was 80% compared to a defensive grant rate of only 31% [3].

Detention of asylum seekers in the USA has been on the rise [4]. Many are detained mandatorily upon arrival, while others are detained once already in the USA, and, while uncommon, some are even detained after applying for asylum. Detention centers are jail-like facilities that house asylees while their asylum applications are pending or until they are deemed safe to be released into the community on parole. Estimates of average detention times range; according to a study by Human Rights First, the average length of detention was 5–6 months, with some detentions lasting years [4].

Asylum is also more likely to be granted if the applicant is represented by a lawyer familiar with the relevant laws and regulations. Pro-bono services are available in some cities and providers are encouraged to become familiar with organizations that provide free legal services to forced migrants (see Table 11.1).

Forced Migrant Mental Health

In general, forced migrants have higher rates of psychological distress than do other migrant groups [5]. Among the most common psychological symptoms are post-traumatic stress, depression, chronic pain, and somatic symptoms [6–9]. These symptoms are often related to trauma exposure [5], although a history of trauma often fails to account for the multiple dimensions that contribute to psychological distress over time. For instance, advocates of a psychosocial approach to mental health emphasize the role of social and material conditions in forced migrants' countries of origin, such as poverty, malnutrition, disease, and chronic stress [10]. Such conditions can lead to poor physical health, which in turn can negatively impact psychological functioning. In addition, post-migration factors are known to significantly impact mental health. In the treatment and care of forced migrants it is therefore essential to understand the

complex and multiple dimensions that contribute to long-term mental and physical health outcomes (see Fig. 11.1).

Pre-migration stressors play an important role in the long-term mental health of forced migrants. These can include events or conditions associated with the period before displacement, and commonly include acute traumatic events (e.g., imprisonment, torture, and rape), chronic discrimination, war, and/or threats to life or livelihood. Additional stressors may include poverty, malnutrition, and an overall paucity of vital resources. Research has demonstrated that greater pre-migration trauma exposure is associated with worse long-term mental health outcomes, including post-traumatic stress disorder, anxiety, and depression [11–13]. In addition, exposure to particular types of traumatic events has been associated with worse psychological distress, including witnessing the disappearance of family members [12, 13], being close to death [12], or being wounded [12, 13], tortured [14], or sexually assaulted [15–18]. A history of head injury has also been shown to be associated with worse mental and physical health outcomes [13, 19–21]. An individual's adjustment to traumatic events is also impacted profoundly by exposure to chronic discrimination on the basis of religious, ethnic, sexual, or other minority group identity. In addition, stressful social and material conditions such as poverty, malnutrition, and destruction of social networks may also contribute to worse long-term psychological distress [10].

Post-migration stressors have been shown to moderate the impact of pre-migration trauma on mental health [15]. Post-migration stressors are events or conditions that occur in the country of resettlement, and several studies have shown that they are more predictive of the severity of mental health problems than is pre-migration trauma [15]. Post-migration factors that can contribute to poor mental health include lack of social support, lack of economic opportunity [5], limited access to healthcare, unstable immigration status [15], lack of basic needs (e.g., housing, food, clothing) [5], the challenges of adjusting to different linguistic and cultural environments, and discrimination and persecution on the

Contributors to the Mental Health of Migrant Individuals

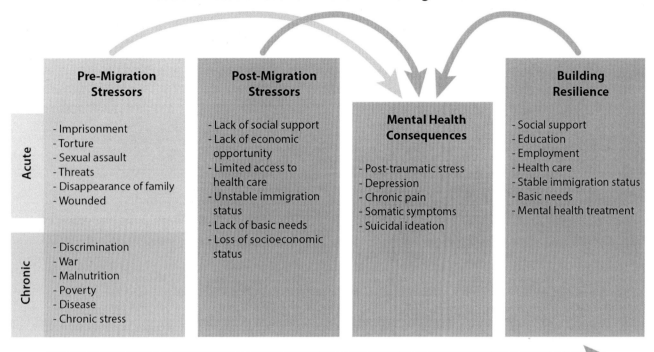

Fig. 11.1 Conceptual model of contributions to forced migrant mental health

basis of one's identification as a migrant, particularly if one remains undocumented. Changes of socio-economic status upon resettlement can also be a source of stress. For this reason, persons with higher education and higher pre-displacement socio-economic status are more likely to experience the worst mental health problems [5, 13, 15]. Unstable immigration status has also been a significant predictor of poor mental health outcomes, including suicidal ideation [17]. For example, the most salient problems for survivors of torture seeking treatment in New York are a lack of a stable immigration status and fear of being deported back to the countries where they were persecuted.

LGBT Forced Migrants

Immigration Status for LGBT Forced Migrants

Among forced migrants, there is a subpopulation of individuals who fled their countries of origin for fear of persecution due to their sexual orientation or gender identity. Currently at least 72 countries have laws that criminalize homosexuality [22]. Most of these countries are in Africa, Asia, Latin America, and Caribbean and Oceania. Thirteen of them have instituted the death penalty for homosexual acts: Mauritania, Sudan, Iran, Saudi Arabia, and Yemen [22]. To evade persecution or even death, persons in these nations who identify as LGBT may flee to Western countries such as the USA and Canada.

In the USA, the rights of LGBT immigrants have only recently been considered. It was not until 1994 that LGBT individuals were officially considered a social group eligible for asylum, and since then a growing number of LGBT asylum seekers have been entering the country every year [23]. However, because the government does not collect data specifying sexual orientation or gender identity among asylum seekers, there is no reliable data about this group of migrants [24].

Despite this limitation, the Center for American Progress released a report in June of 2015 that attempted to describe the status of LGBT people applying for asylum in the USA [24]. The report used data collected by two non-profit organizations that helped LGBT forced migrants apply for asylum: Immigration Equality (www.immigrationequality. org) and Human Rights First (www.humanrightsfirst.org). Briefly, the report found LGBT migrants were negatively impacted by the 1-year filing deadline and more likely to be granted asylum if they applied affirmatively (before being in the process of deportation); transgender people seeking asylum applied affirmatively less often than others. For instance, the report recounted the stories of two transgender women who missed the filing deadline by years due to fear of coming out as transgender to government officials and were subsequently barred from receiving asylum despite their well-founded fear of persecution. They also found that detention hurts LGBT applicants' chances of being granted asylum. The report suggested that LGBT asylum seekers might encounter greater obstacles obtaining information about and/or applying for asylum status than other forced migrants.

LGBT migrants face special immigration challenges. First, they experience the stress of having multiple minority identities, which can include immigrant, LGBT, and possibly racial or ethnic minority status as well. Second, they often feel isolated from LGBT groups within their new country due to cultural expectations and norms within these groups, as well as language barriers [24, 25]. Furthermore, they may have spent many years trying to keep their sexual identities secret, while now, for the purpose of immigration and seeking asylum, they are asked to identify and disclose. Unlike ethnic identity, religion, or political affiliation, it can be difficult to demonstrate sexual orientation in court. Typically, migrants must provide their own affidavits, as well as letters from prior romantic relationships or sexual partners, and evidence of engagement in LGBT groups in their home countries. It also helps if they appear to meet cultural stereotypes of LGBT identities in the USA, which may make their claim that they are part of a particular social group and would be persecuted as such more "believable" to the judge.

However, in the cases of forced migrants, many came from countries where all of these activities would have put their lives at risk, and they may not have engaged in any of them. They may have been married to an opposite-sex partner, or completely avoided or hidden romantic relationships; if they had the opportunity to participate in LGBT groups, which do not exist in all countries, they may have done so quietly to avoid reprisal. Thus, multiple factors make disclosure a stressful experience, including differences in cultural expectations and the meaning of identification, as well as fear of harm to family members and/or prior romantic partners in their home countries [25, 26].

LGBT migrants are also more vulnerable to significant health risks during this period of unstable immigration status as they are less likely to rely on established ethnic or national communities than are non-LGBT migrants and are therefore isolated, lacking resources and social supports [26]. Many come from cultures that engender homophobia and they are not likely to be accepted into their national or ethnic cultural communities after arrival in their new country of residence. Because of this exclusion, LGBT forced migrants are not privy to the informal social networks that other migrants are introduced to as a consequence of membership in a particular national, ethnic, or religious group.

Furthermore, most LGBT forced migrants have been persecuted not only by government entities but also by close relations including neighbors, peers, and even family members [27, 28]. Thus, LGBT forced migrants may have limited financial or emotional support from family members back home in nations that maintain homophobic beliefs.

LGBT Forced Migrant Mental Health

Although information on LGBT forced migrants is sparse, one study reporting on the persecution experiences and mental health of treatment-seeking forced migrants who were persecuted for their sexual orientation found that 66% of the 61 participants surveyed had experienced sexual violence as part of their persecution history, 46% had been persecuted by family members, and 69% had experienced persecution before the age of 18 years [27]. Histories of sexual violence were associated with higher scores on a measure of PTSD. The study compared the persecution histories and indicators of mental health between clients persecuted for their sexual orientation (LGBT group) and those who were persecuted for other reasons (e.g., religious identity, ethnic identity, political affiliation; controls). Statistically significant differences between the two groups of 35 clients who were matched by gender, country of origin, and age included: (1) 67% of the LGBT group had experienced sexual violence compared to 24% of the controls, (2) 39% of the LGBT group had been persecuted by family members compared to none of the controls, and (3) 63% of the LGBT group had experienced their first persecution before the age of 18 compared to 37% of the controls. In addition, while PTSD symptom severity was high across both groups, LGBT survivors of torture had significantly higher rates of suicidal ideation. These results demonstrate that forced migrants persecuted for sexual orientation have a greater risk of child abuse, sexual violence, and interpersonal trauma (e.g., persecution by family members). All three factors, as well as the prolonged and repeated trauma they represent, have been associated with higher rates of symptoms and worse outcomes in a variety of studies [28–33].

These study results point to a unique mental health profile among LGBT asylees that involves PTSD and elevated levels of suicidal ideation. This profile can include multiple symptoms that do not fit well into a single Diagnostic and Statistical Manual of Mental Disorders, 5th edition (DSM-5) diagnosis, and can include but are not limited to difficulties with trust, relational conflicts, personality changes, depression, anxiety, symptoms of PTSD, dissociation, and somatic symptoms [25, 28–33].

Resilience Among Forced Migrants

Forced migrants are rarely portrayed as resourceful individuals with agency and resilience. Instead, common narratives portrayed in the media and propagated by international aid agencies include themes of victimization, helplessness, and neediness. This representation overlooks the skills and important contributions migrants can make to society [34]. While it is unclear if this depiction causes any internalized sense of hopelessness, in our clinical experience, certain terms are best avoided because of the negative images they convey; for example, the word "survivors" could be seen as implying that asylees are barely making it in life. While this might appear to be true from an outsider perspective, use of this word diminishes the ability of asylees to overcome the magnitude of the challenges faced in order to get where they are.

When considering this population, it is important to remember that despite numerous challenges related to medical, legal, communication, and basic needs, LGBT forced migrants travel a long distance against imposing odds. Clinicians will rarely encounter more resilient, determined, and admirable people as asylum seekers. Leaving all they possess behind them, migrating to a new and unknown country, often with no resources or connections, these are incredibly courageous individuals.

Even the act of applying for asylum requires courage. The process of applying for asylum includes declaring oneself rather than remaining under the radar, preparing for court, which means telling and retelling the story of one's trauma, and going before a judge, usually multiple times, with the ultimate risk of being returned to the country from which one fled. Truly, there is no way to care for these individuals without gaining enormous respect for their courage and perseverance.

From the author's own work with migrants, what has been quite striking is the near complete lack of external resilience factors, such as supportive family and community. More often than not, what allowed an LGBT asylum seeker to come to this country appears random: an act of kindness from an employer or friend, a rare opportunity seized, a stroke of luck. Thereafter, they have had to survive of their own ingenuity. LGBT asylum seekers display a diversity of resilience factors that are mainly internal, such as true grit and determination. Caring for this population is a humbling and inspiring experience.

Providing Services to LGBT Forced Migrants

General Considerations

There are many things to keep in mind when treating this heterogeneous and complex group. While guidelines exist for medical screening and treatment, as do evidence-based treatments for mental health concerns, the most important initial considerations involve interpersonal communication and support. Here are some basic guidelines to consider that will help welcome LGBT refugees and trauma victims.

1. Create a safe environment
   The first and most important step in treating those who have survived trauma is to ensure that your office is seen as a safe space. The office's appearance, including the entrance, waiting area, and the bathrooms, is important to making patients feel welcome. LGBT advocacy groups and medical associations offer useful advice regarding these matters. Suggestions include having visible signage demonstrating acceptance to the LGBT community, having forms that do not assume gender or sexual orientation, and having gender-neutral bathrooms [35]. While many symbols of the LGBT movement are Western and thus may not be known or recognized by immigrants, in our experience, immigrants from all areas of the world recognize the rainbow flag as a universal LGBT symbol and a symbol of safety, acceptance, and support.

   Due to fear of maltreatment as identified members of the LGBT population, refugees and survivors of torture may have difficulty trusting authorities and institutions. For example, some have hesitated to enter a hospital building or give their names for fear of being reported and deported. Some have been afraid to use a main entrance due to the presence of security guards or hospital police, which often symbolize persecution. Such factors have caused some potential clients to avoid seeking care altogether. While some of these factors could be difficult to predict or avoid, being thoughtful about the appearance and procedures of the clinical environment can encourage patient trust.

2. Use interpreter services
   Interpreter services should always be available when caring for undocumented immigrants and asylum seekers; family members or friends should not be asked to interpret for the client given the potential for confidential information to be disclosed, sensitive information to be withheld, or information to be misinterpreted. This is especially important for individuals who are LGBT who may not be out to their families/friends, or who may have experienced trauma that they are ashamed of and unwilling to share with friends or family. Interpreters can serve an important role as cultural ambassadors, helping clients understand cultural barriers to care and assist in explaining Western ideas and medical diagnoses that may be difficult to understand or translate [9, 36].

3. Allow enough time for assessment
   When assessing LGBT refugees for symptoms related to trauma, including physical and emotional symptoms, providers should remember that discussion of these matters is often difficult or shameful for refugees. An assessment may therefore require significant time investment, and an individual may need rest breaks during the history-taking process. It can also be helpful to know

some calming strategies to use if patients become overwhelmed while sharing their stories of trauma, as emotional overload can adversely affect their willingness to return for additional care. For example, emotional regulation may be aided by abdominal breathing exercises, progressive muscle relaxation, or having water available to sip or with which to wash one's hands and face [37, 38]. Maintaining a caring, supportive, and empathic rapport, as well as communicating to the patient that the provider wants to hear their stories and does not judge their client for the things that happened to them, is vital when working with any trauma survivor.

4. Establish a trusting relationship

   Once clients are engaged in care, they must continue to feel safe, supported, and helped throughout the treatment process to ensure they will continue to return for necessary medical care. Because asylees often have understandable difficulty with trust and interpersonal relationships, creating rapport is of utmost importance. Healthcare providers should introduce themselves and explain the purpose of the visits and what clients can expect. Further, medical providers should be willing and expect to address clients' doubts or fears about medical care, provide reassurance, and individualize strategies for building trust with clients to assist them in feeling safe.

5. Attend to the hierarchy of needs

   While a medical checklist may be uppermost in a doctor's mind, it is important to remember that the priorities of an individual, and what may be affecting their health to the greatest extent, may include basic needs such as shelter, adequate food, access to a job, extreme lack of social connections and social support, legal challenges, and, of course, lack of ability to pay for care. These needs can be difficult to obtain: as undocumented immigrants without legal standing, asylees are ineligible for government support that is available to citizens, such as affordable housing, welfare, and healthcare. However, until these needs are addressed, it is unlikely that a client will be able to focus on health behaviors and may even engage in high-risk behaviors such as involvement in an abusive relationship or unprotected sex in exchange for money, food, or shelter. Thus, asking about basic needs is a vital part of the medical assessment, and having knowledge about available resources in your area or access to informed social workers can be crucial.

6. Document findings

   Common diagnoses caused by trauma include PTSD, anxiety disorders, and depression, but individuals may also have extensive somatic symptoms as well as scars or physical complications from abuse. [36] It can be very helpful to the client to clearly and meticulously document these symptoms, as physical and emotional signs and symptoms can be useful in court when attempting to obtain asylum. Chapter 16 provides details about how to document such findings in members of LGBT populations.

7. Facilitate social connections

   A major area of concern for many clients is intense loneliness and lack of social support. LGBT individuals may struggle to find a peer group in which they feel safe, experiencing a lack of understanding from members of local LGBT groups due to their migration status and torture histories, while also feeling unsafe with refugees from their own countries, who can be a source of discrimination [26].

   Similarly, having knowledge of local groups that provide support for undocumented migrants can be crucial to providing access to social support, as is being familiar with local LGBT organizations that may provide services such as group therapy or avenues to become involved with the LGBT community. In our experience, supportive therapy groups focused specifically on the needs of LGBT forced migrants can help alleviate isolation. Such groups can serve as social support networks that encourage patients to maintain contact and support each other outside of group [38, 39].

8. Treat with respect for their person and their experience

   As discussed previously, migrants come from diverse backgrounds, had previous lives in which they have been successful, and have a wealth of experience. They also are determined, resilient, and have incredible strengths and fortitude of character. It is important to treat them as such, with respect for their experience and knowledge. While they are in need of services and aid at this time in their lives, this is a temporary circumstance. Given the proper supports, including legal status and permission to work, they will be able to care for themselves and their families independently.

Medical Assessment

Asylum-seekers and other undocumented immigrants have a higher risk of suffering from many medical conditions. The list of specific conditions to consider in each circumstance varies depending on where individuals are from and what illnesses are common in their region, as well as what experiences they encountered prior to immigration, during migration, and also after arrival in this country. While refugees are screened prior to arrival to the USA, undocumented immigrants may not have had prior medical care or screening. A medical exam is required when applying for asylum.

The assessment begins by obtaining a thorough medical history, review of systems, physical exam, and blood screening [9, 36, 40]. The Centers for Disease Control and Prevention provides guidelines for domestic medical screening for newly arriving refugees, including a checklist [40]. Forced migrants may be susceptible to vaccine-preventable diseases that are seen rarely in the USA, and are more likely to be exposed to hepatitis B virus and tuberculosis [41]. Obtaining proper vaccination and health records can help avoid duplicate testing, but these are often unavailable. A higher overall burden of infectious illness and chronic health conditions may result from lack of medical care and high base rates of illness in the country of origin, as well as exposure to illness during migration and crowded living conditions upon arrival in the new country of residence.

Recommended screening includes testing for parasites, sexually transmitted infections, tuberculosis, anemia and nutritional deficiencies, and infections for which individuals may not have been vaccinated. The following tests should be considered: Complete blood count (CBC), serologies for hepatitis B and C, rubella, syphilis, and HIV; nucleic acid testing for gonorrhea and chlamydia; PPD and chest radiograph; stool ova and parasite examination; plus dental, vision, and hearing screenings. Other tests may be included based on the review of systems [36, 42]. Other considerations can include cancer screenings, and lead poisoning screening for children. [43].

In addition, it is important to screen for a history of traumatic brain injury, as high rates of head injuries caused by persecution have been reported among survivors of torture, and have been associated with psychiatric symptoms and worse physical health [16, 19–21]. Torture survivors may have fractures or soft tissue damage from beatings, neuropathies or muscle weakness from hanging by appendages, and cognitive impairment, seizures, or damage to ears and eyes resulting from head trauma [7]. Many individuals will also experience somatic symptoms that are worsened by their emotional distress.

It is of utmost importance to screen for sexual violence, which is particularly common among LGBT forced migrants. This is often a painful, shameful topic that the patient may not want to broach on the first meeting; however, it is important to ask. Providers should make this a standard part of their history taking, introducing relevant questions after some rapport has been established during the visit (i.e., this should not be the first question asked during the encounter). When asking about trauma, use a neutral, compassionate but matter-of-fact tone with a normal volume, similar to how one would ask other medical screening questions. This demonstrates that the provider is capable of discussing these matters without shame, and conveys to the patient that there is nothing for them to be ashamed of either. Even if an individual does not disclose initially, this approach will make it easier for them to disclose in the future. If the patient does disclose, it is also important to display a lack of judgment or assumption about how they feel or should feel about what happened to them. Instead, when told about a trauma, it is appropriate to state that you are sorry that that happened to them. They may also convey guilt over actions that they perceive contributed to or caused what happened to them. It is also appropriate to say that it is not their fault, and very important to avoid statements that could convey blame to the client for what happened to them.

Finally, forced migrants also may have substantial socioeconomic needs including housing, access to food, employment opportunities, language learning courses, assistance with immigration concerns, social support, and community integration. These questions should be included in the assessment.

Mental Health Assessment

Part of the medical evaluation should include a screen for psychiatric illness, emotional distress, and the need for support. It is also important to remember that asylum seekers have undergone a great deal of pain and loss, and having an adverse reaction is normal. Many individuals will be grieving the many losses appropriately and may not need psychiatric care. However, research suggests that the rates of PTSD, depression, and anxiety, as well as psychotic disorders, are higher than in the general population [6, 44–47] and these conditions require careful screening. The practitioner should explore the level of functioning, severity and duration of symptoms, presence of psychosis, and whether an individual is having suicidal thoughts.

Identifying and treating mental health problems among forced migrants is complicated by linguistic and cultural factors. The common practice is to screen and treat for specific psychiatric diagnoses, such as PTSD and depression; however, research has shown that Western-developed psychological constructs may not have cross-cultural validity [47]. Rasmussen et al. [47] reviewed the literature on non-Western post-traumatic reactions and found a variety of manifestations and explanatory models that ranged widely in presentation and included panic, anger, and vegetative symptoms. In addition, spirit possession has been reported in several trauma-specific reactions across African and Latin American studies [47]. Remaining sensitive to culturally appropriate symptoms of distress will prevent overlooking or misinterpreting a potential need for care. For example, patients from cultures that do not have the same understanding of depression may present instead with physical ailments such as pain or gastrointestinal distress rather than the psychological complaints that we express in Western society.

Although post-traumatic reactions vary significantly across cultures, there is evidence that symptoms of PTSD are endorsed by individuals affected by trauma across multiple geographic origins [48–51]. The Harvard Trauma Questionnaire [52] is the most widely used measure of PTSD across various cultures and its validity has been tested in many ethnic groups with varying success [53–55]. If using this measure, be aware that standard clinical cut-offs for PTSD may not hold globally [56]; practitioners are encouraged to research clinical cut-offs appropriate for the populations they serve. Measures of depression that have been validated in several languages and cultural groups include the Hopkins Symptom Checklist-25 (HSCL-25) and the HSCL-37 [53, 55, 57–59].

Mental Health Interventions

For practitioners interested in treating mental health symptoms, there are many evidence-based treatments (EBTs) for mental health problems including depression and PTSD. Division 12 of the American Psychological Association (APA) has resources and links to evidence-based treatments for psychological disorders [60]. However, the efficacy of these treatments in non-Western populations is not well known. In addition, cultural adaptations of these EBTs may be challenging as it can be difficult to balance adherence to treatment standards while modifying treatments appropriately for a specific client [61]. Existing research suggests that among adult and adolescent forced migrants, narrative exposure therapy and cognitive-behavioral therapy show the most promise for treating PTSD [62, 63].

There is no current literature on the efficacy of treatments for LGBT forced migrants; thus, relevant treatments must be extrapolated for this population. However, supportive group therapy has been described [38, 39, 64]. Such treatment is not uncommon in treatment centers for refugee or asylee populations, as it both expands the ability to provide care for multiple clients and provides them with a positive social setting from which to gain support. One such group exists in Ottawa, Canada; this is an open group that allows members to attend between five and 10 sessions, with the goal of processing grief, complications of coming out, and difficulties and barriers encountered in the legal/immigration system and the intersection of multiple minority statuses [25]. Another such group can be found at an LGBT community center in New York City, which has the goal of promoting safety and peer support, mitigating the stress of the asylum-seeking process, addressing cultural challenges, and engendering community [64]. These groups tend to be supportive in nature and community-building, rather than trauma-processing [37, 38]. Care must be taken when utilizing group therapy for this population, as some factors, such as group composition and type of treatment, can prevent improvement and cause worsening symptoms [65, 66].

In our clinical experience, a group provided for our LGBT forced migrant clients was a necessary treatment model and all members (admittedly self-selecting by those who continued to attend) expressed appreciation for the social support. In particular, they appreciated meeting people who, like them, fit into multiple minority classifications. They also appreciated aspects of the group that contributed to their feeling of safety, which included having a predictable structure upheld by designated group leaders, a flexible content designed to meet their immediate needs, and constraints on content that could be perceived as traumatizing to members of the group.

Case Example

Aleksi is a 25-year-old gay man who immigrated to the USA approximately 1 year ago from a country bordering Russia (Fig. 11.2). He plans to apply for asylum based on the abuse he suffered in his home country.

Prior to his arrival in the USA, he was a graduate student who became involved in a political organization that advocates for LGBT rights. After attending a local pride parade he was harassed by neighbors. In his hometown, a small village one hour outside of the capitol, his family was also harassed and his younger sibling was bullied. As a result, his family publicly disowned him. He was tormented

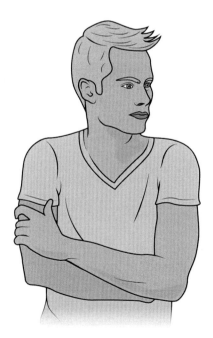

Fig. 11.2 Aleksi is a 25-year-old gay man who immigrated to the United States approximately 1 year ago from a country bordering Russia

daily in school, until he decided that he could no longer tolerate it, stopped attending, and dropped out.

One night, while walking home from teaching a class, he was accosted by a skinhead gang who beat and sexually assaulted him. When he attempted to report the incident to the police, he was harassed by the officers and told that he deserved it. He was later arrested while leaving a gay bar and beaten by the police while in custody. Fearing for his life and seeing no opportunity for recourse, he decided to flee.

Aleksi presents to a torture treatment program in a major metropolitan area on the advice of his immigration lawyer, who found that he was unable to participate in his own defense, as he became emotionally dysregulated when trying to tell his story.

On presentation, Aleksi is tearful and shaky. He often dissociates when reporting his history and requires external help to return to a present state of awareness. With gentle coaxing, he reports symptoms of insomnia, nightmares, flashbacks, and panic attacks. He has back pain and frequent nausea, sometimes with vomiting. He has contemplated ending his life, as he finds it unbearable, and has intense feelings of worthlessness, hopelessness, and constant tension and fear. He is afraid to leave his house due to fear of further harassment. He has been unwilling to seek employment for fear it might compromise his case and risk deportation. He had been living on the street prior to meeting his current boyfriend. The behaviors he reports from the boyfriend are concerning for exploitation. Overall, Aleksi feels powerless to change his life circumstance as he has no resources, no legal status, and no community to lean on.

He refuses psychotherapy because he is reluctant to further discuss his trauma, and believes that engaging in psychotherapy means that he is mentally ill, as this is not done in his country. However, he becomes actively engaged in a peer support group, and his situation improves over time. At his next visit, Aleksi reports that his life has improved significantly in this country, and he hopes things will continue to get better. He is grateful for the help that has been provided, and relies on support by his peers in the torture treatment program, who have helped him to feel safe and supported enough to consider making steps toward health and self-advocacy. He has become involved in a local LGBT organization, and advocates for himself by providing feedback to the torture program on how they could be more welcoming to LGBT minorities, recommending that a rainbow flag be placed in the waiting area of the treatment center.

Discussion Questions

1. What pre- and post-migration challenges are unique to LGBT forced migrants?

2. What cultural differences and challenges may you face in providing treatment to LGBT forced migrants?

3. How can we best address and provide for the complex challenges and health problems presented by LGBT forced migrants?

4. What can be done to foster resilience in LGBT forced migrants?

Summary Practice Points

1. LGBT forced migrants are more likely to have been rejected by multiple people in their communities, including family members, and are more likely to have suffered sexual assault than other forced migrant populations.

2. Removal from the home country can be a relief and provide a sense of safety, but also creates challenges such as cultural differences, lack of community, lack of legal status, and lack of resources. As LGBT forced migrants belong to multiple minority groups, effective communication includes recognizing and welcoming of each of their respective identities. This can be accomplished by simple gestures such as providing LGBT-specific signage in waiting and treatment areas.

3. Attending to the hierarchy of survival needs and addressing multiple aspects of health including medical, mental, social, and legal status are the most effective ways to address the complex challenges of forced migrants.

4. Despite challenges and severe symptoms, LGBT forced migrants' resilience can be facilitated through providing basic human resources such as medical care and access to a supportive community.

References

1. Eastmond M. Stories as lived experience: narratives in forced migration research. J Refug Stud. 2007;20(2):248–64.
2. Martin DC, Yankay JE. Refugees and asylees: 2013. East Asia. 2014;16(18,000):19-000.
3. Office of Planning, Analysis, and Statistics, Executive Office of Immigration Review. FY 2015 statistics yearbook. Falls Church: US Department of Justice; 2016. p. J1–K3.
4. Acer E, Chicco J. US detention of Asylum seekers: Seeking protection, finding prison. Human Rights First; 2009. Available from: https://www.humanrightsfirst.org/wp-content/uploads/pdf/090429-RP-hrf-asylum-detention-report.pdf.
5. Porter M, Haslam N. Predisplacement and postdisplacement factors associated with mental health of refugees and internally displaced persons: a meta-analysis. JAMA. 2005;294(5):602–12.
6. Steel Z, Chey T, Silove D, Marnane C, Bryant RA, Van Ommeren M. Association of torture and other potentially traumatic events with mental health outcomes among populations exposed to mass

conflict and displacement: a systematic review and meta-analysis. JAMA. 2009;302(5):537–49.

7. Burnett A, Peel M. Health needs of asylum seekers and refugees. Br Med J. 2001;322(7285):544.

8. Fazel M, Wheeler J, Danesh J. Prevalence of serious mental disorder in 7000 refugees resettled in western countries: a systematic review. Lancet. 2005;365(9467):1309–14.

9. Kirmayer LJ, Narasiah L, Munoz M, Rashid M, Ryder AG, Guzder J, Hassan G, Rousseau C, Pottie K. Common mental health problems in immigrants and refugees: general approach in primary care. Can Med Assoc J. 2011;183(12):E959–67.

10. Miller KE, Rasmussen A. War exposure, daily stressors, and mental health in conflict and post-conflict settings: bridging the divide between trauma-focused and psychosocial frameworks. Soc Sci Med. 2010;70(1):7–16.

11. Steel Z, Silove D, Phan T, Bauman A. Long-term effect of psychological trauma on the mental health of Vietnamese refugees resettled in Australia: a population-based study. Lancet. 2002;360 (9339):1056–62.

12. Sabin M, Cardozo BL, Nackerud L, Kaiser R, Varese L. Factors associated with poor mental health among Guatemalan refugees living in Mexico 20 years after civil conflict. JAMA. 2003;290 (5):635–42.

13. Fazel M, Reed RV, Panter-Brick C, Stein A. Mental health of displaced and refugee children resettled in high-income countries: risk and protective factors. Lancet. 2012;379(9812):266–82.

14. Silove D, Steel Z, McGorry P, Miles V, Drobny J. The impact of torture on post-traumatic stress symptoms in war-affected Tamil refugees and immigrants. Compr Psychiatry. 2002;43(1):49–55.

15. Chu T, Keller AS, Rasmussen A. Effects of post-migration factors on PTSD outcomes among immigrant survivors of political violence. J Immigr Minor Health. 2013;15(5):890–7.

16. Goldfeld AE, Mollica RF, Pesavento BH, Faraone SV. The physical and psychological sequelae of torture: symptomatology and diagnosis. JAMA. 1988;259(18):2725–9.

17. Lerner E, Bonanno GA, Keatley E, Joscelyne A, Keller AS. Predictors of suicidal ideation in treatment-seeking survivors of torture. Psychol Trauma. 2016;8(1):17–24.

18. Oosterhoff P, Zwanikken P, Ketting E. Sexual torture of men in Croatia and other conflict situations: an open secret. Reprod Health Matters. 2004;12(23):68–77.

19. Keatley E, Ashman T, Im B, Rasmussen A. Self-reported head injury among refugee survivors of torture. J Head Trauma Rehabil. 2013;28(6):E8–13.

20. Keatley E, d'Alfonso A, Abeare C, Keller A, Bertelsen NS. Health outcomes of traumatic brain injury among refugee survivors of torture. J Head Trauma Rehabil. 2015;30(6):E1–8.

21. Mollica RF, Lyoo IK, Chernoff MC, Bui HX, Lavelle J, Yoon SJ, Kim JE, Renshaw PF. Brain structural abnormalities and mental health sequelae in South Vietnamese ex–political detainees who survived traumatic head injury and torture. Arch Gen Psychiatry. 2009;66(11):1221–32.

22. Itaborahy LP, Zhu J. State-sponsored homophobia. ILGA. 2016;11:36–37.

23. Landau J. Soft immutability and imputed gay identity: recent developments in transgender and sexual-orientation-based asylum law. Fordham Urban Law J. 2004;32:237.

24. Gruberg S, West R. Humanitarian diplomacy: The U.S. asylum system's role in protecting global LGBT rights. Center for American Progress; 2015. Available from: https://cdn.americanprogress.org/wp-content/uploads/2015/06/LGBTAsylum-final.pdf.

25. Nerses M, Kleinplatz PJ, Moser C. Group therapy with International LGBTQ+ clients at the intersection of multiple minority status. Psychol Sex Rev. 2015;6(1):99–109.

26. Shidlo A, Ahola J. Mental health challenges of LGBT forced migrants. Forced Migr Rev. 2013;1(42):9.

27. Hopkinson RA, Keatley E, Glaeser E, Erickson-Schroth L, Fattal O, Nicholson Sullivan M. Forced migrants persecuted for lesbian, gay, bisexual, and transgender identity. J Homosex. Under Review. 2016 (In press) http://www.tandfonline.com/doi/full/10.1080/00918369.2016.1253392

28. Herman JL. Complex PTSD: A syndrome in survivors of prolonged and repeated trauma. J Trauma Stress. 1992;5(3):377–91.

29. Ryan C, Huebner D, Diaz RM, Sanchez J. Family rejection as a predictor of negative health outcomes in white and Latino lesbian, gay, and bisexual young adults. Pediatrics. 2009;123(1):346–52.

30. Brewin CR, Andrews B, Valentine JD. Meta-analysis of risk factors for posttraumatic stress disorder in trauma-exposed adults. J Consult Clin Psychol. 2000;68(5):748.

31. Briere J, Kaltman S, Green BL. Accumulated childhood trauma and symptom complexity. J Trauma Stress. 2008;21(2):223–6.

32. Cloitre M, Stolbach BC, Herman JL, Kolk BV, Pynoos R, Wang J, Petkova E. A developmental approach to complex PTSD: childhood and adult cumulative trauma as predictors of symptom complexity. J Trauma Stress. 2009;22(5):399–408.

33. Cook, A, Blaustein, M, Spinazzola, J, van der Kolk, B, editors. Complex trauma in children and adolescents. National Child Traumatic Stress Network. Substance Abuse and Mental Health Services Administration, U.S. Department of Health and Human Services; 2003. Retrieved from: http://www.nctsn.org/sites/default/files/assets/pdfs/ComplexTrauma_All.pdf.

34. Grove NJ, Zwi AB. Our health and theirs: forced migration, othering, and public health. Soc Sci Med. 2006;62(8):1931–42.

35. GLMA. Guidelines for care of lesbian, gay, bisexual, and transgender patients. San Francisco: Gay and Lesbian Medical Association; 2006.

36. Adams KM, Gardiner LD, Assefi N. Healthcare challenges from the developing world: post-immigration refugee medicine. BMJ. 2004;328(7455):1548–52.

37. Kim SH, Schneider SM, Kravitz L, Mermier C, Burge MR. Mind-body practices for posttraumatic stress disorder. J Investig Med. 2013;61(5):827–34.

38. Akinsulure-Smith AM. Using group work to rebuild family and community ties among displaced African men. J Spec Group Work. 2012;37(2):95–112.

39. Kira IA, Ahmed A, Wasim F, Mahmoud V, Colrain J, Rai D. Group therapy for refugees and torture survivors: treatment model innovations. Int J Group Psychother. 2012;62(1):69–88.

40. Pottie K, Greenaway C, Feightner J, Welch V, Swinkels H, Rashid M, Narasiah L, Kirmayer LJ, Ueffing E, MacDonald NE, Hassan G. Evidence-based clinical guidelines for immigrants and refugees. Can Med Assoc J. 2011;183(12):E824–925.

41. Center for Disease Control and Prevention. Summary checklist for domestic medical examination for newly arrived refugees. Atlanta; 2012. http://www.cdc.gov/immigrantrefugeehealth/guidelines/domestic/checklist.html.

42. Bertelsen NS, Selden E, Krass P, Keatley ES, Keller A. Primary care screening methods and outcomes among Asylum seekers in New York City. J Immigr Health Under Rev. 2016 (In Press). doi:10.1007/s10903-016-0507-y

43. Olson CK, Stauffer WM, Barnett ED. Newly arrived immigrants & refugees. Atlanta: Centers for Disease Control and Prevention; 2015 [cited 2015 Jul 10]. Available from: http://wwwnc.cdc.gov/travel/yellowbook/2016/advising-travelers-with-specific-needs/newly-arrived-immigrants-refugees.

44. Keller A, Lhewa D, Rosenfeld B, Sachs E, Aladjem A, Cohen I, Smith H, Porterfield K. Traumatic experiences and psychological distress in an urban refugee population seeking treatment services. J Nerv Ment Dis. 2006;194(3):188–94.

45. Silove D. The psychosocial effects of torture, mass human rights violations, and refugee trauma: toward an integrated conceptual framework. J Nerv Ment Dis. 1999;187(4):200–7.

46. Silove D, Sinnerbrink I, Field A, Manicavasagar V, Steel Z. Anxiety, depression and PTSD in asylum-seekers: associations with pre-migration trauma and post-migration stressors. Br J Psychiatry. 1997;170(4):351–7.
47. Rasmussen A, Keatley E, Joscelyne A. Posttraumatic stress in emergency settings outside North America and Europe: a review of the emic literature. Soc Sci Med. 2014;109:44–54.
48. De Jong JT, Komproe IH, Van Ommeren M, El Masri M, Araya M, Khaled N, van De Put W, Somasundaram D. Lifetime events and posttraumatic stress disorder in 4 postconflict settings. JAMA. 2001;286(5):555–62.
49. Tang SS, Fox SH. Traumatic experiences and the mental health of Senegalese refugees. J Nerv Ment Dis. 2001;189(8):507–12.
50. Ichikawa M, Nakahara S, Wakai S. Cross-cultural use of the predetermined scale cutoff points in refugee mental health research. Soc Psychiatry Psychiatr Epidemiol. 2006;41(3):248–50.
51. Sachs E, Rosenfeld B, Lhewa D, Rasmussen A, Keller A. Entering exile: trauma, mental health, and coping among Tibetan refugees arriving in Dharamsala, India. J Trauma Stress. 2008;21(2):199–208.
52. Mollica RF, Caspi-Yavin Y, Bollini P, Truong T, Tor S, Lavelle J. The Harvard Trauma Questionnaire: validating a cross-cultural instrument for measuring torture, trauma, and posttraumatic stress disorder in Indochinese refugees. J Nerv Ment Dis. 1992;180 (2):111–6.
53. Lhewa D, Banu S, Rosenfeld B, Keller A. Validation of a Tibetan translation of the Hopkins Symptom Checklist–25 and the Harvard Trauma Questionnaire. Assessment. 2007;14(3):223–30.
54. Myer L, Smit J, Roux LL, Parker S, Stein DJ, Seedat S. Common mental disorders among HIV-infected individuals in South Africa: prevalence, predictors, and validation of brief psychiatric rating scales. AIDS Patient Care STDs. 2008;22(2):147–58.
55. Oruc L, Kapetanovic A, Pojskic N, Miley K, Forstbauer S, Mollica RF, Henderson DC. Screening for PTSD and depression in Bosnia and Herzegovina: validating the Harvard Trauma Questionnaire and the Hopkins Symptom Checklist. Int J Cult Ment Health. 2008;1(2):105–16.
56. Rasmussen A, Verkuilen J, Ho E, Fan Y. Posttraumatic stress disorder among refugees: measurement invariance of Harvard Trauma Questionnaire scores across global regions and response patterns. Psychol Assess. 2015;27(4):1160.
57. Kaaya SF, Fawzi MC, Mbwambo JK, Lee B, Msamanga GI, Fawzi W. Validity of the Hopkins Symptom Checklist-25 amongst HIV-positive pregnant women in Tanzania. Acta Psychiatr Scand. 2002;106(1):9–19.
58. Lavik NJ, Hauff E, Solberg Ø, Laake P. The use of self-reports in psychiatric studies of traumatized refugees: validation and analysis of HSCL-25. Nord J Psychiatry. 1999;53(1):17–20.
59. Bean T, Derluyn I, Eurelings-Bontekoe E, Broekaert E, Spinhoven P. Validation of the multiple language versions of the Hopkins Symptom Checklist-37 for refugee adolescents. Adolescence. 2007;42(165):51.
60. Anderson NB. Evidence-based practice in psychology. Am Psychol. 2006;61(4):271–85.
61. Castro FG, Barrera Jr M, Steiker LK. Issues and challenges in the design of culturally adapted evidence-based interventions. Annu Rev Clin Psychol. 2010;6:213.
62. Crumlish N, O'Rourke K. A systematic review of treatments for post-traumatic stress disorder among refugees and asylum-seekers. J Nerv Ment Dis. 2010;198(4):237–51.
63. Ehntholt KA, Yule W. Practitioner review: assessment and treatment of refugee children and adolescents who have experienced war-related trauma. J Child Psychol Psychiatry. 2006;47 (12):1197–210.
64. Reading R, Rubin L. Advocacy and empowerment: group therapy for LGBT asylum seekers. Traumatology. 2011;17(2):86–98.
65. Cloitre M, Koenen KC. The impact of borderline personality disorder on process group outcome among women with posttraumatic stress disorder related to childhood abuse. Int J Group Psychother. 2001;51(3):379–98.
66. Rose S, Bisson J, Churchill R, Wessely S. Psychological debriefing for preventing post traumatic stress disorder (PTSD). Cochrane Database Syst Rev. 2002;2(2):2.

Lesbian and Bisexual Women

Katie Imborek, Dana van der Heide, and Shannon Phillips

Introduction

Lesbian and bisexual women experience chronic societal stress and stigma-related discrimination that can lead to disparities in mental and physical health outcomes. Understanding the minority stress model and the health impact of maladaptive and adaptive coping mechanisms helps to identify factors that may lead either to increased disease severity or provide sexual minority women with the resilience to adapt successfully to adversity. A social ecological model (SEM) is used to illustrate the interconnected realms of support that can promote good health and a sense of well-being among lesbian and bisexual women.

Minority Stress Model

The minority stress model, described in detail in Chap. 4, is a useful theoretical framework for understanding increased rates of negative health outcomes among lesbian, gay, and bisexual (LGB) women [1]. Briefly, this model defines stress processes experienced by minority populations on a continuum that extends from a distal location (i.e., the environment) to a proximal location (i.e., the self). Distal processes are objective occurrences of overt discrimination that may be acute and/or chronic. Proximal processes include an individual's subjective perceptions and appraisals of environmental events.

The core distal stressors affecting LGB populations include anti-LGB victimization, discrimination, and structural bias. Up to 75% of self-identified lesbian and bisexual women report exposure to anti-LGB verbal harassment. Furthermore, 13% report being physically assaulted and 12% report being sexually assaulted on the basis of their known or assumed sexual orientation [2]. Additionally, one in ten self-identified sexual minority women reports loss of employment because of anti-LGB discrimination. Sexual minority women with children may incur additional discrimination or harassment from their children's schools in the context of their role as nontraditional parents [3].

While not exclusively anti-LGB in nature, several studies show that aggregate rates of physical and sexual trauma (including childhood physical abuse, childhood sexual abuse, intimate partner physical abuse, and adult sexual assault) are higher among sexual minority women as compared to heterosexual women [3–5]. The association between childhood sexual abuse and sexual orientation must be interpreted with caution and not used to perpetuate the cultural myth that same-sex attraction or behavior is caused by a history of traumatic experiences with men, particularly when there is no evidence to suggest that such potential childhood sexual abuse precedes development of one's sexual orientation. Women who have sex with women and men (WSWM) may be at highest risk for intimate partner physical and sexual abuse [3]. Sexual minority youth may also be more vulnerable to victimization as compared to their heterosexual counterparts. Often, this is influenced by gender nonconforming appearances and/or behaviors; however, gender nonconformity alone is associated with victimization independent of sexual orientation and it is important not to conflate the two. Race and ethnicity may play a role in risk for victimization, illustrating the intersectionality of discriminatory forces. For example, African American and Latina sexual minority

K. Imborek, MD (✉)
Department of Family Medicine, University of Iowa Hospitals and Clinics, 200 Hawkins Drive, Iowa City, IA 52242, USA
e-mail: katherine-imborek@uiowa.edu

D. van der Heide, MPH
Carver College of Medicine, University of Iowa, 375 Newton Road, Iowa City, IA 52242, USA
e-mail: dana-vanderheide@uiowa.edu

S. Phillips, PA-C
Denver Health, 777 Bannock St., Denver, CO 80203, USA
e-mail: sraephill@gmail.com

© Springer International Publishing AG 2017
K.L. Eckstrand, J. Potter (eds.), *Trauma, Resilience, and Health Promotion in LGBT Patients*,
DOI 10.1007/978-3-319-54509-7_12

women report increased rates of trauma as both children and adults compared to their white counterparts [3, 6].

The least proximal process described in the minority stress model is the individual's subjective experience of stigma. Stigma is defined as "the co-occurrence of labeling, stereotyping, separation, status loss, and discrimination in a context in which power is exercised" [7]. While societal acceptance of gay and lesbian sexual orientations has greatly improved recently, bisexual-identified women have unique experiences of stigma because of their perceived lack of acceptance by both heterosexual and lesbian-identified women and feelings of not being taken seriously due to their bisexual identities [8]. LGB people who have experienced societal stigma related to their identities may start to expect rejection and discrimination. For example, nearly 50% of self-identified lesbian and bisexual adolescents and young adults in one study expressed fear of losing friends because of their sexual orientation, and more than one in three expressed fear of verbal and/or physical abuse at school and verbal abuse at home [2]. As increased perception of stigmatization increases, so does one's need to be continually alert or "on guard" when interacting with the majority culture. This constant vigilance reinforces a tension between self-perception and others' perception that may lead to instability and vulnerability with regard to one's self-concept.

Concealing one's identity is often used as a coping strategy to avoid objective discriminatory experiences; however, it has also been shown to increase psychological distress. Hiding one's identity – often by modifying behavior, dress, mannerisms, and discussion topics – is a substantial cognitive burden and precludes the healthy sharing of emotions and aspects of one's self with others. Concealment of identity often prevents LGB people from affiliating with others in the community and failing to reap potential benefits of formal and informal LGB-related support resources.

Finally, internalized homophobia – the assimilation of society's negative anti-LGB attitudes into one's own self-concept – is a particularly damaging proximal stressor because it is insidious and may be present even in the absence of bias-related victimization and even if an individual has concealed their sexual minority identity. Not surprisingly, therefore, internalized homophobia has been shown to correlate with mental health disorders including depression, anxiety, substance use, and suicidal ideation [9–11]. Internalized homophobia has been inversely related to the duration of the coming out process, with higher levels seen in the beginning stages of coming out. However, even if an LGB person has fully reconciled their sexuality, because of continued exposure to anti-LGB attitudes, internalized homophobia remains a relevant variable in the LGB person's psychological adjustment throughout life.

In addition to elucidating the pivotal role that chronic, socially based stress can have on the mental and physical health of sexual minority individuals, the minority stress model also helps to explain the syndemic theory of disease – how multiple health problems interact and co-occur within a given population. For example, among young sexual minority women, experiences of sexual orientation discrimination have been associated with a cluster of syndemic problems that includes heavy episodic drinking, drug use, depressive symptoms, and high-risk sexual behavior [12].

Development of Coping Mechanisms

An individual's development of coping mechanisms is impacted by the presence or absence of supportive or deleterious interpersonal, organizational/community, and policy constructs that will be discussed in this chapter. Coping mechanisms may be distinguished along a spectrum that extends from adaptive or protective behavioral strategies, on the one hand, to maladaptive or harmful strategies on the other. Identification of factors that promote overall development of coping mechanisms and the adoption of specific strategies that are ultimately beneficial rather than harmful builds a context in which healthcare providers can better support lesbian and bisexual women in developing and increasing resilience and healthy lifestyle behaviors.

Research has demonstrated three coping strategies utilized on an individual level that decrease the overall impact of stressors on health: a sense of personal control over one's circumstances, high self-esteem or perception of one's goodness or value, and social support, which includes family, friends, co-workers, etc. The first two strategies drive the latter by increasing an individual's capacity to both problem-solve and perceive social support, thereby decreasing both the physiologic and emotional heightened arousal to environmental stressors [13].

In contrast to the resources drawn upon to develop protective strategies, internalized homophobia can lead to poor self-regard, emotional conflict and discomfort with oneself. High levels of internalized homophobia mediate increased psychological distress and increase the likelihood that an individual will develop maladaptive coping strategies, including avoidant and concealment behaviors, which then in turn increase psychological distress. This creates a vicious cycle that is perpetuated by social constructs that guide the individual level of belief, which then guides behavior [10].

A recent study by Kaysen et al. examined the relationship between internalized homophobia, coping strategies, and psychological stress among self-identified lesbian and bisexual women. General adaptive coping skills included active

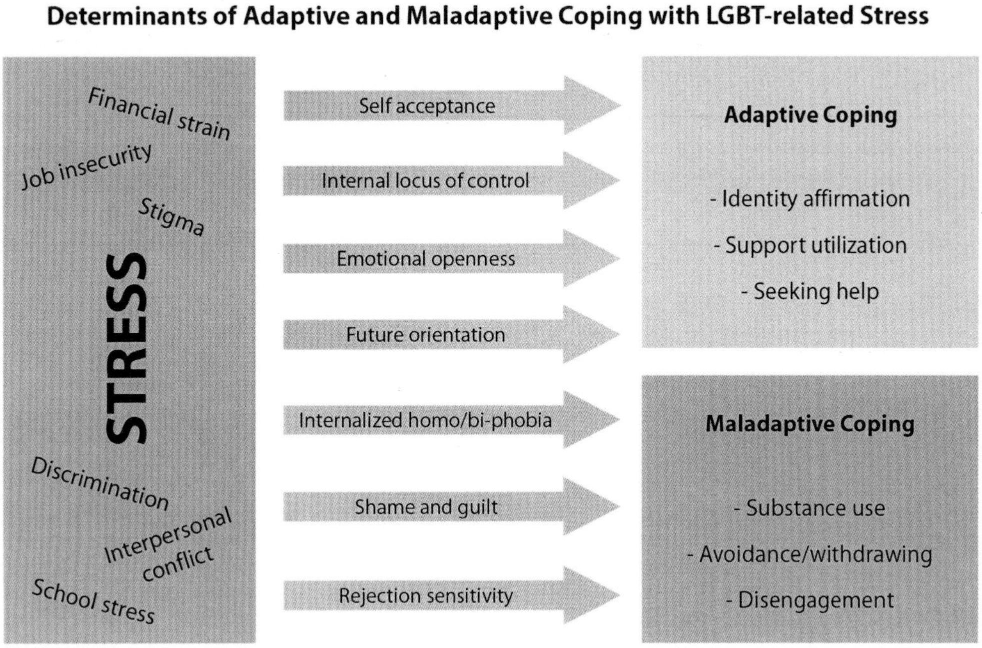

Determinants of Adaptive and Maladaptive Coping with LGBT-related Stress

Fig. 12.1 Development of LGB-specific coping mechanisms. Adaptive vs. maladaptive coping strategies and the factors that influence their development

coping, planning, instrumental support, acceptance, and positive reframing. LGB-specific coping strategies included confronting homophobia, avoidance, self-acceptance, spirituality, and online support. Maladaptive coping strategies included behavioral disengagement, denial, self-blame, self-distraction, and substance use (Fig. 12.1) [14]. Internalized homophobia, on the other hand, was related to maladaptive coping behaviors, and that behavior mediated the correlation between internalized homophobia and psychological distress. Additionally, higher levels of maladaptive coping strategies were associated with lower utilization of sexual minority-specific coping [14].

This literature is just part of a growing field of research investigating the vital role of an individual's development of adaptive vs. maladaptive coping strategies and identification of the unique barriers faced by lesbian and bisexual women that impact the development of these skills. Incorporating these concepts into healthcare conversations may foster the development of adaptive and sexual minority-specific coping strategies critical to improving health outcomes among sexual minority women. Recognition of the unique and broad range of coping skills available to assist sexual minority women is just as vital as recognizing the barriers they must navigate in the face of everyday social and societal expectations and norms [15]. Acquisition of adaptive coping skills builds increased resilience and the ability to successfully navigate other types of adversity.

Health Disparities in Lesbian and Bisexual Women

A growing body of literature demonstrates significant differences in health outcomes of lesbian and bisexual women compared to their heterosexual counterparts. While a large proportion of studies have focused on simply quantifying health disparities among sexual minority women, efforts are being made to delineate the complex causes underlying these inequalities. The CDC's *Healthy People* series of objectives first acknowledged sexual minority women as a health disparate population in 2010 and created a separate topic heading for lesbian, gay, bisexual, and transgender health in *Healthy People 2020*; however, significant advances have yet to be made in addressing the complex etiologies of health disparities among sexual minority women [16, 17].

The majority of national studies in the field have focused on mental health outcomes among sexual minority women, particularly those that occur as a direct consequence of discrimination, victimization, stigmatization, vigilance, and expectations of rejection [16, 18]. When compared with heterosexual individuals, LGB individuals consistently display higher levels of depression, anxiety disorders, substance abuse, and suicidal ideation and attempts, with lesbian and bisexual women at particular risk for generalized anxiety disorder and substance abuse when compared to heterosexual women [18–26]. Additionally, when compared to lesbian-identified women, bisexual women have an even higher risk of experiencing mental distress and poor overall health [16]. Between-group comparisons have further identified significant physical health disparities between sexual minority women and heterosexual women (both self-identified and based on sexual behavior) in a number of different parameters. Most of these unique disparities are modifiable; thus, interventions require incorporation of resilience factors in sexual minority women.

Maladaptive substance use is an area of particular concern, in that higher rates of drug use, heavy alcohol use, and tobacco use are observed among sexual minority women compared to heterosexual women [16, 20, 27–31]. Tobacco use is a particularly significant issue, with a 2004 study demonstrating the smoking rate among lesbian women to be 25.3%, a remarkable 70% higher than that of heterosexual women [32]. The high rate of smoking in sexual minorities has been postulated to have several etiologies. Internalized homophobia and individuals' reactions to disclosing sexual orientation may contribute to the high rates of tobacco use [33]. Second, bars have historically been centers of advocacy and socialization for sexual minority groups and, although empiric evidence has not been demonstrated, the historical relationship between tobacco use and bars is thought to contribute to a cultural acceptance of tobacco use within sexual minority communities. In addition, substance use is thought to be a potential coping mechanism in the face of depression and victimization [33]. Importantly, the disparity in smoking prevalence is not due to a lack of knowledge or education, as lesbian and bisexual women have demonstrated similar attitudes and knowledge about tobacco control [34]. Alcohol use is another issue of concern for lesbian and bisexual women, who are more likely to report alcohol-related social consequences, dependence, and help-seeking for alcohol problems, as well as lower abstention rates than heterosexual women. While this difference disappears above the age of 50, alcohol abuse in the 26–35-year-old population remains a significant concern for young adults as well as older LGB women, as sequelae of long-term alcohol use of older LGB women have not been studied [28].

Another significant difference is seen in weight, with sexual minority women having higher rates of obesity than the general population. Despite some studies showing a greater amount of physical activity among lesbian and bisexual women, obesity continues to be a significant problem [27, 28]. Like other health disparities observed among sexual minorities, the etiology of obesity is believed to be multifactorial, stemming from increased heavy drinking and depressive symptoms [35]. Evidence suggests that obesity differentially affects sexual minority women compared to sexual minority men, with one study demonstrating an increased likelihood of white and African American sexual minority women being overweight compared with heterosexual women of the same race or ethnicity, whereas sexual minority status was actually protective against unhealthy weight among sexual minority men [36]. Interestingly, a positive correlation has been found between overweight and obesity and degree of outness as a lesbian, as well as longer relationship length. This correlation may be a product of a greater acceptance of diverse body types, an attitude that has been repeatedly demonstrated [37, 38]. A higher body mass index (BMI) is associated with an increased risk for multiple cancers, diabetes, and cardiovascular disease; indeed, a commensurate increase in cardiovascular disease has been observed among sexual minority women [20]. Given the disparities in tobacco use, another risk factor for cardiovascular disease, this association is not surprising, but the increased risk persists even when adjusting for smoking status. Importantly, the disparity in risk for cardiovascular disease is significant only among self-identified lesbian and bisexual women, not in women categorized by sexual behaviors, consistent with the explanatory basis of the minority stress model [39].

National disease databases and registries do not collect data on sexual minority status, so there is a relative paucity of data on a number of conditions with the potential to affect lesbian and bisexual women [40]. This is particularly salient when considering the higher prevalence of risk factors for breast and cervical cancer in lesbian women, including high alcohol intake, smoking status, obesity, and higher rates of nulliparity [20, 29, 41]. The literature on relative mammography rates and breast cancer incidence in lesbian and bisexual women has thus far been inconsistent. However, in general, sexual minority women report less healthcare access and regular medical care, and more frequent delaying of care and use of emergency departments [28, 29, 42–45]. The exception is mental health services, which are used more frequently among sexual minority women than among heterosexual women [23]. Lesbian women in particular have shown less willingness to disclose sexual orientation to healthcare providers than gay men and have more difficulty communicating with their healthcare providers [46]. This hesitancy to disclose sexual orientation may have particular importance in early detection of cervical cancer, as lesbians who are out to their healthcare provider are more likely to have had a recent Pap test than those who have not disclosed their sexual orientation [40]. Lower rates of initiation of HPV vaccination have been demonstrated in sexual minority women compared with heterosexual women, though there are limited published large-scale data on HPV vaccination in sexual minority women [47]. Healthcare providers must be aware of the recommendations for cervical cancer screening in sexual minority women and facilitate open discussion of sexual orientation and practices, in order to avoid disparities in detection and treatment.

In general, sexual minority women report lower health-related quality of life than heterosexual women. However, it is important to note that bisexual women report even poorer health-related quality of life than lesbian women, as well as higher rates of significant mental distress. Unfortunately, the small sample sizes in studies of sexual minority women have led many studies to simply combine lesbian and bisexual women into a single group; therefore, data is lacking on some areas and inconsistent in others. For example, heavy alcohol use was reported in one study to be significantly higher only among lesbian women, but elsewhere, bisexual women have been reported to be more likely to smoke and drink excessively [16, 29]. Furthermore, bisexual women have been shown to have fewer attempts at smoking cessation, younger age of first cigarette, and higher nicotine dependence in comparison to heterosexual women [48]. Bisexual women have significantly higher demonstrated rates of intimate partner violence compared to both lesbian and heterosexual women [49–51]. Additional research is needed to explain the disparities between bisexual and lesbian women, particularly the greater sociodemographic risks, health risk behaviors, and decreased access to care [16].

The disparities between sexual minority women and heterosexual women are clearly multifactorial, stemming from differential access to healthcare, cultural norms regarding obesity and substance use, and victimization throughout the life course. It is daunting to consider all of the physical and mental health disparities present in this population. Importantly, however, studies suggest that physical health disparities in sexual minority women are a direct consequence of psychological distress; that is, when distress is taken into account, physical health disparities are no longer significant [16, 22]. Furthermore, the majority of risk factors leading to health outcome disparities among sexual minority women are modifiable [20]. These observations suggest that enhancing the ability to cope with minority stress may help decrease the disparities seen among sexual minority women, and highlights the importance of supporting resilience development in this population.

Resilience Factors in Lesbian and Bisexual Women

Social Ecological Model

First described in 1988 by McLeroy et al., and based on the work of Urie Bronfenbrenner [52], the social ecological model (SEM) focuses on the interaction between the social environment and resilience factors intrinsic to an individual and the importance of the interplay between multiple levels in effecting change. Emergence of the SEM occurred in the context of a new understanding of the limitations of individual-level interventions and programs and the potential for a victim-blaming ideology underlying these strategies. The SEM examines environmental influences on behavior at individual (intrapersonal), interpersonal, institutional/organizational, community, and policy levels; while each of these levels is distinct, interactions between the levels also occur. For the purpose of our review, we will combine organizational and community levels, as many contributing factors can be classified into both realms. While traditionally used to develop and assess public health programs, the divisions of the SEM can also be used to delineate the numerous levels at which both trauma can occur and resilience factors can develop (Fig. 12.2) [53].

Individual Level

Variations in intrapersonal factors, including attitudes, behavior, and skills, contribute to the development of resilience in lesbian and bisexual women. These factors arise early in development and both shape and are shaped by the individual's life experiences [53].

Coming Out

Coming out is a process unique to each individual and has been associated with both trauma and resilience. It is a complex, continuous process in which the multidimensional aspects of self-awareness, self-identification of sexual orientation, self-expression, and self-disclosure intersect. While most literature supports the conclusion that greater levels of outness, earlier self-awareness, and self-disclosure are positively associated with better mental health [54], other research has shown that disclosure at a younger age can also be associated with an increased risk of sexual, physical, and verbal victimization, which may in turn increase levels of intrapersonal stress [2]. An individual's perception of the potential consequences of coming out is based on their expectation of increased vs. decreased social support, and can be predicted by both the level of comfort they have with their self-identity and whether or not they have access to a supportive environment [55].

Several aspects of sexual identity (lesbian vs. bisexual identification, years self-identified, and level of involvement in the LGB community) may predict the degree of outness of an individual. The degree of outness is positively correlated with decreased psychological distress, specifically a decrease in suicidality [54]. Lesbian-identified women are more likely to be out than their bisexual counterparts for multiple reasons that are driven by higher levels of acceptance vs. nonacceptance at the interpersonal and organizational/community levels. Years of self-identification are also positively associated with greater levels of outness. The

Fig. 12.2 Social ecological model of resilience factors in sexual minority women. Circles denote individual spheres of potential factors. Reciprocal causation is assumed among all dimensions

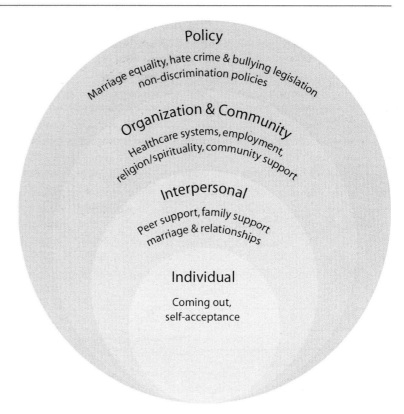

development of self-identification has been extensively studied in lesbian women, and there are milestones that delineate the process from initial awareness to eventual self-identification. The further along a woman is in this journey, the greater her experienced level of outness [56].

There is some variance, however, between different ethnic and racial groups of sexual minority women, which highlights the impact of cultural norms on an individual's coming out experience [54]. For example, African American lesbian and bisexual women have overall lower levels of outness and more years of self-identification compared to European and Latina populations. This may highlight the "triple threat" concept that black sexual minority women also face higher levels of gender and race discrimination, making them more cautious to come out, even if they have self-identified as lesbian or bisexual for years. Latina women have relatively high levels of outness; however, levels of psychological distress are not proportionately lower in this population. Asian American women, on the other hand, tend to have significantly increased levels of psychological distress compared to other ethnic groups [54].

Overall, greater levels of intrapersonal outness have been associated with reduced levels of depression and anxiety, more positive outlook and higher self-esteem, and on broader levels, higher relationship satisfaction, greater social support and more regular use of healthcare [57–59]. Providers should develop strategies to address the multifaceted and intersecting forces that influence an individual's

level of sexual identity disclosure in order to improve the overall mental and physical health outcomes of sexual minority women.

Self-Acceptance

Self-acceptance must be distinguished from self-identity and even self-disclosure. As previously discussed, the foundation of an individual's development of her value and worth, or acceptance of self, is built with "bricks" of messages she receives from her interpersonal relationships, local community, religious experience, and government. These messages begin at a young age, often before awareness of sexual orientation, and can create a discrepancy between how she feels/behaves and how she is expected to feel/behave.

Deconstructing these external messages using self-acceptance, specifically emotional acceptance and processing, as a sexual minority-specific coping mechanism has been shown to effectively mitigate the relationship between internalized homophobia and psychological distress. Using pragmatic language to describe traumatic events has been shown to decrease the psychological and physical stress responses, allowing people to both recognize and distance themselves from the trauma [60]. These findings are relevant to lesbian and bisexual women who have increased exposure to stressful situations.

Thus, self-acceptance is a critical mediator for not only the level of outness but overall levels of psychological health. Greater social support is associated with increases in both the level of outness and self-acceptance [55]. However, research examining the differences in levels of self-acceptance among different ethnic and racial groups, as well as in lesbian vs. bisexual individuals, shows significant differences in levels of psychological distress in relationship to coming out [54]. Additional research investigating specific ethnic and cultural barriers and facilitators to coming out and development and implementation of community, psychotherapeutic support, and policy services tailored specifically to the unique challenges faced by each group are needed to foster greater levels of self-acceptance among diverse populations of sexual minority women.

Interpersonal Level

In the SEM, processes at the interpersonal level are enacted via relationships between members of "primary groups" – family, friendships, work groups, and other formal and informal social support systems and networks [53]. Social support comprises the key resilience variable for LGB individuals [60]. This level of support often manifests as day-to-day emotional support, shared social activities, and decision-making advice. In the event of a major life transition or trauma, support at the interpersonal level may also include material, financial, housing, or home health support.

Family of Origin Support

Family support is an important protective factor associated with decreased depression and suicidality among sexual LGB young adults [61]. Support from family may be even more critical for LGB youth who rely on parents for financial and housing support. Family acceptance is associated with higher self-esteem, less substance use, improved mental health, and decreased internalized homophobia among LGB adolescents and young adults [62]. As is true of other sexual minority groups, lesbian and bisexual women are at risk for rejection from their families of origin because of their sexual orientation. Family rejection may lead to homelessness, substance abuse, and mental health symptoms including suicidality [63, 64]. Fear of such rejection may lead to delayed or non-disclosure of one's sexual identity. Sexual minority women who retain family connections in the context of non-disclosure may still derive the benefits of familial support. If lesbian and bisexual youth and adults decide to disclose, they have been shown to discuss their sexual orientation with their mothers more frequently than their fathers. Even though the majority of parents were found to be less than fully accepting, disclosure of one's sexual identity may in itself protect against mental health symptoms such as suicidality

[2]. Unlike gay and bisexual men who rely more on friends or co-workers, lesbian and bisexual women may rely more on family members for major support (financial, housing, home healthcare) [65]. This finding may be explained by sexual minority women experiencing less frequent familial rejection and/or greater focus on maintaining relationships with their families as compared to sexual minority men.

Peer Support

Many LGB individuals experience nonacceptance or even rejection from their families of origin. In response, some may form "chosen families" of intentionally selected individuals who play a significant role in each other's lives. Spending time with others who share the same sexual orientation, or are willing to listen to the experiences of being a sexual minority, allows for discussion of discriminatory experiences with a shared understanding of heterosexist societal structures. Additionally, lesbian and bisexual women serve as role models for each other when facing unique challenges regarding coming out, dating, marriage, family building, and end of life care. However, finding and/or selecting friends based on a similar sexual orientation is less applicable, and is more challenging, for adolescent girls with a preexisting friend group who are in the process of self-actualizing and disclosing their lesbian or bisexual orientation and identity. Nonetheless, the support from peers is still quite integral to their overall health, as adolescent girls who lose friends because of their sexual orientation are at risk for lower self-esteem and more mental health problems [2]. Similarly, in studies of support networks for lesbian and bisexual women, support from friends, regardless of their sexual orientation, is a stronger predictor of reduced depressive symptoms than support from family of origin [66].

The social support networks of sexual minority women often include peers that also identify as lesbian or bisexual. Additionally, it has been shown that lesbian and bisexual women of color construct support networks of individuals with the same race/ethnicity [65]. This tendency for sexual minority women of color to surround themselves with individuals who are most like themselves may help to ameliorate the minority stress experienced from the intersection of racism, heterosexism, and sexism.

One opportunity to promote the health of sexual minority women may be the utilization of community health workers or peer supporters. Peer supporters have been used within multiple healthcare contexts including chronic disease management, HIV-related care, mental healthcare, and breastfeeding. Lesbian- and bisexual-identified women in the role of peer supporters may provide sexual minority women with emotional, social, and practical assistance in a culturally appropriate manner.

Marriage/Recognized Intimate Relationships

As compared to heterosexual couples, women in same-sex relationships have been shown to have similar amounts of overall and sexual satisfaction with their partners [67]. Intimate relationships can provide a deep sense of emotional support. The benefits of such relationships can be profound because women in a same-sex relationship may have more egalitarian division of labor, power differential, and gender roles, leading to improved relationship quality, compatibility, and intimacy and less conflict as compared to married heterosexual couples [68].

Similar to individuals in heterosexual relationships [69], individuals in same-sex relationships experience less psychological distress and more well-being as compared to single LGB adults [70]. Additionally, same-sex and heterosexual couples experience increased stability and personal well-being as the level of commitment and perceived investment in a relationship increases [71]. Marriage confers additional protection, as evidenced by improved mental health of legally married same-sex women as compared to non-married cohabiting partners, domestic partners, and those who entered into civil unions [72]. These protective effects include reduced stress and internalized homophobia, decreased depressive symptoms, and perceived more meaning in life [70].

In the United States, lesbian and bisexual women in a same-sex relationship had few options for legal recognition of their partnerships (civil unions, legal marriage at the discretion of individual states) until the Supreme Court's *Obergefell v. Hodges* marriage equality decision in June of 2015. In the years leading up to this decision, research indicated that the denial of full marriage rights to same-sex couples had negative mental and physical health implications for all LGB people regardless of their relationship status [73]. While the opportunity to marry will not in and of itself eliminate health disparities among lesbian and bisexual women, it will hopefully promote health by decreasing structural stigmatization as described in the minority stress model.

Organization/Community Level

The organizational level of the SEM – also referred to as the institutional level – adds the dimension of "rules and regulations" found in organized social institutions. Community factors expand upon organizational interactions to include relationships among different organizations and institutions, as well as larger informal networks [53]. Because resilience factors develop as a product of both intra- and inter-organizational and network-based factors, these two spheres will be considered together in this evaluation.

Healthcare Systems

There is much literature, as previously discussed, demonstrating significant disadvantages in access to a regular source of healthcare and preventive services experienced by lesbian and bisexual women. Stigma leading to discrimination and maltreatment within medical settings may lead to decreased disclosure and delayed utilization of healthcare resources. On the other hand, disclosure of one's sexual orientation in the context of healthcare settings has also been associated with more regular utilization of healthcare [59]. Rate of disclosure of one's sexual orientation to providers varies from urban to rural settings and with an individual's perception of the provider's comfort discussing sexual orientation and sexual health. An increased level of outness is associated with better patient-provider rapport and may be a key factor leading to increased utilization of healthcare by lesbian and bisexual individuals and enhanced rates of screening and prevention [74].

Decreased access to healthcare has been repeatedly demonstrated among sexual minority women [16, 29, 42, 43, 75]. While much of this disparity has been attributed to a greater proportion of un- or underinsurance, disparities in healthcare utilization still persist when controlling for pre-ACA insurance status [28]. While it is unclear what other factors contribute to decreased access to care, sexual minority women are more likely to report unmet healthcare needs than heterosexual women, heterosexual men, and sexual minority men; in fact, men in same-sex relationships have been demonstrated to have equivalent or greater access to healthcare than men in opposite-sex relationships [43]. This fact suggests that access to care is a multifactorial issue perhaps related to socioeconomic disparities, prejudice, and minority stress, reflecting the fluid and interdependent nature of the levels of the SEM [41, 42]. Sexual minority women who perceive greater acceptance will increase utilization of healthcare. Providers can enhance access to care by using inclusive language, signage, and training staff to help foster an environment of acceptance.

Employment/Workplace

Discrimination in the workplace remains present even with social and cultural shifts toward acceptance and increased legal protection for sexual minority individuals. Just as with racial and ethnic minority populations, despite an overall decrease in overt discrimination, the presence of microaggressive gestures makes the decision of being "out" at work a difficult one for many LGB individuals today [76]. Critical factors shown to drive an individual's decision to be out at work include the existence of social support from co-workers to supervisors in the workplace as well as the presence of institutional nondiscrimination policies and LGB-affirmative activities. Increased interpersonal and organizational support is correlated with greater outness and overall life satisfaction; thus, it is important for providers to support legislation and policies at all levels which support sexual minority women [77].

Religion/Spirituality

Multiple studies conducted in the general population have shown that religiosity (standardized practices, beliefs, and spiritual activity) and spirituality (sense of connection and engagement with the sacred) can promote mental health and psychological well-being. For many individuals, religion promotes resilience by acting as a framework to explain and make meaning out of difficult or painful experiences in the context of a congregational support network. However, because of the long-standing history of Judeo-Christian churches promoting anti-gay messages and, in extreme cases, endorsing conversion therapy (treatment that attempts to change one's sexual orientation or behavior), lesbian and bisexual women may not universally benefit from religious affiliation or participation. In fact, engagement in such activities may in certain instances increase internalized homophobia and shame, and decrease perceived social support.

Even though religion and sexual minority status are often perceived to be incompatible and this belief has translated into lower rates of affiliation with organized denominations, sexual minority women have been shown to manifest increased levels of spirituality as compared to the general population [78]. While undefined in this study, spirituality among lesbian and bisexual women may include a connection with a personal "God" in the traditional Judeo-Christian model or a focus on Wiccan practices, feminist spirituality, meditation or yoga. There is evidence that religiosity and/or spirituality can promote resilience in self-identified lesbian and bisexual women. For example, LGB individuals who experienced affirmation in the context of a faith group, by feeling accepted in the faith community, seeing openly LGB members of the congregation, and being affiliated with a denomination that affirmed same-sex marriage; experienced less internalized homophobia, decreased depressive symptoms, greater levels of spirituality, and improved over-all psychological health [79, 80].

The benefits of spiritual connection for sexual minority women depend upon the ability to reconcile one's religious faith and sexual identity, usually by reframing scripture and religious tradition and finding safe religious communities [81]. For some women, resolution of this religious/sexuality identity conflict is accomplished by choosing to leave one religious community and affiliating with a congregation or denomination that affirms same-sex relationships and sexual minority identity [82]. Religious groups that have been recognized as more accepting of LGB individuals include the United Church of Christ, Episcopal Church, Unity, Quaker Friends Meetings, and Unitarian Universalists. In addition, two Christian denominations have been founded specifically for lesbian, gay, bisexual, and transgender congregants – the Metropolitan Community Church and the Unity Fellowship Church Movement. However, there are diverse paths toward identity integration. Some individuals find support within their current religious community even if it does not explicitly affirm sexual minorities. For women in these "supportive but not affirming" communities, the process of reintegrating one's religious and sexual minority identity is in itself a form of resilience. Additionally, these women may be empowered by making a commitment to work toward social justice by transforming the church from within.

A complex interplay exists between religiosity, spirituality, internalized homophobia, poor mental health outcomes, and resilience. There is evidence that religious affiliation can both mediate harmful outcomes and promote health and psychological well-being among LGB individuals, depending on a number of variables. Providers working with lesbian and bisexual women should consider the possibly of religion/spirituality as a resilience factor by investigating the importance of faith and spirituality to each individual, and paying particular attention to identity integration and the presence of affirming experiences in that person's current or prospective faith environments.

Community Support Structures

One way that sexual minority women can cope with societal and structural discrimination is to connect with the larger LGB community. The size and vitality of this community is dependent upon the geographic region, size of the LGB population, political climate, and community resources. In many larger metropolitan areas, there are dedicated LGB community centers which may provide specific support in the areas of housing, education, healthcare, legal needs, employment, mentoring, and parenting. These community centers provide services tailored to the needs of members of the LGB community and may offer resources not readily available to heterosexual individuals. For example, the mental health benefits of support found through specialized resource centers was perceived to be more accessible to sexual minority women with HIV as compared to heterosexual women with HIV [4]. However, it is important to remember the limitations of some of these LGB organizations, as there has been some indication that they are largely utilized by and perceived to cater to gay-identified white men [83]. - Non-urban areas, while not often having the breadth of community services available, may still have organized support groups for the LGB community (including PFLAG [formerly Parents and Friends of Lesbians and Gays] chapters and school-based gay-straight alliances (GSA)) as well as nonformalized community networks comprised of self-identified sexual minority individuals. Healthcare organizations serving sexual minority women may ask women involved in these community groups to serve as community advisory board members or community health workers.

Another source of community-level support for lesbian and bisexual girls and women may be organized sports. In general, participation in high school athletics has been associated with decreased depressive symptoms, improved self-reported general health, and increased collegiate graduation rates among adolescent girls [84–86]. Unfortunately, the high school and collegiate athletic environment has also been found to be especially homophobic, leading to overall decreased participation in competitive level sports by lesbian- and bisexual-identified youth [87, 88]. This exclusionary climate can have long-lasting effects on the amount of physical activity, rates of obesity, and overall health outcomes of adolescent and adult sexual minority women. However, lesbian and bisexual women have long been known to enjoy recreational organized sports, and some communities may have sexual minority women-specific sports teams available. Additionally, there is a promise of a more accepting competitive athletic environment with the increased visibility of openly lesbian- and bisexual-identified female professional athletes. Healthcare providers should be familiar with athletic opportunities available in their community as participation on an athletic team may serve an important role of social connection and support for sexual minority women.

Policy Level

This outermost circle of the SEM is influenced by factors from all other dimensions of the SEM, and in turn exerts influence at all levels. Public policy is itself a multilevel factor, governed at local, state, and national levels [53]. Healthcare providers should be aware of the downstream health effects of supportive legislation and advocate for the rights of sexual minority women as health-promoting factors.

Marriage Equality and Health Outcomes: Impact of *Obergefell v. Hodges*

Changes in marriage legislation over the last decade have provided vital opportunities to quantify the impact of discrimination on health in LGB individuals. After the 2004–2005 elections and subsequent passage of constitutional marriage bans in 16 states, several studies were conducted to examine the relationship between these amendments and the psychiatric health of LGB residents of those states. A groundbreaking study by Hatzenbuehler et al. used data from the National Epidemiologic Survey on Alcohol and Related Conditions to assess psychiatric disorders as diagnosed by the DSM-IV before and after the elections. The results showed significant increases in psychiatric

disorders including mood disorders, generalized anxiety disorder, alcohol use disorders, and psychiatric comorbidities. Significantly, none of these disorders had a significant increase in LGB individuals in states without such amendments, nor did they increase in heterosexual residents of states with new marriage bans [89]. Another study conducted a survey after the November 2006 elections, in which a number of political campaigns intended to further deny civil marriage to same-sex couples, and found an increase in psychological distress and minority stress among LGB individuals [90]. Such disparities have been rigorously studied in order to determine causation; legal recognition of relationships is associated with psychological benefits including less internalized homophobia, decreased depressive symptoms and stress, and more self-reported meaning in one's life [70]. These results suggest that social policy changes may reduce mental health disparities in LGB people, likely mediating improvements in physical health disparities as well [89].

The Supreme Court's *Obergefell v. Hodges* marriage equality decision in 2015 determined that (1) all states must recognize the marriage between two same-sex individuals in their state and (2) must recognize marriages of same-sex couples performed in other states [91]. This decision impacted health-related policies in a number of ways, including employer-provided benefits for same-sex spouses in all 50 states, nationwide family and medical leave for LGB couples, and recognition of spousal surrogate decision-making rights and healthcare proxies [92]. Although quantitative research on the health outcomes of marriage equality has yet to be published, it is widely believed to have the potential to improve mental and physical health beyond the proximal effect of expanding health benefits [73].

Nondiscrimination Policies and Hate Crime Legislation

As a marginalized population, LGBT individuals are at risk for hate-motivated crimes, and gender-based violence disproportionately affects women [93]. Hate crimes are typically more violent than non-hate-motivated crimes and are more likely to be unprovoked and have greater long-term mental health consequences [94]. Furthermore, internalized homophobia has been demonstrated to mediate the relationship between hate crime victimization and psychiatric symptoms – that is, hate crime victims with significant internalized homophobia are more likely to have long-lasting mental health sequelae [95]. These health effects extend to sexual minority individuals who are not direct victims of LGBT-motivated hate crimes. Sexual minority youth living in neighborhoods with high rates of sexual orientation-motivated hate crimes are significantly more likely to report suicidal ideation, suicide attempts, and drug use; this relationship does not exist for overall violent crime and petty crimes [96–98].

The existence of these relationships lends strong support to the development of hate crime and nondiscrimination legislation. This is a complex area of policy, facing the challenges of intersectionality and defining marginalized groups [99]. However, significant progress has been made in this area, as evidenced by the release of the 2013 update to the Violence Against Women Act (VAWA) which contains specific provisions for LGBT individuals. Prior to 2013, VAWA had already made a significant impact on gender-based violence in the United States, and these new provisions support increased protection and resources for LGB women [51]. Furthermore, states without policies against hate crimes and employment discrimination have been shown to have a higher prevalence of psychiatric disorders among LGB individuals [100]. Using the minority stress model, this suggests that existence of such policies may improve psychiatric and overall health by decreasing stigma and internalized homophobia. In the coming years, advocacy must focus on maintaining women's rights, as well as promoting legal protections on housing and employment for LGB people [73].

Bullying as a Health Risk

Sexual minorites, particularly youth, have higher levels of minority stress resulting in depressive symptoms and suicidality, therefore making it imperative to advocate for public policies to reduce bullying and hate crimes [19]. While civil rights protections against harassment in school do exist, these have been criticized for applying only to children in certain protected groups, including students with disabilities, racial and ethnic minorities, and victims of gender harassment or religious discrimination [101]. There is evidence that extending such protections to include sexual minority youth may improve mental health outcomes. Pooled data on sexual orientation and suicidal thoughts showed fewer past-year suicidal thoughts among LGB students in schools with safe spaces and/or gay-straight alliances [102]. Even after controlling for exposure to peer victimization, policies that include sexual orientation can reduce the risk for suicide attempts [103]. Policies that recognize and promote the right of all children to a public education, including a safe environment with protection against bullying, are necessary to improve the psychological health of LGB youth.

Promoting Resilience in Lesbian and Bisexual Women

Caring for Self

Research has shown that many lesbian and bisexual women do not disclose their sexual orientation to their healthcare providers, feeling this information has no bearing on their health. Promoting openness and positive patient-provider relations in healthcare settings through displayed nondiscrimination policies, utilization of intake forms that do not assume heterosexual orientation, and training of providers and staff to increase awareness of population-specific terminology and healthcare may lead to increased identity disclosure by lesbian and bisexual women. An open dialogue initiated by providers with lesbian and bisexual women which emphasizes the benefits of disclosure and the important relationship between lifestyle behaviors and overall health outcomes gives the individual a tangible way to understand and enhance their self-care [74].

When discussing particular health behaviors with sexual minority women, it is important to inquire about and consider their unique cultural perspective. A focus group-based study with sexual minority women indicated that programs to encourage healthy eating and exercise ought to focus on health and fitness rather than beauty, given expressed ambivalence toward dominant attitudes about appearance, weight, and size. Functional fitness, in particular, is a dimension of importance to sexual minority women, and health and fitness goals should be tailored to fit within the lifestyle of sexual minority women [37]. Effective counseling to promote regular exercise in sexual minority women may include messages about "getting stronger" and "increasing endurance," rather than focusing on weight loss and appearance.

Caring for Others

Altruism may be an important resilience factor for lesbian and bisexual women. This may take the form of serving as positive role models for other sexual minority women and becoming involved in social justice movements. This activism increases a sense of connection with the broader LGB community and may in turn increase social support and improve health outcomes. Additionally, altruism may be related to increased hope and optimism for the future, both of which can serve as important resilience factors [60].

Lesbian and bisexual women have long been integral to feminist movements. Sexual minority women have fought valiantly for the right to vote, civil rights, and legal recognition of marriage. Many of them became caretakers for their gay brothers suffering from HIV/AIDS in the darkest days of the crisis. Black women identifying as lesbian or bisexual have formed strong coalitions rooted in their shared experience of discrimination at the intersection of gender, race, and sexual identity. Working toward social justice in the context of larger feminist movements may be an important source of resilience for sexual minority women.

Building Families

Lesbian and bisexual women have been at the forefront of changing the face of family. For years, these women have been pioneers by breaking down the "traditional" notion of genetics and bloodlines, building alternative families intentionally and uniquely.

Some women partner in parenting biological children conceived during a relationship with a previous male partner. Integration for these families may be complex, and result from delayed coming out of lesbian individuals, or having parented with a previous male partner in the case of bisexual women. Adoption is another path women choose to build a family. There are unique challenges in the adoption selection process lesbian and bisexual women must face and overcome at many levels including facing prejudice in the selection process of adopting together, as well as one parent adopting a child from her partner's previous relationship.

The significant increase use of sperm donors, both known and anonymous, reflects an increasing acceptance of alternative family building at the community and policy level, allowing for a shared experience of the process of pregnancy, childbirth, and growing a family. Some choose to know their donor and may have continued involvement with the donor and encourage relationships with their children. Others choose anonymous donors. Regardless of the many different paths to forming families and the depth of complexity that may be involved, creating alternative family structures promotes increased self-acceptance and family support for lesbian and bisexual women and ultimately leads to more authentic living. It is important for providers to gain knowledge about the different options for family building to ensure that lesbian and bisexual women are provided with counseling that supports them in this important process.

Bisexual Pride

An identifiable and supportive peer group made up of women of the same sexual identity may be especially influential in increasing the overall health of bisexual women. Bisexual women living in urban areas report increased high-risk behaviors and decreased self-reported health as compared to lesbian women [16]. This discrepancy is postulated to result from the relative lack of a defined group or community. Furthermore, the finding of greater mental distress experienced by bisexual-identified women in urban areas as compared to those in non-urban areas may be explained by an increased awareness of the relative lack of support, especially from within the lesbian and gay community, as compared to that available to lesbian-identified women. The possible shifting of identities of bisexual women throughout the life course may add to the complexities of finding consistent peer support [16]. Providers should be aware of relevant support services specifically serving bisexual women to help connect them with similarly identified peers.

Conclusion

Lesbian and bisexual women experience a myriad of factors across the spectrum of the SEM (i.e., at individual, interpersonal, organizational/community, and policy levels) that may either foster or impede attainment of their full health potential. At each level, there are specific clinical interventions or opportunities for social justice advocacy that should be considered by providers caring for sexual minority women. Shifting focus from the traditional disease-based model to a resilience-based model helps to promote empowerment and a sense of agency among lesbian and bisexual women, and is integral to supporting the health and well-being of these populations.

Case Scenario

Jude is a 23-year-old female who presents to establish primary healthcare with you after recently moving to your area (Fig. 12.3). On the electronic intake form, Jude endorses symptoms of depression and anxiety including past hospitalizations for suicidal ideation. As part of the social history section, she reports having both male and female lifetime partners and notes that her current partner is a woman.

Upon entering the exam room, you find Jude to be mildly anxious and immediately notice the row of scars in parallel covering her left forearm. After discussing her past medical

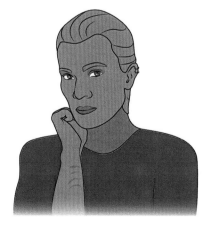

Fig. 12.3 Jude is a 23-year-old female who presents to establish primary healthcare

history, family history, and current medications, you feel that you have begun to establish rapport with Jude and she seems more at ease.

You then say, "Jude, I understand that you have been sexually active with both men and women in the past, is there a particular term or label that you feel best describes your sexual identity?"

Jude seems somewhat surprised by your question and states, "Wow, I haven't ever been asked this question by my doctor. But you are correct, I have had sex with men in the past, but it was a number of years ago. For the past 2 years I have been in a committed relationship with my current girlfriend; though I think if I had to label myself, it would be as bisexual."

"Thanks for sharing that information with me, Jude," you reply. "Who are your sources of support in terms of your sexuality?"

"Well, my family is a big support now, although they weren't great initially," Jude explains. "My parents are pretty religious and when I came out to them it was pretty hard. They accept my girlfriend and now that I've moved, they are understanding of how hard it is that she's 6 hours away. I had a great group of friends before I moved, but I am feeling really disconnected and lonely since having to relocate here for graduate school."

Discussion Questions

1. What are the different processes involved in minority stress theory?
2. How does the intersectionality of multiple identities relate to trauma and victimization, stigma, and health?
3. How might religious beliefs, degree of outness, parental acceptance, and integration in the LGB community highlight strengths and vulnerabilities in lesbian and bisexual women?
4. What strategies can health professionals use when attempting to promote health among bisexual women?
5. What community-level resources are available to support emerging adults who identify as sexual minority women?

Summary Practice Points

1. Stress processes involved in minority stress theory include experiences of anti-LGB discrimination, the expectation of rejection, concealing one's sexual identity, and internalized homophobia.
2. It is critical for providers to consider how racism, sexism, classism, heterosexism, biphobia, and ableism may

increase risks of victimization, structural stigma, and poor mental and physical health outcomes.
3. Increased affirmation within multiple social constructs can decrease internalized homophobia and improve overall health and well-being.
4. Tailored health promotion strategies must acknowledge and identify the stressors, health behaviors, and outcomes unique to bisexual women.
5. It is vital to be aware of the different organizations and resources serving LGB individuals in your community.

Resources

1. GLAAD Bisexual Resource Center: http://www.glaad.org/tags/bisexual-resource-center
2. National Black Justice Coalition: http://nbjc.org
3. Fredriksen-Goldsen KI, Simoni JM, Kim H, Lehavot K, Walters KL, Yang J, Hoy-Ellis CP. The Health Equity Promotion Model: reconceptualization of lesbian, gay, bisexual, and transgender (LGBT) health disparities. Am J Orthopsychiatry. 2014 Nov;84(6):653–63.
4. Kwon P. Resilience in lesbian, gay, and bisexual individuals. Pers Soc Psychol Rev. 2013;17(4):371–83.
5. PFLAG: http://community.pflag.org

References

1. Meyer IH. Prejudice, social stress, and mental health in lesbian, gay, and bisexual populations: conceptual issues and research evidence. Psychol Bull. 2003;129(5):674–97.
2. D'Augelli AR. Lesbian and bisexual female youth aged 14 to 21: developmental challenges and victimization experiences. J Lesbian Stud. 2003;7(4):9–29.
3. Morris JF, Balsam KF. Lesbian and bisexual women's experiences of victimization: mental health, revictimization, and sexual identity development. J Lesbian Stud. 2003;7:67–85.
4. Cooperman NA, Simoni JA, Lockhard DW. Abuse, social support, and depression among HIV-positive heterosexual, bisexual, and lesbian women. J Lesbian Stud. 2003;7(4):49–66.
5. Balsam KF, Rothblum ED, Beauchaine TP. Victimization over the life span: a comparison of lesbian, gay, bisexual, and heterosexual siblings. J Consult Clin Psychol. 2005;73(3):477–87.
6. Balsam KF, Blayney JA, Molina Y, Dillworth T, Zimmerman L, Kaysen D. Racial/ethnic differences in identity and mental health outcomes among young sexual minority women. Cultur Divers Ethnic Minor Psychol. 2015;21(3):380–90.
7. Link BG, Phelan JC. Conceptualizing stigma. Annu Rev Sociol. 2001;27:363–85.
8. Bostwick W. Assessing bisexual stigma and mental health status: a brief report. J Bisex. 2012;12(2):214–22.
9. DiPlacido J. Minority stress among lesbians, gay men, and bisexuals: a consequence of heterosexism, homophobia, and stigmatization. Herek GM, editor. Thousand Oaks: Sage Publications; 1998.

10. Meyer IH, Dean L. Stigma and sexual orientation: understanding prejudice against lesbians, gay men, and bisexuals. Thousand Oaks: Sage; 1998.

11. Williamson I. Internalized homophobia and health issues affecting lesbians and gay men. Health Educ Res. 2000;15:91–107.

12. Coulter RWS, Kinsy SM, Herrick AL, Stall RD, Bauermeister JA. Evidence of syndemics and sexuality-related discrimination among young sexual-minority women. LGBT Health. 2015;2 (3):250–7.

13. Thoits PA. Stress and health: major findings and policy implications. J Health Soc Behav. 2010;51(Suppl):S41–53.

14. Kaysen D, Kulesza M, Balsam KF, Rhew IC, Blayney JA, Lehavot K, et al. Coping as a mediator of internalized homophobia and psychological distress among young adult sexual minority women. Psychol Sex orientat Gend Divers. 2014;1(3):225–33.

15. Balsam KF. Trauma, stress, and resilience among sexual minority women: rising like the phoenix. J Lesbian Stud. 2003;7(4):1–8.

16. Frederiksen-Goldsen KI, Kim HJ, Barkan SE, Balsam KF, Mincer SL. Disparities in health-related quality of life: a comparison of lesbians and bisexual women. Am J Public Health. 2010;100 (11):2255–61.

17. Healthy People 2020 [Internet]. U.S. Department of Health and Human Services. Available from: http://www.healthypeople.gov.

18. Warner J, McKeown E, Griffin M, Johnson K, Ramsay A, Cort C, et al. Rates and predictors of mental illness in gay men, lesbians and bisexual men and women: results from a survey based in England and Wales. Br J Psychiatry. 2004;185:479–85.

19. Burton CM, Marshal MP, Chisholm DJ, Sucato GS, Friedman MS. Sexual minority-related victimization as a mediator of mental health disparities in sexual minority youth: a longitudinal analysis. J Youth Adolesc. 2013;42(3):394–402.

20. Case P, Austin B, Hunter DJ, Manson JE, Malspeis S, Willett WC, et al. Sexual orientation, health risk factors, and physical functioning in the Nurses' Health Study II. J Womens Health (Larchmt). 2004;13(9):1033–47.

21. Cochran SD, Mays VM. Relation between psychiatric syndromes and behaviorally defined sexual orientation in a sample of the US population. Am J Epidemiol. 2000;151(5):516–23.

22. Cochran SD, Mays VM. Physical health complaints among lesbians, gay men, and bisexual and homosexually experienced heterosexual individuals: results from the California Quality of Life Survey. Am J Public Health. 2007;97(11):2048–55.

23. Cochran SD, Sullivan JG, Mays VM. Prevalence of mental disorders, psychological distress, and mental health services use among lesbian, gay, and bisexual adults in the United States. J Consult Clin Psychol. 2003;71(1):53–61.

24. Fergusson DM, Horwood J, Beautrais AL. Is sexual orientation related to mental health problems and suicidality in young people? Arch Gen Psychiatry. 1999;56(10):876–80.

25. Gilman SE, Cochran SD, Mays VM, Hughes M, Ostrow D, Kessler RC. Risk of psychiatric disorders among individuals reporting same-sex sexual partners in the National Comorbidity Survey. Am J Public Health. 2001;91(6):933–9.

26. Sandfort TGM, de Graaf R, Bijl RV, Schnabel P. Same-sex sexual behavior and psychiatric disorders. Arch Gen Psychiatry. 2001;58 (1):85–91.

27. Aaron DJ, Markovic N, Danielson ME, Honnold JA, Janosky JE, Schmidt NJ. Behavioral risk factors for disease and preventive health practices among lesbians. Am J Public Health. 2001;91 (6):972–5.

28. Boehmer U, Miao X, Linkletter C, Clark MA. Adult health behaviors over the life course by sexual orientation. Am J Public Health. 2012;102(2):292–300.

29. Diamant AL, Wold C, Spritzer K, Gelberg L. Health behaviors, health status, and access to and use of care. Arch Fam Med. 2000;9:1043–51.

30. Gruskin EP, Hart S, Gordon N, Ackerson L. Patterns of cigarette smoking and alcohol use among lesbians and bisexual women enrolled in a large health maintenance organization. Am J Public Health. 2001;91(6):976–9.

31. Scheer S, Parks CA, McFarland W, Page-Shafer K, Delgado V, Ruiz JD, et al. Self-reported sexual identity, sexual behaviors and health risks: examples from a population-based survey of young women. J Lesbian Stud. 2008;7(1):69–83.

32. Tang H, Greenwood GL, Cowling DW, Lloyd JC, Roeseler AG, Bal DG. Cigarette smoking among lesbians, gays, and bisexuals: how serious a problem? Cancer Causes Control. 2004;15 (8):797–803.

33. Blosnich J, Lee J, Horn K. A systematic review of the aetiology of tobacco disparities for sexual minorities. Tob Control. 2013;22 (2):66–73.

34. Pizacani BA, Rohde K, Bushore C, Stark MJ, Maher JE, Dilley JA, et al. Smoking-related knowledge, attitudes and behaviors in the lesbian, gay and bisexual community: a population-based study from the U.S. Pacific northwest. Prev Med. 2009;48 (6):555–61.

35. Mason TB, Lewis RJ. Minority stress, depression, relationship quality, and alcohol use: associations with overweight and obesity among partnered young adult lesbians. LGBT Health. 2015;2 (4):333–40.

36. Deputy NP, Boehmer U. Weight status and sexual orientation: differences by age and within racial and ethnic subgroups. Am J Public Health. 2014;104(1):103–9.

37. Bowen DJ, Balsam KF, Diergaarde B, Russo M, Escamilla GM. Healthy eating, exercise, and weight: impressions of sexual minority women. Women Health. 2006;44(1):79–93.

38. Heffernan K. Eating disorders and weight concern among lesbians. Int J Eat Disord. 1996;19(2):127–38.

39. Farmer GW, Jabson JM, Bucholz KK, Bowen DJ. A population-based study of cardiovascular disease risk in sexual-minority women. Am J Public Health. 2013;103(10):1845–50.

40. Quinn GP, Sanchez JA, Sutton SK, Vadaparampil ST, Nguyen GT, Green BL, et al. Cancer and lesbian, gay, bisexual, transgender/transsexual, and queer/questioning populations (LGBTQ). CA Cancer J Clin. 2015;65(5):384–400.

41. Kerker BD, Motashari F, Thorpe L. Health care access and utilization among women who have sex with women: sexual behavior and identity. J Urban Health. 2006;83(5):970–9.

42. Everett BG, Mollborn S. Examining sexual orientation disparities in unmet medical needs among men and women. Popul Res Policy Rev. 2014;33(4):553–77.

43. Heck JE, Sell RL, SheinfeldGorin S. Health care access among individuals involved in same-sex relationships. Am J Public Health. 2006;96(6):1111–8.

44. Mays VM, Yancey AK, Cochran SD, Weber M, Fielding JE. Heterogeneity of health disparities among African American, Hispanic, and Asian American women: unrecognized influences of sexual orientation. Am J Public Health. 2002;92(4):632–9.

45. McNair R, Szalacha LA, Hughes TL. Health status, health service use, and satisfaction according to sexual identity of young Australian women. Womens Health Issues. 2011;21(1):40–7.

46. Klitzman RL, Greenberg JD. Patterns of communication between gay and lesbian patients and their healthcare providers. J Homosex. 2002;42:65–75.

47. Agénor M, Peitzmeier S, Gordon AR, Haneuse S, Potter JE, Austin SB. Sexual orientation identity disparities in awareness and initiation of the human papillomavirus vaccine among US women and girls: a national survey. Ann Intern Med. 2015;163 (2):99–106.

48. Fallin A, Goodin A, Lee YO, Bennett K. Smoking characteristics among lesbian, gay, and bisexual adults. Prev Med. 2015;74:123–30.

49. Goldberg NG, Meyer IH. Sexual orientation disparities in history of intimate partner violence: results from the California health interview survey. J Interpers Violence. 2013;28(5):1109–18.

50. Messinger AM. Invisible victims: same-sex IPV in the National Violence Against Women Survey. J Interpers Violence. 2011;26(11):2228–43.

51. Modi MN, Palmer S, Armstrong A. The role of Violence Against Women Act in addressing intimate partner violence: a public health issue. J Womens Health (Larchmt). 2014;23(3):253–9.

52. Bronfenbrenner U. The ecology of human development: experiments by nature and design. Cambridge, MA: Harvard University Press; 1979.

53. McLeroy KR, Bibeau D, Steckler A, Glanz K. An ecological perspective on health promotion programs. Health Educ Behav. 1988;15(4):351–77.

54. Morris JF, Waldo CR, Rothblum ED. A model of predictors and outcomes of outness among lesbian and bisexual women. Am J Orthopsychiatry. 2001;71(1):61–71.

55. Levitt HM, Puckett JA, Ippolito MR, Horne SG. Sexual minority women's gender identity and expression: challenges and supports. J Lesbian Stud. 2012;16(2):153–76.

56. Garnets LD, Kimmel DC. Psychological perspectives on lesbian and gay male experiences. New York: Columbia University Press; 1993.

57. Jordan KM, Deluty RH. Coming out for lesbian women: its relation to anxiety, positive affectivity, self-esteem and social support. J Homosex. 1998;35(2):41–63.

58. Caron SL, Ulin M. Closeting and the quality of lesbian relationships. Fam Soc. 1997;78:413–9.

59. Steele LS, Tinmouth JM, Lu A. Regular health care use by lesbians: a path analysis of predictive factors. Fam Pract. 2006;23(6):631–6.

60. Kwon P. Resilience in lesbian, gay, and bisexual individuals. Pers Soc Psychol Rev. 2013;17(4):371–83.

61. Ryan C, Huebner D, Diaz R, Sanchez J. Family rejection as a predictor of negative health outcomes in white and Latino lesbian, gay, and bisexual young adults. Pediatrics. 2009;123:346–52.

62. Ryan C, Russell ST, Huebner D, Diaz R, Sanchez J. Family acceptance in adolescence and the health of LGBT young adults. J Child Adolesc Psychiatr Nurs. 2010;23:205–13.

63. D'Augelli AR, Hershberger SL, Pilkington NM. Suicidality patterns and sexual orientation-related factors among gay, lesbian, and bisexual youth. Suicide Life Threat Behav. 2001;31:250–65.

64. Savin-Williams R. Verbal and physical abuse as stressors in the lives of lesbian, gay male, and bisexual youths: associations with school problems, running away, substance abuse, prostitution, and suicide. J Consult Clin Psychol. 1994;62:261–9.

65. Frost DM, Schwartz S, Meyer IH. Social support networks among diverse sexual minority populations. Am J Orthopsychiatry. 2016;86(1):91–102.

66. Alaya J, Coleman H. Predictors of depression among lesbian women. J Lesbian Stud. 2000;4:71–86.

67. Patterson CJ. Family relationships of lesbians and gay men. J Marriage Fam. 2000;62(4):1052–69.

68. Balsam KF, Beauchaine TP. Three-year follow up of same-sex couples who had civil unions in Vermont, same-sex couples not in civil unions, and heterosexual married couples. Dev Psychol. 2008;44(1):102–16.

69. KampDush CM, Amato PR. Consequences of relationship status and quality for subjective well-being. J Soc Pers Relat. 2005;22:607–27.

70. Riggle ED, Rostosky SS. Psychological distress, well-being, and legal recognition in same-sex couple relationships. J Fam Psychol. 2010;24(1):82–6.

71. Cox CL, Wexler MO, Rusbult CE, Gaines SO. Prescriptive support and commitment processes in close relationships. Soc Psychol Q. 1997;60:79–90.

72. Kornblith E, Green RJ, Casey S, Tiet Q. Marital status, social support, and depressive symptoms among lesbian and heterosexual women. J Lesbian Stud. 2016;20(1):157–73.

73. Perone AK. Health implications of the Supreme court's Obergefell v. Hodges marriage equality decision. LGBT Health. 2015;2(3):196–9.

74. Whitehead J, Shaver J, Stevenson R. Outness, stigma, and primary health care utilization among rural LGBT populations. PLoS One. 2016;11(1):1–17.

75. Marrazzo JM, Koutsky LA, Kiviat NB, Kuypers JM, Stine K. Papanicolaou test screening and prevalence of genital human papillomavirus among women who have sex with women. Am J Public Health. 2001;91(6):947–52.

76. Colgan F, Creegan C, McKearney A, Wright T. Equality and diversity practices at work: lesbian, gay, and bisexual workers. Equal Oppor Int. 2007;26:590–609.

77. Huffman AH, Watrous-Rodriguez K, Kine EB. Supporting a diverse workforce: what type of support is most meaningful for lesbian and gay employees? Hum Resour Manag. 2008;47:237–53.

78. Barnes DM, Meyer IH. Religious affiliation, internalized homophobia, and mental health in lesbians, gay men and bisexuals. Am J Orthopsychiatry. 2012;82(4):505–15.

79. Gattis MN, Woodford MR, Han Y. Discrimination and depressive symptoms among sexual minority youth: is gay-affirming religious affiliation a protective factor? Arch Sex Behav. 2014;443:1589–99.

80. Lease SH, Horner SG, Noffsinger-Frazier N. Affirming faith experiences and psychological health for Caucasian lesbian, gay, and bisexual individuals. J Couns Psychol. 2005;52:378–88.

81. Foster KA, Bowland SE, Vosler AN. All the pain along with all the joy: spiritual resilience in lesbian and gay Christians. Am J Community Psychol. 2015;55:191–201.

82. Bowland SE, Foster K, Vosler AN. Culturally competent and spiritually sensitive therapy with lesbian and gay Christians. Soc Work. 2013;58(4):321–32.

83. Ward F. White normativity: the cultural dimensions of whiteness in a racially diverse LGBT organization. Sociol Perspect. 2008;51:563–86.

84. Gore S, Farrell F, Gordon J. Sports involvement as protection against depressed mood. J Res Adolesc. 2001;11(1):119–30.

85. Troutman KP, Dufur MJ. From high school jocks to college grads. Youth Soc. 2007;38(4):443–62.

86. Steiner H, McQuivey RW, Pavelski R, Pitts T, Kraemer H. Adolescents and sports: risk or benefit. Clin Pediatr. 2000;39:161–6.

87. Gill DL, Morrow RG, Collins KE, Lucey AB, Schultz AM. Perceived climate in physical activity settings. J Homosex. 2010;57(7):895–913.

88. Mereish EH, Poteat P. Let's get physical: sexual orientation disparities in physical activity, sports involvement, and obesity among a population-based sample of adolescents. Am J Public Health. 2015;105(9):1842–8.

89. Hatzenbuehler ML, McLaughlin KA, Keyes KM, Hasin DS. The impact of institutional discrimination on psychiatric disorders in lesbian, gay, and bisexual populations: a prospective study. Am J Public Health. 2010;100(3):452–9.

90. Rostosky SS, Riggle ED, Horne SG, Denton FN, Huellemeier JD. Lesbian, gay, and bisexual individuals' psychological reactions to amendments denying civil access to marriage. Am J Orthopsychiatry. 2010;80(3):302–10.

91. Obergefell v. Hodges, 576 U.S. ___ .2015.

92. Lyon SM, Moore N, Douglas IS, Cooke CR. Update on the Affordable Care Act: *King v. Burwell* and *Obergefell v. Hodges*. Ann Am Thorac Soc. 2016;13(3):324–8.

93. UNFPA strategy and framework for action to addressing gender-based violence 2008–2011 [Internet]. United Nations Population Fund. 2009. Available from: http://www.unfpa.org/publications.

94. Hein LC, Scharer KM. Who cares if it is a hate crime? Lesbian, gay, bisexual, and transgender hate crimes – mental health implications and interventions. Perspect Psychiatr Care. 2013;49:84–93.

95. Burks AC, Cramer RJ, Henderson CE, Stroud CH, Crosby JW, Graham J. Frequency, nature, and correlates of hate crime victimization experiences in an urban sample of lesbian, gay, and bisexual community members. J Interpers Violence. 2015;pii 0886260515605298 [Epub ahead of print].

96. Duncan DT, Hatzenbuehler ML. Lesbian, gay, bisexual, and transgender hate crimes and suicidality among a population-based sample of sexual-minority adolescents in Boston. Am J Public Health. 2014;104(2):272–8.

97. Duncan DT, Hatzenbuehler ML, Johnson RM. Neighborhood-level LGBT hate crimes and current illicit drug use among sexual minority youth. Drug Alcohol Depend. 2014;135:65–70.

98. Hatzenbuehler ML, Jun HJ, Corliss HL, Austin SB. Structural stigma and sexual orientation disparities in adolescent drug use. Addict Behav. 2015;46:14–8.

99. Chakraborti N. Re-thinking hate crime: fresh challenges for policy and practice. J Interpers Violence. 2015;30(10):1738–54.

100. Hatzenbuehler ML, Keyes KM, Hasin DS. State-level policies and psychiatric morbidity in lesbian, gay, and bisexual populations. Am J Public Health. 2009;99(12):2275–81.

101. Cornell D, Limber SP. Law and policy on the concept of bullying at school. Am Psychol. 2015;70(4):333–43.

102. Hatzenbuehler ML, Birkett M, van Wagenen A, Meyer IH. Protective school climates and reduced risk for suicide ideation in sexual minority youths. Am J Public Health. 2014;104(2):279–86.

103. Hatzenbuehler ML, Keyes KM. Inclusive anti-bullying policies and reduced risk of suicide attempts in lesbian and gay youth. J Adolesc Health. 2013;53(10):S21–6.

Institutionalization and Incarceration of LGBT Individuals

13

Erin McCauley and Lauren Brinkley-Rubinstein

Lesbian, gay, bisexual, and transgender (LGBT) populations are highly diverse; however, they share a common history of marginalization, stigma and discrimination, and violence [1], and some groups—particularly LGBT youth—also experience disproportionate rates of institutionalization and incarceration [2]. Experiences of social exclusion, stigma, and discrimination have had a sizable impact on both the unique mental health issues that members of the LGBT community face and their health-seeking behavior and access to care [1]. Additional injustices experienced by LGBT people who are institutionalized and/or incarcerated further contribute to the burden of trauma accumulated across the life course and must be appropriately addressed during the recovery process. An understanding of the prevalence, impact, and forces leading to increased rates of institutionalization and incarceration in LGBT communities is therefore crucial to providing competent healthcare to these groups.

Drivers of Incarceration/Institutionalization

LGBT and gender nonconforming (GNC) individuals experience elevated rates of incarceration and institutionalization; both a history of and current experience of incarceration and institutionalization have profound influences on everyday health needs. While the drivers of incarceration and institutionalization within and across

E. McCauley, MEd
Department of Policy Analysis and Management, College of Human Ecology, Cornell University, Ithaca, NY, USA

L. Brinkley-Rubinstein, PhD (✉)
Department of Social Medicine, University of North Carolina-Chapel Hill, 333 S. Columbia Street, Chapel Hill, NC 27514, USA

Center for Health Equity Research, University of North Carolina-Chapel Hill, Chapel Hill, NC, USA
e-mail: Lauren_Brinkley@med.unc.edu

diverse and often multifaceted LGBT and GNC communities can be difficult to tease apart, Fig. 13.1 offers a pictorial representation to organize our discussion.

Pathologization of LGBT and GNC Status

Both historical and the modern pathologization of LGB sexualities and transgender and GNC gender expressions lie at root of much of the discrimination and oppression of LGBT and GNC people and expose them to ongoing inhumane and immoral treatment. Categorization of nontraditional sexual orientations and gender expressions as illnesses established a seemingly rational pathway whereby discrimination in mental healthcare was sanctioned, with lasting societal implications. Pathologization of LGBT and GNC identities and expressions contributed to the creation of negative archetypes (which have often been used in the criminalization process as well), exposed LGBT and GNC people to traumatizing "treatments" such as conversion therapy, and acted as a barrier to access appropriate healthcare (either through LGBT and GNC people avoiding medical and psychiatric care or not disclosing their status to medical care providers) [3].

Effect of Pathologization

The pathologization of LGBT and GNC sexuality and gender expression has had many negative consequences, including increased incarceration and institutionalization. Mogul, Ritchie, and Whitlock argued that one of the initial and core functions of imprisonment in the USA has been the regulation and punishment of sexualities and gender expressions considered "deviant" [4]. Using archetypes of criminality, predation, disease, and sexuality imprisonment, the criminal justice system in the USA has focused on punishing "deviance" through forced sex/gender segregation, violence, isolation, and the denial of sexuality and gender expression in

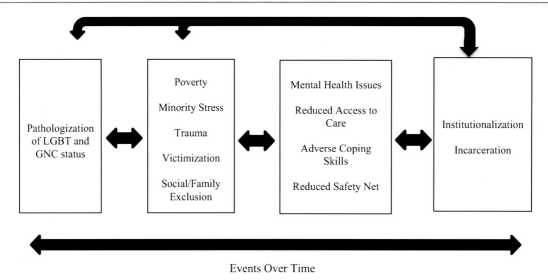

Events Over Time

Fig. 13.1 Drivers of institutionalization and incarceration for LGBT people

prisons and jails [4]. Laws that unjustly targeted LGB people, such as the sodomy laws (which were struck down in 2003), contributed to the criminalization of homosexuality [4]. Mogul, Ritchie, and Whitlock argued that sodomy laws gave "renewed legal weight to the message that queer people are immoral, sinful, and deserving of criminal punishment" [1, p. 72]. They also point to the sumptuary laws—laws limiting expenditures on food, clothing, and personal items—which ended in the 1980s and required people to wear three or more articles of clothing associated with their birth gender, as another form of gender and sexuality policing that contributed to the criminalization of sexuality and gender expression [4].

The pathologization of sexuality and gender expression also led indirectly to increased criminalization and institutionalization through several other mechanisms including poverty, minority stress, victimization, trauma, and social/familial exclusion. By conceptualizing some sexuality and gender identities and expressions as illnesses, these characteristics became "othered," exposing LGBT and GNC people to a plethora of risks. In turn, increased risks of poverty, minority stress, victimization, trauma, and exclusion led both directly and indirectly to increased incarceration and institutionalization. Because of these risks, LGBT and GNC people were and are more likely to experience reduced access to care and mental health issues, develop maladaptive coping skills, and have a diminished safety net which leaves them more vulnerable to incarceration and institutionalization. Poverty is linked to access to care among LGBT and GNC populations. Fredriksen-Goldsen found that 22% of older transgender and GNC people were unable to access medical care due to cost, and 15% of LGBT people fear seeking medical care by a provider outside of the LGBT community [3]. Lack of access to care is associated with increased self-medication through maladaptive coping

behaviors, such as drug and alcohol use. Older adult LGB people are more likely to drink heavily and smoke cigarettes than their heterosexual counterparts [3]. Fredriksen-Goldsen also found that older LGBT adults have a high prevalence of depression and mental distress (31%) and 82% of LGBT people had experienced victimization [3]. People with mental health issues are overrepresented in the criminal justice system and mental health issues can lead to institutionalization, particularly for those who experience social rejection and therefore have a reduced safety net of people to provide care. Research has found that LGBT people are more likely to rely on the support of a friend than a family member [3, 5]. The reduced safety net experienced by many LGBT people can be even more significant for youth. Hunt and Moodie-Mills found that LGBT youth face higher risks of incarceration due to homelessness because of family rejection [6]. The many risks and barriers that LGBT and GNC people face which put them at increased likelihood of incarceration and institutionalization frequently overlap and intersect, leading to a complex web of risks with no simple solution or intervention. Furthermore, the experience of incarceration then exposes LGBT and GNC people to further traumatization and victimization which can lead to persistence of or development of more adverse coping mechanisms, with further social exclusion and a further decreased safety net and an increase in survival crimes. This vicious cycle of traumatization, institutionalization, and incarceration is also affected by events over time.

Events Over Time

Several events over time have influenced the incarceration and institutionalization of LGBT people. Two highlighted here—transinstitutionalization and the War on Drugs—have

Phase	Decade	Information
Institutionalization	1840s	Dorothea Dix, after witnessing incarcerated people with mental illnesses chained naked to beds, left without heat, bathrooms, and in some cases, lights, started a campaign to improve conditions (7). She succeeded in advocating for the development of mental health hospitals run by state governments in the U.S.and Europe (7).
	1870s	A study of sexual behavior defines a "third sex"—homosexuality-- to describe same-sex relations and transgender/gender non-conforming behavior. Homosexuality was considered morally neutral and the result of "inversion"—changes in the brain while in the womb (8).
	1930s	Throughout the early 1900's, Freud developed the theory that homosexuality is a result of early childhood experiences (8). Shock therapy and lobotomy became popular treatments for "curing" mental illness.
	1940s	The National Institutes of Mental Health (NIMH) was established 1949, aimed at preventing, curing, or aiding in the recovery of mental illnesses (10). Homosexuality was conceptualized as an "illness" that needed treatment in institutions and via psychoanalysis, a belief which continued through the 1970s (8).
	1950s	The first effective anti-psychotic drugs were introduced, behavioral therapy was implemented on a broad scale, and the number of people in mental health institutions reached its peak (560,000 in 1955) (11). The first Statistical Manual of Mental Disorders (DSM) was published, which classified homosexuality alongside other sexual "disorders" (8).
Deinstitutionalization	1960s	The Mental Retardation Facilities and Community Mental Health Centers Construction Act provided federal money to develop community-based mental health services (7) . Public opinion of institutionalization suffered (11). The gay rights movement garnered more publicity and public attention (8).
	1970s	Due to increased symptom management by drugs and therapy, newly prevalent community-based mental health services, and the changing cultural perception of mental health institutions, the number of people institutionalized started to decline (11). Many people who left institutions were met with inadequate housing and follow-up care.
	1980s	LGBT and GNC people became disproportionately represented among the homeless. Rates of mental illnesses among homeless populations increased. An estimated 1/3 of all people experiencing homelessness were found to suffer from a serious mental illness (11). Homosexuality was no longer classified as a mental disorder in the DSM-III; however, Gender Identity Disorder was added (63).
Incarceration	1990s	Many people suffering from serious mental illnesses were unable to find adequate housing or mental health care, and ended up incarcerated (11). Series of policies criminalized substance abuse, leading to an increase in the number of people incarcerated for nonviolent drug law violations from 50,000 in 1980 to 400,000 in 1997 (12). Conversion therapies aimed at changing homosexual orientation continued despite criticism (8).
	2000s	High rates of mental illness among incarcerated populations continued. By midyear in 2005, more than half of the incarcerated population in the U.S. suffered from a mental illness (11). According to Bureau of Justice Statistics, between 2002 and 2004 56% of people incarcerated in State prisons, 45% of people incarcerated in Federal prisons, and 64% of people incarcerated in jails suffered from a mental illness (13).
	Current	In 2012, one in every 35 adults in the U.S. was on probation, parole, or incarcerated in prison or jail, with 6,937,600 adults under the supervision of the correctional system (14). Currently, half of males and 75% of females who are incarcerated in state prisons and 63% of males and 75% of females incarcerated in jails experience mental health problems that merit services each year (13). LGBT and GNC people (particularly youth) have a higher likelihood of having mental health issues and being incarcerated (2). While we have seen a slight decrease in incarceration, rates remain high.

Fig. 13.2 A brief history of mental healthcare

had particularly adverse effects on the lives of LGBT and GNC people. The history of mental healthcare in the USA can be considered in three distinct phases: institutionalization, deinstitutionalization, and incarceration; the term transinstitutionalization refers to the transition from treating mental health issues via institutionalization to incarceration. Figure 13.2 provides a brief history of mental healthcare in the USA, highlighting the three stages of transinstitutionalization.

The Shift from Mental Health Hospitals to Incarceration

The stated goal of deinstitutionalization was to allow people suffering from mental illnesses the ability to live more independent and full lives; the reality of deinstitutionalization, however, has been far different. The closure of mental health hospitals overwhelmed communities and families with individuals who had complex psychosocial and healthcare needs and eventually contributed to high rates of incarceration through a process often referred to as transinstitutionalization. Several factors contributed to transinstitutionalization, including the cost of healthcare for families and communities and high rates of dual diagnoses of substance use disorder and mental illness. These general trends were exacerbated among LGBT and GNC people, coinciding with a period of zero tolerance, as well as increased criminalization of LGB sexuality and transgender and GNC gender expression. Furthermore, the pathologization of LGBT and GNC individuals that contributed to high rates of institutionalization had far-reaching consequences that contributed to their later incarceration—such as the archetypes of "deviant" sexuality in need of treatment which were repurposed as "deviant" sexuality in need of punishment [4] through the process of transinstitutionalization.

Cost for Families and Communities

When institutions for people suffering from mental health diagnoses were closed, families often took on the burden of paying for and providing care [11]. The expectation that families could or would take on the financial and interpersonal burdens of mental healthcare was particularly unrealistic for LGBT and GNC people. For example, Hunt and Moodie-Mills have found that LGBT youth are far more likely to have experienced family rejection and are forced to fend for themselves financially [6]. According to the Substance Abuse and Mental Health Services Administration (SAMHSA), the estimated total costs associated with treating people with serious mental illnesses in 2014 were $239 billion [15]. The process of deinstitutionalization caused a shift of the financial burden of care from the government to the families and communities to which individuals were released [11, 16]. This burden was particularly difficult for lower-income families or families from historically marginalized populations, such as genderqueer individuals who already faced barriers to access for healthcare [17]. The end result was that some families were unable to afford or did not have suitable access to adequate mental healthcare services. Furthermore, families who were unable to attain adequate care were more likely to

be from low-income communities in which there were insufficient resources for community healthcare provision. This resulted in a disproportionate number of people suffering from mental illnesses in low-income areas, or from historically marginalized populations, to go untreated or to self-medicate with substances. This in turn contributed to increased criminalization of these communities and subsequent incarceration rates.

Dual Diagnosis with Substance Use Disorders

Many people who suffer from a mental illness have a dual diagnosis with substance use disorder. According to the National Alliance on Mental Illness (NAMI), approximately one third of people experiencing mental illness and half of people experiencing severe mental illness also struggle with substance misuse issues [18]. Additionally, approximately one third of people who abuse alcohol and half of people who misuse drugs suffer from a mental illness [18]. In 2005, the Bureau of Justice Statistics reported that over one third (37%) of individuals with mental health diagnoses in state prisons were using drugs at the time of offense, compared to around a quarter (26%) of individuals without mental health problems [13]. One study looking at "postbooking" jail diversion programs for adults with dual diagnoses of mental health illness and substance misuse in Hawaii found that substance misuse was a more significant causal factor for criminal offenses [19]. This indicates that substance use increases the likelihood of incarceration, meaning that someone with a mental health issue who has lower access to healthcare, such as an LGBT or GNC-identified individual, is at increased risk of being incarcerated for misusing illicit substances. Another study comparing offending and violence rates between patients with dual diagnoses and patients with mental illness alone found that those in the group with dual diagnoses were more likely to have a criminal history, although there were no significant group differences as far as history of violence specifically [20].

The Current State of Mental Healthcare

Simultaneous with the closure of mental health institutions and the increasing criminalization of mental health disorders, access to quality mental healthcare was difficult to attain. A recent study found that between 2012 and 2013, 57.2% of adults suffering from a mental illness received no treatment, with Vermont reporting the lowest prevalence of untreated adults with serious mental illnesses (41.7%) and Nevada reporting the highest (70.7%) [21]. In addition, more than 20% of adults in the USA with a mental illness reported that they were unable to access necessary treatment [21].

LGB individuals report experiencing discrimination at a higher rate than their heterosexual counterparts and, additionally, perceived discrimination is positively correlated with indicators of psychiatric morbidity, meaning that LGB individuals are more likely to experience mental health issues as a result of discrimination [22]. These findings have been confirmed in several other studies; for example, Meyer found that experiences of stigma, prejudice, and discrimination contribute to a stressful social environment and subsequent high rates of mental health problems [23]. LGBT individuals are at even higher risk than heterosexual, cisgender individuals of experiencing mental health issues. LGBT youth are more than twice as likely to take drugs or alcohol, and only 37% of LGBT youth report being happy (compared to 67% of non-LGBT youth) [24]. In addition, LGB youth are four times more likely to attempt suicide than their heterosexual peers [25].

Unfortunately, currently available options for provision of mental healthcare may be particularly inaccessible to or problematic for LGBT and GNC individuals. We will consider three loci in which mental healthcare is rendered in the USA today: (1) community-based mental health services, (2) institutions for the mentally ill, and (3) the criminal justice system.

Community-Based Mental Health Services

The current trend in mental healthcare favors community-based services over institutional care, such that community-based mental health services are considered the standard of care in the USA [26]. Unfortunately, however, cost is often a barrier to accessing care in community-based settings. A recent study reported that 8 million adults with mental illnesses (18.5%) were uninsured between 2012 and 2013 [21]. In 2014, 27% of uninsured Americans did not seek needed treatment due to cost [27]. Furthermore, having insurance does not necessarily grant access to mental healthcare. People with mental health issues in certain regions, like Massachusetts or Washington, DC, reported being unable to access care due to the inadequacy of their health insurance [21]. Of adults with a disability in the USA, 25.5% (1.2 million) were unable to see a healthcare provider due to cost [21]. The rates of access to mental healthcare are even lower for youth. Nearly 65% of youth with major depression do not receive any mental health treatment, and of those who do, many do not receive the level of care they need [21]. In fact, Mental Health America found that only 21.7% of youth with severe depression received "consistent treatment" (defined as 7–25+ visits per year) [21]. While the treatment of mental illnesses may ideally be delivered in community-based settings, several factors prohibit access and lead individuals to seek care in less desirable venues.

LGBT populations are also likely to find cost a barrier to community mental health treatment. Four in ten of LGBT people who had an income under 400% of the federal poverty level delayed engagement in care because of cost [28]. In addition, those who identify as LGB more often report unmet medical needs and less often report having a usual source of care [29]. Transgender individuals specifically are much less likely to be covered by health insurance, have access to care, and, even if insured, to have coverage for transgender-specific health services such as surgical treatment for gender transition and hormone therapy [28].

Institutions for the Mentally Ill

While most institutions that provide mental healthcare were closed during deinstitutionalization, around 200 state hospitals remain open and operational today. Despite the small number of state-run psychiatric hospitals, they accounted for nearly one third of state mental health agency (SMHA) budgets in 2006, totaling $7.7 billion [26]. A recent study found that the current role of state psychiatric hospitals is to house "populations deemed inappropriate for other settings" (p. 679), targeting three primary populations: forensic patients (people deemed incompetent to stand trial or not guilty by reason of insanity), sexually dangerous persons, and difficult-to-discharge patients [26]. This same study argued that the diminishing economic climate at the turn of the twenty-first century complicates efforts to close the last psychiatric hospitals. Community-based healthcare services do not have enough funding to accommodate mentally ill patients with extremely high needs [26]. Additionally, psychiatric hospitals do not have enough staff to prepare patients for successful discharge [26]. A study in Washington State found that 44% of people discharged from mental health hospitals were readmitted within 540 days [30]. While information on currently institutionalized LGBT and GNC people is difficult to come by, a study by Orel found that middle- to older-aged LGBT participants expressed the legality of their relationships as a primary concern, fearing that their living wills and power of attorney would not be sufficient to guarantee them in-home care as opposed to institutionalization [31]. Institutionalization remains a pressing concern for LGBT and GNC communities.

Criminal Justice System

While the criminal justice system was not intended or designed to serve as a method of healthcare provision, it currently does provide healthcare for the growing population of people who are currently incarcerated, including disproportionate numbers of LGBT and GNC people. Incarceration is associated with a variety of negative outcomes, such as higher occurrences of mental and physical health concerns [32], economic immobility [33], high rates of discrimination [34], and high rates of future or lifetime incarceration [35]. Beginning in the late 1970s, the USA began to experience an unprecedented era of incarceration. While due in part to changes in mental healthcare (as noted previously), this was largely due to the "War on Drugs."

Policies related to mass incarceration, including the War on Drugs, have had dramatic implications for people who suffer from mental illness, including those who are LGBT and/or GNC. The strict policies associated with the War on Drugs have been credited, in part, for the criminalization of mental illness in the USA. Criminologists continue to debate the roles of these various policies in the process of increasing incarceration rates, and have been unable to provide robust evidence as to the root cause [36] because these policies are highly embedded within a complex context that makes it difficult to tease apart cause and effect. However, there is an agreement in the literature that several key policies, including the War on Drugs, influenced both the criminalization of mental illness and sentencing policies and that these policies also influenced the disproportionate incarceration of LGBT and GNC people. Drug and alcohol use rates are higher among LGBT people than the general population. A review of the existing literature on drug and alcohol rates for LGBT people by SAMHSA found that 30% of lesbians struggle with alcohol abuse, that 20–25% of LG people are heavy alcohol users (as opposed to 3–10% of heterosexual people), that gay men are more likely to use drugs (including marijuana, psychedelics, hallucinogens, stimulants, and cocaine), and that LGBT people are more likely to use so-called party drugs, such as ecstasy and ketamine [37]. A meta-analysis of studies looking at sexual minority drug use found that LGB youth were nearly twice as likely to use substances [38]. A study that sought to explore the relationship between sexual and gender minority stress, substance use, and suicidality found that LGBT substance use was an insidious coping response to victimization on the basis of LGBT identity and had deleterious effects on suicidality [39]. Russel, Driscoll, and Truong found that LGB youth were more likely to use substances, and had different trajectories of substance use [40]. Additionally, SAMHSA found that LGBT people who are struggling with substance use disorders may be less likely to seek treatment for fear of discrimination from treatment providers or compounding discrimination if their sexual orientation, gender identity, and substance use disorders were to be discovered [37].

Incarceration and Mental Health

In 2015, the Los Angeles County Jail was reported to be the largest provider of mental healthcare in the USA [41]. People suffering from mental illnesses are three times more likely to be in jail or prison than in mental health facilities and 40% of people with a diagnosis of severe mental illness are under the supervision of the criminal justice system [42]. Some people with mental illnesses also end up in diversion programs, such as drug court, or referral out to community-based mental health courts [16]. Others are not as fortunate. According to a 2003 report by Human Rights Watch, which may still have some applicability in the current criminal justice system, "in the most extreme cases, conditions [in jail/prison] are truly horrific: mentally ill prisoners locked in segregation with no treatment at all; confined in filthy and beastly hot cells; left for days covered in feces they have smeared over their bodies; taunted, abused, or ignored by prison staff" [43, p. 2]. The current state of healthcare provision relies disproportionately upon the criminal justice system as a provider of care, especially for LGBT people who experience disproportionately high levels of trauma, victimization, and mental health illness. Furthermore, LGBT adults and youth experience social isolation and family exclusion, and this diminished safety net increases the risk of incarceration. Unfortunately, the health care received in justice settings can be inadequate [43], and the disadvantage associated with incarceration can have deleterious effects on long-term health [44] and economic mobility and gain [33]. These issues will be discussed at length later in the chapter.

Prevalence and Impact of Incarceration on LGBT People

Mass incarceration, coupled with transinstitutionalization, has had adverse effects on the health and well-being of LGBT people. Mass incarceration is a term that describes the rise in incarceration rates in the USA by more than 300% over the past 30 years [45]. Mass incarceration disproportionately impacts marginalized populations, such as people who identify as African American [46], Latino or Hispanic [47], or those who identify as LGBT [48]. Mogul, Ritchie, and Whitlock argue that the regulation of sexualities and gender expressions that are considered "deviant" by the dominant cultural narrative has always been a paramount feature of the justice system in the USA, making incarceration a highly dangerous proposition for LGBT people in particular [4]. To illustrate, these authors state, "prisons are places where deviance from gender and sexual norms is punished through sexual systemic violence, forced segregation, and denial of sexual and gender expression and failure to provide medically necessary treatment for the conditions deemed queer" [4, p. 95–96].

Prevalence of Incarceration Among LGBT Individuals

Identifying the number of LGBT individuals involved in the criminal justice system is challenging [49]. When gender identity or sexual orientation is queried (some data collection systems do not include LGBT or GNC status), data collection often relies on self-report, which can be highly unreliable, especially in coercive and controlled settings. Justice-involved individuals may hide their LGBT status for fear of punishment or discrimination by other inmates or correctional staff.

Arrest and Incarceration of LGBT Adults

Adults who identify as LGBT are more likely to be questioned by the police, engage in what is often referred to as "survival crime" such as sex work, and be incarcerated. The National Center for Transgender Equality [50] found that one in six transgender people has been incarcerated (16%), whereas the Bureau of Justice Statistics estimates that only 5.1% of all persons in the USA will be incarcerated during their life [51]. In addition, 21% of transgender women and 47% of Black transgender people have been incarcerated in their lifetime [50]. Another recent study found that 19.3% of transgender women reported being incarcerated during their lifetime [52]. This same study also reported that transgender women who were Black and Native American/Alaskan Native were more likely than their White (non-Hispanic) counterparts to report a history of incarceration [52]. Mandatory minimum sentencing (which disproportionately affects racial minorities and the poor, both of which have high representation among transgender people), the federalization of crimes, and the abolishment of parole for people reentering the community from prison are factors that have influenced the disproportionately high representation of transgender people in the criminal justice system [50].

Juveniles

LGBT youth are significantly overrepresented in the juvenile justice system, with an estimated 300,000 LGBT youth having contact with the juvenile justice system each year. While LGBT youth comprise 13–15% of justice-involved youth, they only represent five to seven percent (5–7%) of the youth population [6]. In addition, LGBT youth are disproportionately arrested and/or detained for nonviolent crimes [49]. Research has found that youth who identify as LGBT are twice as likely to be arrested and detained for nonviolent crimes than their heterosexual peers [48, 53]. One study identified detainment for truancy, warrants, probation

violations, running away, and prostitution as key areas of disproportion [48]. There were no differences in detention rates for LGBT youth for serious violent crimes, however, indicating that the overrepresentation of LGBT youth in the criminal justice system centers around nonviolent offenses.

Several possible reasons for the disproportionate rate of incarceration among LGBT youth have been proposed. For instance, a study by Majd, Marksamer, and Reyes identified several factors that may be associated with the increased risk of detention among LGBT youth [54]. They found that disproportionate detention centered around juvenile justice professionals (including judges and court personnel) perceiving that LGBT youth lack family support, misperceptions that LGBT youth are "aggressive," and misconceptions that LGBT youth are more likely to reoffend [54]. Hunt and Moodie-Mills argue that family rejection, homelessness, and failed safety nets put LGBT youth at a higher risk of incarceration and that family rejection specifically can lead to homelessness and being pushed into the justice system [6]. Furthermore, youth who are experiencing homelessness and can no longer depend on their families to provide for them may be emotionally and physically vulnerable to abuse, coercion, and engaging in and becoming victims of survival crimes [6]. Stanley and Smith also illuminate survival crimes as a key contributor to the criminalization of LGBT youth. Survival crimes are nonviolent crimes that are committed out of desperation to survive, such as shoplifting food or prostitution in order to pay for food and shelter. Twenty-six percent (26%) of LGBT youth leave their homes at some point during their adolescence, and LGBT youth account for 40% of the youth population experiencing homelessness, despite being only 5–7% of the overall youth population [6]. These data are particularly significant because homelessness is one of the strongest predictors of contact with the juvenile justice system among LGBT youth [6]. Heightened levels of police contact can also have a disproportionate impact on LGBT youth. Police are often able to arrest and detain youth for violations that would not be considered crimes if committed by adults, such as running away or breaking curfew, leading to increased contact between the police and LGBT youth [48]. The increased risk of incarceration observed among LGBT youth is enormously troubling, as youth detention has been found to dramatically reduce educational attainment and increase long-term adult incarceration rates [55].

Specific Health-Related Concerns Relevant to LGBT Inmates

People who identify as LGBT face numerous difficulties in the carceral environment, including emotional abuse and harassment, physical abuse, sexual assault, and prolonged periods of isolation. In addition, research has shown that LGBT individuals in correctional facilities often also have issues related to the provision of medication, housing policies, discrimination and abuse by correctional staff and other inmates, and access to support systems.

Provision of Medication

While those who are incarcerated represent one of the only groups in the USA with a constitutional guarantee of medical care, gaining access to necessary medical care and medication is still a persistent issue for LGBT people [50].

Hormone Therapies

Most prisons and jails in the USA deny transgender people access to hormone therapies, despite the medical necessity of these medications for this population [4]. For example, some states have ruled that hormone therapies are "cosmetic," despite the DSM-V classification of "gender dysphoria" that categorizes hormone therapies as medically necessary. Even in states where transgender people can access their hormone therapies from prison health facilities, such prescription is under a strict regulation. Typically, a transgender person must prove that they had a legal prescription for hormones and were taking them prior to being incarcerated, which can be exceedingly difficult given the poor access to healthcare that transgender people face overall [4]. Also, hormone therapies for express purpose of gender affirmation are often not covered by medical insurance, making a prescription for hormone therapies economically unfeasible [4]. Therefore, many transgender people obtain their hormone therapies through unregulated markets, and therefore lack the documentation necessary to continue receiving treatment while incarcerated [4]. Denying hormone therapies to transgender people is associated with "extreme mental distress and anguish, leading to an increased likelihood of suicide attempt, as well as depression, heart problems, and irregular blood pressure" [4, p. 112]. In some cases, even when a transgender person is approved to receive hormone therapy while incarcerated, it is provided sporadically, inconsistently, at inappropriate doses, and without psychological support [4]. Furthermore, the irregular administration of hormone therapies, created by the denial or mismanagement of hormone therapies while incarcerated, and the inconsistent supply of hormones that incarcerated transgender people sometimes access from the black market, may lead to adverse health effects such as an elevated risk of cancer, liver damage, depression, hypertension, and diabetes [4].

Treatment of HIV/AIDS

HIV and AIDS disproportionately affect transgender people, and men who have sex with men [56]. Although data are not comprehensive, it is believed that transgender people have the highest rate of HIV/AIDS in the world [56]. In 2010, transgender people had the highest rate of newly identified HIV-positive test results in the USA (2.1%), compared to females (0.4%) and males (1.2%) [57]. From 2007 to 2011, there were 191 new diagnoses of HIV among transgender people in New York City, and 99% of those infections were among transgender women [57]. Additionally, 51% of those transgender women had a documented history of substance misuse or incarceration [57]. The testing for and treatment of HIV/AIDS for incarcerated transgender people or men who have sex with men is important for the health and well-being of these populations. Some LGBT people have been denied treatment or testing while incarcerated [4]. Historically, people who are HIV positive have suffered discrimination, and HIV-positive people have also died at higher rates by preventable diseases [4]. Mogul, Ritchie, and Whitlock describe circumstances at the Limestone Correctional Facility in Alabama between the late 1980s and early 2000s in which HIV-positive people were housed in a segregated unit which was crowded and vermin infested [4]. Many of the people in this separated unit were suffering from chronic health conditions and an outbreak of staphylococcus infections, and were essentially abandoned in this segregated unit until the Southern Center for Human Rights sued the Alabama Department of Corrections and the private prison healthcare service company [4]. An infectious disease specialist reviewed the case and found that nearly all of the 43 people who died in this unit between 1999 and 2003 died of preventable illnesses because of the failure to provide proper medical care [4]. Lastly treatment and testing for HIV and AIDS often comes with a violation of confidentiality for LGBT people [4]. Because LGBT people often already face elevated rates of discrimination and inadequate healthcare, added stigmatization resulting from prison employees and other inmates knowing that an LGBT person has HIV or AIDS can be particularly dangerous.

Housing Policies

The evaluation of LGBT status during jail or prison intake can be used in housing decisions to separate individuals who are LGBT from the general population [58]. Depending on the circumstance and the individual, separate housing may be either beneficial (i.e., afford protection) or punitive (i.e., result in further stigma and isolation). Unfortunately, such housing decisions, made at the sole discretion of prison officials, are frequently used to punish and regulate what is considered by dominant cultural narratives to be "deviant" sexuality or gender expression. Housing incarcerated adults who identify as LGBT in separate units can increase the risk of abuse depending on what other individuals are also housed in these separate units [4]. On the other hand, many LGBT people suffer extremely high rates of abuse (physical and sexual) in general population housing. Mogul, Ritchie, and Whitlock describe the story of one Black gay man, Roderick Johnson, who was incarcerated in 1999 [4]. Originally placed in safe housing, he was eventually transferred to a maximum-security prison where he was housed in the general population, where he experienced repeated rapes which were not investigated and was traded as a commodity, masturbated on, and physically assaulted when he refused to perform sexual acts. At one point, he was even punished by loss of recreation and commissary privileges after being forced into performing a sexual act with another inmate. Despite experiencing horrific violence and abuse, Johnson's requests for safe and separate housing were repeatedly denied [4].

In other circumstances, the placement of LGBT people in special "protection" units can be harmful. Some jails and prisons have administrative segregation units for vulnerable or at-risk individuals where people have less access to social interaction with their peers and severely limited access to programs; LGBT people are also subjected to solitary confinement at higher rates than their heterosexual and gender binary counterparts [4]. Tellingly, Mogul, Ritchie, and Whitlock also describe the story of one inmate who explained that the psychological toll of solitary confinement was worse than the experience of rape and abuse that he suffered in the general population [4].

Housing placement is even more influential for transgender and gender nonconforming people. Typically, transgender people are placed in sex-segregated facilities based on their genitalia [4]. This can be particularly dangerous for transgender women, who are often targets of abuse and harassment in male prisons [4]. The primary justification for placing transgender women in male prisons is due to fear that transgender women pose a threat to other women [4]. This fear is underwritten by the dangerous and untrue archetype of transgender women as sexually degraded predators [4]. Transgender people are also more likely to be placed inappropriately in medical wings, as a consequence of untrue archetypes of transgender and gender nonconforming people as mentally ill [4].

Treatment by Correction Staff and Fellow Inmates
The Bureau of Justice Statistics found that of incarcerated adults in federal prisons who identified as bisexual, homosexual, gay or lesbian, or other sexual orientation minority, 11.2% reported being sexually victimized by another inmate (compared to 1.3% of incarcerated adults who identified as being heterosexual) and 6.6% reported being sexually victimized by a staff member (compared to 2.5% of incarcerated adults who identified as heterosexual) [59]. Similarly, among incarcerated adults who identified as bisexual, homosexual, gay or lesbian, or other sexual orientation minority in jails, 7.2% reported being sexually victimized

by another inmate (compared to 1.1% for their heterosexual peers) and 3.5% reported being sexually victimized by staff members (compared to 1.9% of their heterosexual peers) [59]. The Bureau of Justice Statistics found that after controlling for variables, "an inmate's sexual orientation remained an important predictor of (sexual) victimization" [59, p. 15].

Transgender and gender nonconforming people also face high rates of physical abuse and sexual abuse. The Justice Department emphasized in a 2012 report that GNC individuals face particularly high levels of sexual victimization [58]. Mogul, Ritchie, and Whitlock argue that transgender men and women who are perceived as gay or effeminate are at particularly high risk for sexual abuse, as they occupy the bottom rung of the prison hierarchy [4]. These investigators also emphasized that transgender women, in addition to the abuse and discrimination they face as a result of identifying as transgender women, are also exposed to added sexual degradation and harassment that women experience, such as, "excessive, abusive, and invasive searches, groping their breasts, buttocks, or genitalia, repeatedly leering at the while they shower, disrobe, or use the bathroom" [4, p. 101].

Majd, Marksamer, and Reyes found that LGBT youth experienced physical and emotional abuse, sexual assault, harassment by guards and peers, and prolonged periods of isolation [54]. Wesley Ware wrote, "nowhere in the literature regulation and policing of gender and sexuality, particularly of low-income queer and trans youth of color, so apparent than in the juvenile courts and in the juvenile justice system" [48]. The Bureau of Justice Statistics found that youth who identified as nonheterosexual reported disproportionate rates of youth-on-youth sexual victimization compared to their heterosexual counterparts (10.3% versus 1.5%, respectively); however, rates of reported staff-on-youth sexual victimization were similar for both heterosexual and nonheterosexual youth [60].

In response to the high rates of sexual assault and victimization of incarcerated individuals, the Prison Rape Elimination Act (PREA) was signed into law in 2003, and a comprehensive set of regulations was implemented in 2012 [58]. In the final summary of the PREA regulations, the Department of Justice emphasized the particular vulnerability of LGBT individuals in justice settings, especially those whose "appearance and manner does not conform to traditional gender expectations" [58]. Among the protections afforded to transgender people by the PREA is the right to request private showers; such rights are outlined for prison staff in an LGBT training guide [50]. The PREA Resource Center revised the protocol for screening and searching transgender prisoners in 2013 [50]. Although the PREA regulations can be leveraged to reduce the violence that LGBT people face while incarcerated, the ACLU warns that some facilities or systems may not be updated [58]. Furthermore, the PREA regulations require adults to be screened within 72 h of intake to assess their risk of sexual victimization and abuse, which includes an evaluation of the likelihood that an individual may be perceived as LGBT [58].

Access to Support Systems

Prisons and jails in the USA enforce strict rules against any sexual contact—inmate on inmate or staff on inmate. Some argue that while in theory these policies are meant to protect incarcerated people from unwanted sexual contact or attention, in reality the idea of situational homosexuality (sex among same-sex inmates who identify as heterosexual when outside of carceral settings) is considered a threat to the presumption of normalcy and heteronormativity [4]. This "threat" of homosexuality can lead to increased monitoring of LGB nonsexual relationships and forced isolation of LGB people from their peers [4]. Furthermore, LGB people can be cut off from their outside support systems. While heterosexual couples are allowed to embrace during visitation times, homosexual couples are often not permitted to do so and even cited an instance where a homosexual couple embraced and were threatened with loss of future visitation [4]. Furthermore, before the legalization of same-sex marriage, conjugal visits for homosexual partners were not allowed in four out of the five states in which such visits were permissible for other inmates [4].

Specific Mental Health Issues Among Justice-Involved LGBT Individuals

Incarceration has far-reaching effects on both health and health-seeking behaviors [61]. In particular, justice-involved LGBT individuals face specific mental health issues, including increased levels of anxiety and stress, issues of self-esteem, and post-traumatic stress disorder (PTSD).

Increased Levels of Anxiety and Stress

The carceral environment can lead to increased levels of anxiety and stress through stereotype threat—the fear or risk of confirming stereotypes related to a minority group one identifies with, the constant threat of violence, and the strict regulation of gender expression and sexuality. Increased anxiety and stress may also lead to clinical depression [62]. Incarcerated LGBT people may develop psychological adaptations in response to the high levels of stress and anxiety, including distrust, hypervigilance, and isolation [62]. While these adaptations might seem dysfunctional or even pathological in a community context, these psychological processes and coping mechanisms represent normal responses to the pathological context of prison or jail [62].

Issues of Self-Esteem

Transgender people who are denied access to necessary hormone therapies may suffer from issues of self-esteem upon release. The physical and psychological effects of hormone deprivation can leave transgender people trapped in a space between womanhood and manhood, unable to express their true gender identity [4]. The repression of identity is correlated with issues of self-esteem that can lead to social isolation, depression, self-harm, and suicidal ideation. A study by Nuttbrock, Rosenblum, and Bluminstein found that identity affirmation was crucial for the emotional well-being of transgender people [63]. Transgender identity affirmation was conceptualized as the extent to which transgender identity is disclosed and recognized by others, preformed and supported by others, and incorporated successfully in social roles and relationships [63]. The carceral environment for most transgender people limits the ability of identity affirmation through social isolation, regulation of identity, and the denial of hormone therapies.

Post-traumatic Stress Disorder

LGBT people are at an increased risk of being raped or sexually assaulted during incarceration. Additionally, more than two third of people who are raped in prison are raped multiple times, making the negative effects on their health and likelihood of PTSD even higher [64]. Neal and Clements found that people who were sexually assaulted by other prisoners were physically injured 70% of the time, whereas people who were sexually assaulted by correctional staff were physically injured 50% of the time, indicating that prisoner-on-prisoner rape can be particularly traumatic [64]. Furthermore, rape, particularly brutal or repeated rape, has been found to be associated with PTSD [65], meaning that LGBT people who have been sexually assaulted or raped while incarcerated are at risk for PTSD. Moreover, researchers have found a link between PTSD manifestations among people who have been raped and negative social reactions such as coping avoidance [66]. LGBT people who have been raped during incarceration may exhibit additional symptoms beyond PTSD, such as depression, anger, guilt, disruption of belief systems, and sexual dysfunction [64].

Mental Deterioration

Transgender and gender nonconforming people who have been incarcerated in solitary confinement for prolonged periods of time may suffer from mental deterioration due to sensory deprivation [4]. Mogul, Ritchie, and Whitlock described punitive segregation units in which transgender and gender nonconforming people were caged 23 h a day for 7 days a week without television, radio, or personal contact [4]. This extreme level of sensory deprivation, over a prolonged period of time can cause people to lose the ability to concentrate, to hallucinate, and in some cases to lose their aptitude for social interaction [4].

The Future of LGBT Justice-Involved Individuals: Returning to a Public Health Paradigm

Incarceration rates have seen a slight decline over the last few years, but rates remain at historically high levels [67] and LGBT individuals are still disproportionately represented in correctional facilities. However, there is a swelling national movement to identify and understand the harms that incarceration is causing among the most disproportionately impacted populations and to return to a public health paradigm for mental health and substance use disorder treatment. For LGBT populations specifically, numerous policy and legal shifts have facilitated improved access to medical care and health insurance coverage, including passage of the Affordable Care Act and the recent Supreme Court overturning of the Defense of Marriage Act. However, much work remains to be done.

Decriminalization of Substance Use and Mental Illness

Recent initiatives have devoted time and energy to developing programs such as "prebooking" diversion, which gives police officers the discretion to take a person with a substance use or mental health issue to a treatment facility rather than to jail. In addition, drug court and mental health courts have been established in states across the nation and research shows that they work. Findings from Virginia recently showed that on average drug courts cost taxpayers less money and that participants recidivated less often. Other alternatives to incarceration that deploy therapeutic techniques should be used more often as more and more advocates (see decarceration.org) are calling for an expanded era of decarceration. Criminal justice-involved LGBT populations, who often experience worse outcomes while incarcerated, would benefit exponentially from continued progression away from mass incarceration. However, given that correctional facilities are one of the largest "providers" of mental health services in the USA, and that structural change often happens gradually, there is also a need to consider the current context of incarceration and its impact on LGBT individuals specifically. Jails and prisons should engage in training for correctional workers in an attempt to lessen the prevalence of LGBT-related stigma and discrimination. Additionally, housing policies should be thoughtfully considered with an eye toward the collateral consequences of solitary confinement and policies that house

people solely according to their biological sex. Research exploring the specific impact of incarceration on the physical and mental health of LGBT individuals is still nascent and much remains to be learned. Future studies must endeavor to elucidate how best to identify LGBT individuals in carceral settings, effective policies to protect LGBT people, and the impact of incarceration on LGBT populations over the life course. While mental healthcare has evolved for the better over the years, further improvement is still needed. For LGBT persons who suffer from both mental illness and co-occurring substance use, incarceration is a very real possibility, and stigma related to each problem can compound the challenges and result in destabilization. Research and advocacy efforts must continue so that, in the future, mental health and substance use can be addressed concurrently and without inflicting further harm on the lives of already vulnerable populations.

References

1. Ard K, Makadon H. Improving the healthcare of lesbian, gay, bisexual, and transgender (LGBT) people: understanding and eliminating health disparities. Boston: The Fenway Institute, Fenway Health; 2012.
2. National Center for Transgender Equality. Standing with LGBT prisoners: an advocate's guide to ending abuse and combating imprisonment. 2014. Retrieved 6 Mar 2016 from http://www.transequality.org/issues/resources/standing-lgbt-prisoners-advocate-s-guide-ending-abuse-and-combating-imprisonment.
3. Fredriksen-Goldsen KI. Resilience and disparities among lesbian, gay, bisexual, and transgender older adults. Public Policy Aging Rep. 2011;21(3):3–7.
4. Mogul JL, Ritchie AJ, Whitlock K. Queer injustice: the criminalization of LGBT people in the U.S. Boston: Beacon Press; 2011.
5. Muraco A, Fredriksen-Goldsen K. "That's what friends do": informal caregiving for chronically ill midlife and older lesbian, gay, and bisexual adults. J Soc Pers Relat. 2011;28(8):1073–92.
6. Hunt J, Moodie-Mills AC. The unfair criminalization of gay and transgender youth: and overview of the experiences of LGBT youth in the juvenile justice system. Washington, DC: Center for American Progress; 2012.
7. Parry MS. Dorothea Dix (1802–1887). Am J Public Health. 2006;96(4):624–5.
8. Holler J. Pathologizing sexuality and gender: a brief history. Ment Health Addict J. 2010;6(2):7–9.
9. Freeman W, Watts JW, Hunt T. Psychosurgery: intelligence, emotion, and social behavior following prefrontal lobotomy for mental disorders. London: Bailliére, Tindal & Cox; 1942.
10. National Institutes of Health. National Institute of Mental Health (NIMH) mission. 2016. Retrieved 6 Mar 2016 from http://www.nih.gov/about-nih/what-we-do/nih-almanac/national-institute-mental-health-nimh.
11. PBS Online. Timeline: treatments for mental illnesses. Retrieved 4 Feb 2016 from PBS Online: http://www.pbs.org/wgbh/amex/nash/timeline/index.html.
12. Drug Policy Alliance. A brief history of the Drug War. 2016. Retrieved 6 Mar 2016 from http://www.drugpolicy.org/new-solutions-drug-policy/brief-history-drug-war.

13. James DJ, Glaze LE. Mental health problems of prison and jail inmates. Washington, DC: Bureau of Justice Statistics; 2006.
14. Glaze LE, Herberman EJ. Correctional populations in the U.S., 2012. Washington, DC: Bureau of Justice Statistics; 2013.
15. Levit KR, Kassed CA, Coffrey RM, Mark TL, McKusick DR, King E, Vandivort R, Buck J, Ryan K, Strangers E. Projections of national expenditures for mental health services and substance abuse treatment. Rockville: Substance Abuse and Mental Health Services Administration; 2008.
16. Peternelj-Taylor C. Criminalization of the mentally ill. J Forensic Nurs. 2008;4(4):185–7.
17. Richards C, Bouman WP, Seal L, Barker MJ, Nieder TO, T'Sjoen G. Non-binary or genderqueer genders. Int Rev Psyc. 2016;28 (1):95–102.
18. National Alliance on Mental Illness. Public Policy Platform. 2016. Retrieved from http://www.nami.org/getattachment/Learn-More/ Mental-Health-Public-Policy/Public-Policy-Platform-up-to-12-09-16.pdf.
19. Junginger J, Claypoole K, Laygo R, Crisanti A. Effect of serious mental illness and substance abuse on criminal offenses. Psychiatr Serv. 2006;57(6):879–82.
20. Wright S, Gournay K, Glorney E, Thornifcroft G. Mental illness, substance abuse, demographics and offending: dual diagnosis in the suburbs. J Forensic Psyc. 2002;13(1):35–52.
21. Nguyen T, Davis K, Counts N, Fritze D. The state of mental health in America: Mental Health America; 2016.
22. Mays VM, Cochran SD. Mental health correlates of perceived discrimination among lesbian, gay, and bisexual adults in the U.S. Am J Public Health. 2001;91(11):1869–76.
23. Meyer IH. Prejudice, social stress, and mental health in lesbian, gay, and bisexual populations: conceptual issues and research evidence. Psychol Bull. 2003;129(5):674–97.
24. Human Rights Campaign. Growing up LGBT in America: HRC youth survey report key findings. Washington, DC: Human Rights Campaign; 2013.
25. Center for Disease Control and Prevention. Sexual identity, sex of sexual contacts, and health-risk behaviors among students in grades 9–12: youth risk behavior surveillance. Atlanta: Department of Health and Human Services; 2011.
26. Fisher WH, Geller JL, Pandiani JA. The changing role of the state psychiatric hospital. Health Aff. 2009;28(3):676–84.
27. Kaiser Family Foundation. Key facts about the uninsured population. 2015. Retrieved from http://kff.org/uninsured/fact-sheet/key-facts-about-the-uninsured-population/.
28. Center for American Progress. LGBT communities and the Affordable Care Act: findings from a national survey. 2013. Retrieved from https://www.americanprogress.org/wp-content/uploads/2013/ 10/LGBT-ACAsurvey-brief1.pdf.
29. Clift J, Kirby J. Healthcare access and perceptions of provider care among individuals in same-sex couples: findings from the Medical Expenditure Panel Survey (MEPS). J Homosex. 2012;59 (6):839–50.
30. Mancuso D. Quality indicators and outcomes for persons discharged from state psychiatric hospitals. Depart Soc Health Sci Res Data Anal Divi. 2015;3(41):1–10.
31. Orel NA. Investigating the needs and concerns of lesbian, gay, bisexual, transgender older adults: the use of qualitative and quantitative methodology. J Homosex. 2014;61(1):53–78.
32. Brinkley-Rubinstein L. Incarceration as a catalyst for worsening health. Health Justice. 2013;1(3):2–17.
33. Western B. The impact of incarceration on wage mobility and inequality. Am Sociol Rev. 2002;67(4):526–46.
34. LeBel TP. If one doesn't get you another one will: formerly incarcerated persons' perception of discrimination. Prison J. 2011;92(1):63–87.
35. Durose MR, Cooper AD. Recidivism of prisoners released in 30 states in 2005: patterns from 2005 to 2010. Washington, DC: Bureau of Justice Statistics; 2014.
36. Eckholm E. Prison rate was rising years before 1994 law. New York Times. 10 Apr 2016. Retrieved from http://www.nytimes.com/2016/ 04/11/us/prison-rate-was-rising-years-before-1994-law.html?_r=0.
37. Substance Abuse and Mental Health Services Administration. A providers introduction to substance abuse treatment for lesbian, gay, bisexual, and transgender individuals. U.S. Rockville: Department of Health and Human Services; 2012.
38. Marshal MP, Friedman MS, Stall R, King KM, Miles J, Gold MA, Bukstein OG, Morse JQ. Sexual orientation and adolescent substance use: a meta-analysis and methodological review. Addiction. 2008;103(4):546–56.
39. Mereish EH, O'Cleirigh C, Bradford JB. Interrelationships between LGBT-based victimization, suicide, and substance use problems in a diverse sample of sexual and gender minorities. Psychol Health Med. 2014;19(1):1–13.
40. Russell ST, Driscoll AK, Truong N. Adolescent same-sex romantic attractions and relationships: implications for substance use and abuse. Am J Public Health. 2002;92:198–202.
41. Steinberg, D, Mills, D, Romano, M. When did prisons become acceptable mental healthcare facilities? Stanford Law School—Three Strikes Project. 2012. Retrieved from http://law.stanford. edu/wp-content/uploads/sites/default/files/child-page/632655/doc/ slspublic/Report_v12.pdf.
42. Aufderheid, D. Mental illness in America's jails and prisons: toward a public safety/public health model. Health Affairs Blog. 2014.
43. Human Rights Watch. Ill-equipped: U.S. prisons and offenders with mental illness. Washington, DC: Human Rights Watch; 2003.
44. Massoglia M. Incarceration, health, and racial disparities in health. Law Soc Rev. 2008;42(2):275–306.
45. Defina R, Hannon L. The impact of mass incarceration and poverty. Crime Delinq. 2013;59(4):562–86.
46. Alexander M. The new Jim crow: mass incarceration and the age of colorblindness. New York: New Press; 2012.
47. Lopez, H, Light, MT. A raising share: hispanics and federal crime. Pew Research Center; 2009. Retrieved from http://www. pewhispanic.org/2009/02/18/a-rising-share-hispanics-and-federal-crime/.
48. Stanley EA, Smith N, editors. Captive genders: trans embodiment and the prison industrial complex. Oakland: AK Press; 2015.
49. Department of Justice Statistics. LGBTQ youths in the juvenile justice system. Washington, DC: Office of Juvenile Justice and Delinquency Prevention; 2014.
50. National Center for Transgender Equity. Reducing incarceration and ending abuse in prisons. A blueprint for equality: federal agenda for transgender people. Washington, DC: National Center for Transgender Equality; 2015. p. 41–3. It was retrieved from: http://www.transequality.org/sites/default/files/docs/resources/ NCTE_Blueprint_June2015.pdf?quot%3B=
51. Bonczar TP, Beck AJ. Special report: lifetime likelihood of going to state or federal prison. Washington, DC: Bureau of Justice Statistics; 1997.
52. Reisner SL, Bailey Z, Sevelius J. Racial/ethnic disparities in the history of incarceration, experiences of victimization, and associated health indicators among transgender women in the U.S. Women Health. 2014;54(8):750–67.
53. Heck NC, Livingston NA, Flentje A, Oost K, Stewart BT. Reducing risk for illicit drug use and prescription drug misuse: high school gray-straight alliances and lesbian, gay, bisexual, and transgender youth. Addict Behav. 2014;39(4):824–8.
54. Majd K, Marksamder J, Reyes C. Hidden injustice: lesbian, gay, bisexual, and transgender youth in the juvenile courts. San

Francisco: Legal Services for Children and National Center for Lesbian Rights; 2009.

55. Aizer A, Doyle JJ. Juvenile incarceration, human capital and future crime: evidence from randomly-assigned judges. Cambridge, MA: The National Bureau of Economic Research; 2013.

56. The Global Fund. The global fund strategy in relation to sexual orientation and gender identities. 2016. Retrieved from http://www.theglobalfund.org/documents/core/strategies/Core_SexualOrientationAndGenderIdentities_Strategy_en/.

57. Centers for Disease Control and Prevention. HIV among transgender people. 2016. Retrieved 6 Mar 2016 from http://www.cdc.gov/hiv/group/gender/transgender/.

58. ACLU. End the abuse: protecting LGBTI prisoners from sexual assault. Prison Rape Elimination Act (PREA) toolkit. 2014. Retrieved from https://www.aclu.org/sites/default/files/assets/012714-prea-combined.pdf.

59. Beck AJ, Harrison PM, Berzofsky M, Caspar R, Krebs C. Sexual victimization in prisons and jails reported by inmates, 2009–09. Washington, DC: Bureau of Justice Statistics; 2010.

60. Beck AJ, Canton D, Hartage J, Smith T. Sexual victimization in juvenile facilities reported by youth, 2012: national survey of youth in custody, 2012. Washington, DC: Bureau of Justice Statistics; 2013.

61. Bailey ZD, Williams DR, Kawachi I, Okechukwu CA. Incarceration and adult weight gain in the National Survey of American Life. Prev Med Int J. 2015;81:380–6.

62. Haney C. From prison to home: the effect of incarceration and reentry on children, families, and communities. Washington, DC: U.S. Department of Health and Human Services; 2001.

63. Nuttbrock L, Rosenblum A, Blumenstein R. Transgender identity affirmation and mental health. Int J Transgenderism. 2002;6(4). Retrieved from: http://www.symposion.com/ijt/ijtvo06no04_3.htm

64. Neal TMS, Clements CB. Prison rape and psychological sequelae: a call for research. Psychol Public Policy Law. 2010;16(3):284–99.

65. Boeschen LE, Sales BD, Koss MP. Rape trauma experts in the courtroom. Psychol Public Policy Law. 1998;4:414–32.

66. Ullman SE, Townsend SM, Filipas HH, Starzynki LL. Structural models of the relations of assault severity, social support, avoidance coping, self-blame, and PTSD among sexual assault survivors. Psychol Women Q. 2007;31:23–38.

67. Kaeble D, Glaze LE, Tsoutis A, Minton TD. Correctional populations in the United States, 2014. Washington, DC: Bureau of Justice Statistics; 2015.

An Overview of Trauma-Informed Care

14

Andrés Felipe Sciolla

Trauma-informed care (TIC) is a comprehensive approach to clinical practice that evolved from the treatment of mental health and substance misuse among populations of disenfranchised, low-income, ethnic minority women in the 1980s to encompass modifications at individual provider, team and systems levels in provision of healthcare to all patients in all settings. This evolution has been buttressed by a remarkable surge of traumatic stress-related research in multiple disciplines over the last two decades. Both clinical experience and research suggest strongly that patient care should reflect an awareness of the prevalence and impact of trauma in the lives of patients and providers and should offer conditions for recovery from exposure to traumatic experiences, such as feeling safe and minimizing the risk for retraumatization.

This chapter begins with an overview of TIC from an historical perspective, describing the various definitions of TIC that have emerged over the years. The chapter also features a focused discussion on the neurobiology of fear learning, including fear acquired early in life. Research into the neural basis of fear provides an empirical context to explain the emphasis of TIC on the adaptive nature of posttraumatic stress reactions (i.e., "What happened to you?" instead of "What's wrong with you?"), normalizes the persistence of such reactions, and highlights the path to recovery and resilience. In addition, the particular relevance of TIC to provision of healthcare services to LGBT individuals is reviewed while making a case for trauma-informed *approaches* in other settings where LGBT populations receive services, such as education, foster care, and corrections. The chapter closes with a discussion of current practice gaps and a critique of some features of

TIC and resilience, understood to be cultural products of highly individualistic western, educated, industrialized, rich, and democratic societies. From a global perspective, it remains to be seen how collectivistic societies, in which the majority of humans live, can adapt and test the effectiveness of TIC to their populations, including LGBT individuals, their resources, and their needs.

Definitions of TIC

Several definitions of TIC have been advanced over the years. Recently, Elizabeth Hopper and colleagues arrived at a consensus definition from a review of the literature, which contains cross-cutting themes from previous definitions:

> Trauma-Informed Care is a strengths-based framework that is grounded in an understanding of and responsiveness to the impact of trauma, that emphasizes physical, psychological, and emotional safety for both providers and survivors, and that creates opportunities for survivors to rebuild a sense of control and empowerment. [1]

These cross-cutting themes are largely captured and elaborated in the Substance Abuse and Mental Health Administration's (SAMHSA's) influential definition and promotion of a trauma-informed approach to care, which is grounded on four assumptions and six principles (Table 14.1) [2]. This approach includes understanding the definition of trauma, its impact across settings, services, and populations, and appreciating the role of context and culture on individuals' perceptions and processing of traumatic events. A later publication by SAMHSA added several key elements, including the importance of trauma screening and assessment, the difference between trauma-informed (i.e., may not target trauma sequelae) and trauma-specific (i.e., designed to target trauma sequelae) services and steps recommended to build a workforce capable of implementing TIC [3].

A.F. Sciolla, MD (✉)
University of California, Davis, Department of Psychiatry & Behavioral Sciences, 2230 Stockton Bvld, Sacramento, CA 95817, USA
e-mail: afsciolla@ucdavis.edu

© Springer International Publishing AG 2017

K.L. Eckstrand, J. Potter (eds.), *Trauma, Resilience, and Health Promotion in LGBT Patients*,
DOI 10.1007/978-3-319-54509-7_14

Table 14.1 Assumptions and principles of trauma-informed approach (SAMHSA) for human services organizations and systems [2]

Assumptions	Comments
Realize the widespread impact of trauma and potential paths for recovery	The subjective experience and overt behavior of individuals are understood as attempts at coping overwhelming events or circumstances
	Exposure to trauma plays a role in the emergence of health risk behaviors, substance use and mental disorders, as well as medical illness directly linked to (e.g., sexually transmitted infections) or mediated (e.g., cardiovascular disease) by health risk behaviors
	In addition to healthcare, opportunities for recovery are found among individuals seen in other sectors, such as schools, child welfare, criminal justice, and faith-based organizations
Recognize signs and symptoms in patients and members of the healthcare system, including staff and providers	Familiarity and recognition of signs and symptoms of traumatic exposure is achieved through timely screening and assessment, workforce development, supervision, and self-care practices
Respond by fully integrating knowledge about trauma into policies, procedures, and practices	Members at every level of the organization adapt their language, policies, and procedures to conform to the trauma-based needs of the people they serve
	Practitioners in the organization are trained in evidence-based therapies and best or promising trauma practices
	Inclusion of trauma awareness in mission statement
Resist retraumatization	Commitment to an ongoing identification and modification of organizational practices that may retraumatize staff or clients or interfere with recovery
	Maintenance of "universal precautions" (See Fig. 14.2)
Principles	Examples
Safety	The physical environment and interpersonal relationships promote a sense of physical and psychological safety, as defined by those served
Trustworthiness and transparency	Trust between clients and providers is built and maintained through operations and decisions that are transparent
Peer support	To promote recovery and healing, safety and hope, services integrate the mutual self-help and collaboration of those with lived experiences of trauma (often referred as "trauma survivors")
Collaboration and mutuality	Power differences among clients, providers, and organization members are minimized in order to promote meaningful participation in decision-making
Empowerment, voice, and choice	The primacy of the people served is affirmed, strengths are recognized and built upon, resilience and the ability to heal and recover from trauma are intrinsic to individuals, organizations, and communities
	Self-advocacy skills are cultivated and clients are given choices and supported in goal-setting
Cultural, historical, and gender Issues	The organization offers gender culture and sexual orientation-responsive services, understands the impact of historical trauma, and leverages the healing potential of traditional cultural practices

The Origins of Trauma-Informed Care

Throughout the 1980s, as homelessness, poverty, and the use of crack cocaine reached epidemic proportions in larger cities across the USA, providers of substance use and mental health services observed that childhood and adult victimization affected nearly every client they served. Among those clinicians were social worker Helen Bergman and psychologists Maxine Harris and Roger D. Fallot, founders of Community Connections, the largest private, nonprofit agency providing a full range of supportive services in the metropolitan Washington, DC, area. In a series of interviews with 99 homeless individuals, mostly African American women with serious mental illness, Harris and collaborators found extraordinarily high prevalence rates of 87% and 65%

for childhood physical and sexual abuse, respectively, and similarly high rates (87% and 76%, respectively) for adult physical and sexual assault [4]. Sadly, only 3 of the 99 women reported no experience of physical or sexual abuse in either childhood or adulthood [4]. Further analysis revealed that the degree of trauma, as measured by recentness, frequency, and number of types of exposure to violence, was positively associated with the severity of a broad range of psychiatric symptoms. The authors therefore concluded that there was an urgent need for services that would include consideration of the impact of trauma in the lives of women who are homeless [5]. Paradoxically, these women had come to view abuse and violence as normative, not their primary problem, and presented to providers with complaints of physical or mental symptoms, while accepting the psychiatric labels of "sad," "bad," or "mad" as given to them by others [6].

While acknowledging the contributions to the field of contemporary authors in diagnostic challenges [7], treatment [8], and theoretical conceptualizations regarding coping with trauma exposure [9], Harris saw the need for new treatment approaches for the women who sought help at Community Connections, whose substance misuse, and poorer mental and physical health were embedded in socio-economic disadvantage and stigmatization [6]. Because of the complexity of the relationships between trauma exposure, adaptation to trauma, and the larger socioeconomic context, treatment focused primarily on the reduction of symptoms from diagnosed posttraumatic stress disorder (PTSD) was often insufficient [10]. Moreover, these women did not have the resources to access individual therapy, were deemed too disturbed or disruptive for group therapy, and lacked the resources to sustain participation in peer-led or self-help substance recovery programs [6]. In response to these gaps, Harris and Fallot developed the Trauma Recovery and Empowerment Model (TREM), a manualized group intervention in which feminist principles are central to the intervention's empowerment goals [11]. TREM is based on four core assumptions: (1) perceived dysfunctional behaviors and/or symptoms can be legitimate coping responses to trauma; (2) women exposed to child-hood trauma frequently do not develop typical adult coping skills because of the impact of trauma on development; (3) sexual and physical abuse sever core connections to women's families, communities, and sense of self; and (4) women who have been abused repeatedly feel powerless and unable to advocate for themselves [11].

Later, in considering how mental health and substance use treatment *served* individuals exposed to childhood trauma without *treating* the sequelae of that exposure, Harris and Fallot distinguished between trauma-specific services – designed to treat the psychological and behavioral sequelae of trauma – and trauma-informed services [12]. The latter, while not designed to treat trauma sequelae per se, make the necessary accommodations to be responsive to the needs of individuals who have been exposed to trauma across a wide variety of missions (e.g., physical health, mental health, employment counseling, housing supports, etc.)[12]. Harris and Fallot listed structural and organizational conditions required to support the establishment of trauma-informed systems of care, and delineated a set of core principles that should be cultivated and maintained among the people providing services (Table 14.2).

Around the same time that Bergman, Fallot, and Harris made their observations with homeless women, psychiatrists noted a similar high prevalence of histories of abuse and violence among adult psychiatric inpatients, most of which

Table 14.2 Requirements and principles of a trauma-informed system (Harris and Fallot [12])

Requirements	1. Administrative commitment to allocate resources, set priorities, and design programs that acknowledge the role that trauma plays in the presenting problems of consumers 2. Universal screening for trauma history 3. Training and education of all staff members on trauma-related issues 4. Hiring practices that target trauma champions 5. Review policies, procedures, and practices (i.e., client–provider relationships that reenact abusive dynamics) that may retraumatize clients or trigger their trauma-based coping	
Principles	Traditional approach	Trauma-informed approach
1. Understanding trauma	Understood as a single event frequently associated with PTSD impacting predictable areas of functioning (e.g., fear and avoidance of riding or driving a car after a car accident)	Repeated traumas that challenge fundamental assumptions about the self, relationships, and the world that come to define an individual's identity and impact unpredictable areas of functioning (e.g., learning difficulties in a girl repeatedly raped by a babysitter)
2. Understanding the consumer survivor	The appreciation of the whole person is blocked by the importance of the chief presenting problem	The understanding of a problem or symptom is placed in the context of the whole individual and her or his life trajectory and context
3. Understanding services	Services are time-limited, cost-conscious, and risk-aversive, and goals are circumscribed (e.g., stabilization after a crisis)	Services are strengths-based. Emphasis on skills building, promotion of autonomy, and prevention of problematic behavior in the future. Symptom management is secondary. Risks associated with interventions are negotiated between consumers and service providers
4. Understanding the service relationship	Hierarchical relationship between a professional expert and an passive recipient of services. Trust and safety are assumed from the outset of the relationship. Can replicate dynamics of childhood trauma	Collaborative relationship in which the professional expert's recommendations can be questioned and the consumer is an active participant. Emphasis on consumer choice. Trust and safety are earned over time

were not being documented in clinical charts [13]. Among these psychiatrists was Sandra L. Bloom, whose experience adapting the therapeutic community model (or "therapeutic milieu") to this population eventually led her to develop another model of trauma-informed care – the Sanctuary Model – in the early 1990s [14]. This Model is informed by four types of evidence: the neurobiology of trauma, the creation of nonviolent environments, social learning, and the study of complex adaptive systems [15]. Specifically, Bloom and colleagues recognized the challenge of helping individuals recover from trauma when a healthcare team functions in ways reminiscent of family or other systems that caused trauma in the first place [14]. To the extent that the traumatizing system abused power, induced helplessness, manipulated information, and discouraged the expression of positive emotions while engendering negative emotions such as shame and fear, the new approach would mitigate these abuses by distributing power among patients and team members, offering options and choice, sharing information freely, maintaining safety, and avoiding retraumatization [14]. However, in Bloom's opinion, children who grow up in dysfunctional, traumatic environments often understand these systems and behaviors as normative and are more likely to propagate that abuse on themselves or others into adulthood even when the abuse causes additional suffering. As noted by Bloom, "the more dangerous the environment is and the more normalization of that environment has been mandatory to survival, the greater the resistance to change" [14].

In the Sanctuary Model, the view of mental illness itself shifted from a "sickness model" to an "injury model." The injury model encompasses the meaning of symptoms, the role of the patient, and treatment goals. Instead of equating problems to psychopathology, behavioral adaptations were viewed as stemming from developmental trauma; instead of a passive patient meeting a sickness expert, a person presenting for care was considered to be actively seeking to learn about the nature of their injuries and recovery; instead of a magical cure, the goal of treatment was to work on rehabilitation, even if this meant learning to live with limitations [14]. For Bloom, violence "[threatens] the integrity of attachment relationships" and "is broadly defined as anything that hurts the self or the community," while safety includes a moral dimension that "is an attempt to reduce the hypocrisy that is present, both explicitly and implicitly, in our social systems" [14].

In its latest iteration, published in 2013, the Sanctuary Model places even greater emphasis on organizational culture, making a distinction between trauma-organized systems (i.e., those that continuously reproduce the conditions that traumatize its members) and developmentally grounded trauma-informed systems [16]. According to Bloom, "developmentally grounded" refers to a system

built around the implications of attachment theory and neurobiology. Here Bloom expands the traditional view on attachment in psychologically intimate dyads to the relationships that develop among all members of a system or organization. Borrowing computer terminology, Bloom equates metaphorically the attachment relationships that characterize organizational culture to an "operating system" and trauma to a "virus" infecting a trauma-organized organization [16]. The trauma-informed healthy system she proposes entails the commitment to address seven "universals": (1) the inevitability of change, (2) managing power, (3) envisioning safety, (4) emotional intelligence, (5) learning all the time, (6) the constancy of communication, and (7) justice and the common good [16].

Although Bloom's Sanctuary Model has limited empirical evidence [17–19], it inspired what is arguably the most widely known dictum of TIC: a shift from the symptom-oriented, detached questioning of "What's wrong with you?" to the narrative-based, compassionate inquiry of "What happened to you?" [20].

Toward a Synthesis: Raja's Pyramid Model of Trauma-Informed Care

In a scoping review of the literature of TIC in medical settings, Raja and colleagues identified core principles of TIC in medical settings and characterized how providers can apply these principles to maximize patient engagement and empowerment [21]. Principles were divided into two domains: "universal trauma precautions" and "trauma-specific care." Because the former are foundational – used with all patients and in all settings – while the latter are appropriate in a smaller percentage of specific circumstances, these investigators arranged the core principles of TIC into a pyramid, further subdividing the two aforementioned domains to create a total of five key clinical strategies (see Fig. 14.1) [21].

A. *Universal trauma precautions.* The first domain in the pyramid contains two strategies – patient-centered care and cultural competence/humility and understanding the health effects of trauma. Individuals exposed to trauma are frequently sensitive to and react emotionally (e.g., with fear or avoidance) to the power differential that is ubiquitous in healthcare settings and encounters with providers. *Patient-centered* communication and behavioral practices [22] – care that is respectful and responsive to patient beliefs and needs in clinical decision making – are well suited to address such emotional reactions by engendering rapport, trust, and safety. To increase the applicability of patient-centeredness to diverse populations, the concept of *cultural competence*

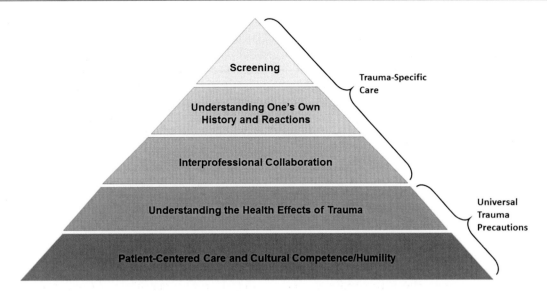

Fig. 14.1 The pyramid model of trauma-informed care. The base of the pyramid is comprised of "universal trauma precautions," the knowledge, skills, and attitudes of healthcare providers that increase the engagement – and ultimately health outcomes – of patients with trauma histories, without requiring screening or knowledge of trauma exposure. The "trauma-specific care" domain is depicted above this base and correspond to the strategies in which healthcare providers engage when a patient's trauma exposure history is known. The shape of the figure represents the recommendation that universal trauma precautions should be used with all patients, while trauma-specific care should be adopted with a smaller percentage of patients and clinical situations. Having screening for trauma on top of the pyramid reflects the fact that this topic is debated and it requires training and appropriate resources for patient referral (Reproduced from Raja et al. [21], with permission from Wolters Kluwer Health, Inc.)

– the behaviors, attitudes, and institutional policies required to effectively provide cross-cultural care – is also included at the foundational level [23]. With its explicit commitment to redressing power imbalances in the patient–provider dynamic and community-based care and advocacy [23], *cultural humility* can synergize patient-centered care, especially for patients from socially disadvantaged or stigmatized backgrounds. Such patients are not only at higher risk for exposure to traumatic events across the lifespan but also are detrimentally affected by microaggressions [24, 25], defined as "indignities, slights or insults that send a message of derogatory or negative status to members of marginalized group" [26]. The second strategy in the universal trauma precautions domain requires an *understanding [of] the health effects of trauma*. Providers commonly feel unprepared to work effectively with patients presenting with psychiatric comorbidity and health risk behaviors in so-called difficult encounters because of the negative attitudes toward or limited training in dealing with psychosocial aspects of patient care [27]. Providers may feel better able to handle this common clinical presentation if they keep in mind the health effects of trauma, which include increased prevalence of health risk behaviors such binge drinking, heavy drinking, smoking, risky HIV behavior as well as medical-psychiatric comorbidity [28]. By linking childhood adversities and self-destructive behaviors, essentially

shifting from "what's wrong with you?" to "what happened to you?" perspective, providers may be more likely to empathize with patients and minimize patient shame and maladaptive behaviors. Training programs can leverage this strategy with patient-centeredness and motivational interviewing techniques.

B. *Trauma-specific care.* The second domain in the pyramid includes three strategies: interprofessional collaboration, understanding one's own history and reactions pertaining to trauma, and trauma-screening practices. *Interprofessional collaboration* in this model underscores the importance of cultivating relationships with other providers, knowledge of their expertise or scope of practice, and education regarding trauma-specific services and resources to which patients can be referred. This includes developing a thorough understanding of professional roles and responsibilities, such as mandated reporting laws. *Understanding one's own exposure history and reactions to trauma* underscores the need for clinicians to acknowledge their own vulnerability as human beings to trauma and its sequelae, including exposure during the course of professional work to so-called vicarious or secondary traumatic stress. Secondary traumatic stress (also called "compassion fatigue") and vicarious traumatization are distress reactions in care providers who, as a result of their work, are exposed to disturbing images, intense affect, and intrusive memories recounted to them by their patients or clients. Although conceptually related, secondary traumatic stress emphasizes symptoms of PTSD while vicarious traumatization highlights changes in cognitive schemas in providers about the self, relationships, and the world. Sitting atop the pyramid, is *screening* for traumatic events. Whether or not and how to offer such screening is a complex decision for both individual practitioners and healthcare systems, and involves careful consideration of patient preferences, the scope of screening (universal versus case-finding) and the availability of resources to which patients who screen positive may be referred.

The Relationship Between the Neurobiology of Trauma and TIC

Research on the neurobiology of trauma in early life has progressed rapidly during the last three decades. Due to space constraints, this section will focus on the manner in which knowledge of threat conditioning and extinction (see Chap. 4 for more detail) informs TIC's emphasis on conveying a sense of safety and avoiding retraumatization. Interested readers can glean additional support of TIC tenets from recent comprehensive reviews in fields such as genetics and epigenetics [29], cellular aging [30], neuroendocrinology [31], neuroimmunology [32], and neuroimaging [33]. By documenting the automatic and nearly instantaneous sequelae of early life trauma in molecular and physiological processes, findings from these fields suggest that the persistence of neurobiological changes long after trauma exposure cannot be reversed simply by individual determination or effort. Indeed, brain systems underlying the executive control necessary to consciously alter behavior to become more adaptive are those that are most compromised by childhood trauma. Appreciation of this body of work may thus facilitate expressions of empathy from providers and the general public and decrease the ongoing discrimination experienced by patients with trauma-related problems. For people exposed to childhood trauma, these research findings may foster development of self-compassion and self-forgiveness through metacognitive processes in which they see themselves as individuals with their own strengths and resilience. Readers may also be interested in sweeping attempts at cross-disciplinary syntheses [34–36] as well as clinical applications of this neurobiological research [37, 38].

The learning and extinction of defensive behaviors evoked by discrete and acutely threatening stimuli and the modulation of those behaviors according to context depend on highly interconnected brain structures in the so-called "fear" circuit. This system detects, interprets, and guides the behavioral response to fear. In PTSD, this circuit reorganizes such that the response to threat is no longer contextual and appropriate to certain threatening stimuli; rather, it is a prolonged and generalized response that shuts down other brain systems important for appropriate behavioral responses and adaptations to emotional stimuli. The circuit includes, among other structures, the hippocampus, amygdala, and medial prefrontal cortex [39]. While the amygdala appears to be crucially involved in detecting and responding to threatening stimuli, the ventromedial prefrontal cortex and the hippocampus appear to be essential in the process of learning and remembering when stimuli that predicted threat before no longer do so [39]. In maladaptive responses to threat like those that occur in PTSD, heightened amygdala activity amygdala and aberrant function of the medial prefrontal cortex and hippocampus are thought to underlie deficits in response discontinuation and contextual processing (i.e., disregard of safety signals) [39]. Figure 14.2 depicts a schematic representation of this circuit.

The anxious anticipation of day-to-day events that evoke previous traumatic experiences (commonly referred to as "triggers") and a low threshold for recurrent posttraumatic "fight, flight, or freeze" reactions are pervasive among individuals exposed to trauma. Many may not know what their triggers are until they encounter them and, even then, may not be aware of their reactions to these triggers. For others, their sense of helplessness can be compounded by knowing that their triggers seem innocuous to most people, and their reactions to them inappropriate. These anecdotal observations can be related to a neuroimaging study of healthy adults exposed to childhood maltreatment. For example, subjects showed activation of the amygdala in response to sad faces presented to them *subliminally* (i.e., the pictures were shown too briefly to permit conscious recognition), and the amygdala activation was positively related to the severity of reported maltreatment [40]. This finding corresponds to the fast, subcortical pathway of threat depicted in Fig. 14.1.

Research [41–44] and anecdotal reports [45] have consistently shown that individuals with trauma histories can experience severe posttraumatic reactions in response to prevalent aspects and practices of healthcare environments that serve as reminders of previous trauma. For example, it has been documented for some time that anxious individuals require significantly higher doses of anesthetics for induction and maintenance of anesthesia during surgical procedures [46]. More recently, a multicenter, prospective cohort study found that accidental awareness during general anesthesia was associated with both the incidence and

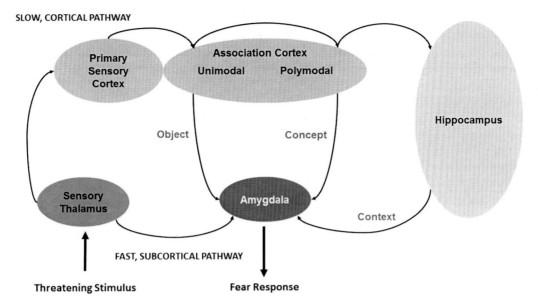

Fig. 14.2 The two pathways of responding to threat. In the fast subcortical pathway, threatening stimuli are routed directly to the amygdala from the sensory thalamus. This is an unconscious process that involves implicit memory systems. In the slow, cortical pathway, threatening stimuli engage higher order cognitive processes that provide the amygdala increasingly more complex appraisal of the stimuli, including the explicit memory context provided by input from the hippocampus (Adapted from The Brain from Top to Bottom, The Two Pathways of Fear, available at http://thebrain.mcgill.ca. The content of the site is under copyleft)

severity of PTSD symptoms 2 years postoperatively, and that prior history of PTSD and perioperative dissociation were independent predictors of PTSD after surgery [47]. A case report of two young male veterans with a history of PTSD who underwent elective surgery contrasts the outcomes of trauma-uninformed and trauma-informed care [48]. While recovering from anesthesia, one patient exhibited flashbacks in the form of a prolonged agitated delirium that did not respond to several attempts to reorient him; indeed, he believed he was in battle and that his buddies needed his help [48]. The other patient had an uneventful emergence from anesthesia after the team followed several trauma-informed modifications. These included avoiding touching the veteran's upper body when waking him up and instead using a "foot touch" (the latter being less likely to trigger a defensive reaction than the former), the use of clonidine (a medication that decreases the release of norepinephrine associated with the fight, flight, or freeze response), and discharge instructions that included referral to a primary care-psychiatry collaborative program [48].

The central argument of this section is that knowledge of the cross-species neural [49] and genetic basis of the fear circuit [50], fear conditioning and extinction [51], stress sensitization [52], and fear generalization [53] makes understandable – indeed, "normalizes" – the distress reactions that patients with trauma histories can experience in response to healthcare practices and features in the physical environment. This normalization is also aided by research showing that fear conditioning can be established or elicited without conscious awareness of being exposed to a threatening stimulus, as evidenced by experiments in patients with hippocampal damage and subliminal exposure [54].

Abnormalities in the acquisition and extinction of responses to threat in PTSD patients have received the most research attention. In contrast to trauma-exposed subjects without PTSD, those with PTSD exhibit both enhanced conditioned responses to a trauma reminder during acquisition as well as impaired extinction [55]. Extinction of a learned threat response depends on the intactness of at least three brain regions, including the prefrontal cortex, hippocampus, and amygdala [51]. Integrity of these structures ensures that the environmental context in which an individual encounters a threatening stimulus is encoded [49]. A meta-analysis of neuroimaging studies found evidence of structural changes of these brain regions in individuals with PTSD [56]. Summarizing a large body of evidence, a recent review concluded that "people suffering from PTSD have difficulty learning and remembering that stimuli that used to predict threat [are] no longer [predictive]" [57]. Since stress itself can impair extinction of conditioned fear responses and PTSD is associated with heightened stress, the conditions for a vicious cycle that perpetuates symptoms and undermines treatment efforts are thus established [58].

The changes in brain structures and failure to discriminate between threat and safety cues documented in PTSD patients have also been observed in maltreatment-exposed children without PTSD [59]. Furthermore, both animal and human models show that early life stress is associated with early appearance of the adult mode of extinction of responses to threat [60]. In contrast to the infant extinction mode, which leads to a permanent reduction in the threat response, the adult system is characterized by greater relapse of fear response after extinction training [60]. These observations are consistent with evidence that exposure to childhood adversities, especially when associated with adult revictimization or trauma, is associated with subsequent development of PTSD [52].

In summary, research on the neurobiological basis of trauma provides a theoretical foundation for some of the tenets (safety) and principles (resist retraumatization) of trauma-informed approaches (Table 14.2) and suggests modifications of practices and the physical environment in healthcare. The impact of these modifications on patient experience, satisfaction with care, and health outcomes can subsequently be empirically tested.

TIC and Trauma-Informed Approaches Outside Healthcare

Besides healthcare settings, individuals exposed to trauma are overrepresented in other human services systems and, consequently, the tenets of trauma-informed approaches may be of benefit to consumers and providers in many settings. Children and adolescents exposed to trauma interact with multiple systems, and members of the National Child Traumatic Stress Network (NCTSN) have made recommendations to make the education, healthcare, corrections, juvenile justice, first responders, and child welfare systems more trauma-informed [61]. In addition to reviewing the literature supporting the adoption of trauma-informed approaches for each of these systems, NCTSN made seven recommendations to help independent practitioners interact with clients and coordinate services from a trauma-informed perspective [61]. The recommendations are:

1. Promote the integration of trauma-focused practices across formal mental health treatment and other service sectors.
2. Identify changes in practice that providers and policymakers in each system view as important to achieving outcomes that matter to them (e.g., school attendance, grades, recidivism, physical health outcomes, service utilization, cost-effectiveness).
3. Rigorously evaluate the benefits of implementing trauma-informed care.
4. Introduce trauma-informed services into the core education and training for every child- and family-serving system.

5. Provide trauma-informed care and traumatic stress interventions early and strategically.
6. Replicate specialized evaluation, assessment, and treatment services provided by programs within the NCTSN.
7. Emphasize interdisciplinary collaboration and relationship-building.

These recommendations have improved care in a variety of settings [62–64]; interested readers are referred to these references for further information.

Another system highly impacted by trauma is the corrections system. A comparative study found a 48% prevalence rate of PTSD in a prison sample, while the corresponding rate in the general population was 4% [65]. Prevalence rates of PTSD represent only one aspect of trauma burden in this population, as the prevalence of childhood sexual abuse in the prison population was 70% for women and 50% for men [65]. The high trauma burden found in this study has been replicated in various samples of incarcerated individuals, such as women [66], youth [67], and older adults [68]. Additionally, a history of childhood maltreatment has been shown to be associated with disciplinary actions while in custody, especially for women [69]. Given the pervasive risk of violence and further retraumatization during incarceration, and the fact that systems of incarceration are separated based on biologic sex, a model of trauma-informed correctional care has been proposed that considers gender-specific responses to trauma [70]. According to this model, treatment for cisgender women needs to emphasize empowerment, emotion regulation, and safety, considering that internalizing behaviors (e.g., anxiety, social withdrawal, and somatic concerns) are more common in cisgender women. For cisgender men, on the other hand, treatment needs to emphasize feelings, relationships, and empathy since externalizing behaviors (e.g., bullying, substance use) are associated with cisgender men. It is worth noting that this model adopts a binary view of gender and, for a gender-based TIC model to be truly comprehensive, transgender individuals must be included. As in trauma-informed approaches in healthcare, the authors of the proposed model argue that trauma-informed principles may be helpful even in the absence of trauma-specific clinical interventions available to inmates [70]. The model also includes specific recommendations to increase buy-in from leaders and administrators, group exercises for staff (e.g., demonstrating how to sensitively talk inmates through pat downs and searches) and encouraging the sharing of stories of trauma healing while keeping trauma details to a minimum to avoid triggering of staff's own traumatic memories or vicarious traumatization [70]. Miller and Najavits' model also considers the integration of trauma-specific treatment, which others have extended to community-based programs available to inmates upon reentry [71], which have promising empirical support [72]. The literature on trauma-informed interventions for incarcerated women has been systematically reviewed, revealing decreases in PTSD symptoms and other outcomes such as drug use and reincarceration [73].

SAMHSA has also published specific recommendations for a trauma-informed criminal justice system and its Gather, Assess, Integrate, Network, and Stimulate (GAINS) Center for Behavioral Health and Justice Transformation offers apropos training for criminal justice professionals (samhsa.gov/gains-center).

TIC for LGBT Healthcare and the Promotion of Wellness Among LGBT Individuals and Communities

Although the topic remains understudied, especially among bisexual, transgender, and gender nonconforming individuals, a meta-analysis of school-based studies showed that sexual minority youth are at increased risk of exposure to abuse and violence, with odd ratios of 1.2, 1.7, 2.4, and 3.8 for physical abuse, violent threat or assault, missing school because of fear, and sexual abuse, respectively [74]. Using the Adverse Childhood Experiences (ACE) Study scale in a probability-based sample from three US states (Maine, Washington, Wisconsin), researchers found a higher rate in the number of reported ACEs as well as increased odds of exposure to each ACE category among LGB respondents [75]. The ACE Study scale inquires about five categories of childhood maltreatment and five categories of household dysfunction (familial mental illness, substance abuse, incarceration, parental discord, and domestic violence) [76]. Likewise, a systematic review of stressful childhood experiences including probing for household dysfunction in addition to maltreatment showed that nearly one in two LGBT individuals reported childhood emotional abuse in both probability (47.5%) and nonprobability samples (48.5%) [77].

Predictably, given that sexual minority groups have an increased likelihood of exposure to early life adversities, prominent disparities have been documented in PTSD prevalence between LGBT and heterosexual populations. Using data from a representative US sample and heterosexual adults without same-sex attraction or partners as comparison, researchers showed that LGB and heterosexual respondents with same-sex sexual partners had significantly elevated risk of exposure to nearly all traumatic events, especially childhood maltreatment and interpersonal violence (risk was not elevated among heterosexuals with same-sex attraction but no same-sex sexual partners, perhaps due to lower stigma levels) [78]. The adjusted odd ratios for PTSD onset were 2.03, 2.06, and 2.13 for lesbian and gay, heterosexual with same-sex sexual partners and bisexual participants, respectively [78]. Further insight into how gender nonconforming behaviors elevate risk for lifetime PTSD has been shed by the Growing Up Today Study, a US population-based longitudinal cohort of children of the Nurses' Health Study II participants. PTSD prevalence was highest among bisexual women (26.6%) and lesbians (18.6%), followed by mostly heterosexual women (13.5%) and men (11.8%) [79]. Between 32.3% and 48.4% of the variance in PTSD risk among sexual minorities in this sample (heterosexual with same-sex contact, mostly heterosexual, bisexual, lesbian/gay) was explained by childhood abuse, which in turn was partly explained by gender nonconformity [79].

LGBT individuals are not only targets of acts of abuse and violence by heterosexual individuals but also their own romantic and sexual partners. A systematic review of US studies of men who have sex with men revealed similar or higher rates of intimate partner violence (IPV) to those documented among presumed heterosexual women [80]. Results from a systematic review of IPV in self-identified lesbians found multiple limitations in the literature, including convenience samples and near-absent consideration of the role of homophobia and heterosexism in the emergence of violence or abuse. Victimization rates of any type of IPV ranged widely from 9.6% to 73.4%, and perpetration rates similarly ranged widely from 17% to 75% [81]. Considering probabilistic samples only, lesbians report lower rates of IPV than bisexual women, whose perpetrators are generally their male partners [81]. In another systematic review, LB women were at higher risk for lifetime and childhood sexual assault than GB men, although the authors cautioned that further studies are needed that disaggregate gay/lesbian from bisexual individuals [82]. Similar to adults, a cross-sectional, school-based study in three US states (Pennsylvania, New Jersey, and New York) showed that, in comparison to heterosexual youth, sexual minority adolescents reported significantly higher rates of all types of dating victimization and perpetration experiences, with the highest rates reported by transgender youth [83].

In addition to various forms of interpersonal violence, indirect forms of chronic stress in the lives of LGBT individuals have been the subject of systematic studies, mostly inspired by the Minority Stress Model [84, 85]. Undeniably, structural stigma, defined as "societal-level conditions, cultural norms, and institutional practices that constrain the opportunities, resources, and wellbeing for stigmatized populations" [86], is a source of chronic psychological stress to LGBT populations, often lying outside conscious awareness [87]. Conceptually, however, structural stigma does not meet a widely accepted definition of trauma that emphasizes the *individual experience* of an event, series of events, or set of circumstances [2]. Nevertheless, as is discussed in more detail in Chap. 4, structural stigma has been shown to be associated with a blunted hypothalamic-pituitary-adrenal axis response in LGB young adults [88], which has also been associated with PTSD [80] and environmental [81] and psychological distress [82]. Moreover, Hatzenbuehler and colleagues have shown that sexual minorities living in communities with high levels of structural stigma exhibit a shorter life expectancy of approximately 12 years due to an excess of suicide, homicide, violence, and cardiovascular disease [86].

The TIC implications of the increased prevalence of abuse, victimization, and structural stigma observed among LGBT populations have been the subject of multiple lines of research. Among the earliest is the association between childhood sexual abuse (CSA) and HIV infection. During the early 1980s, data from a small sample of adult men with a history of CSA (partnered with women at the time of the study) showed that most reported preoccupation with sexual thoughts, compulsive masturbation, and multiple female and male sexual partners [89]. A few years later, a longitudinal study of heterosexual men and women attending an HIV testing and counseling program found that 28% and 15% of the women and men, respectively, reported a history of CSA, and were four and almost eight times more likely, respectively, to have engaged in sex work at some point in their lives [90]. Participants reporting CSA were also more likely to report sex with anonymous partners, a higher average number of partners in a given year and to abuse substances [90]. These findings were replicated in a sample of gay men from three large urban centers in the USA who reported significantly increased HIV risk behaviors, including unprotected anal intercourse, being paid to have sex, positive syphilis serology, and being HIV-positive [91]. Studies since then have been the subject of a meta-analysis indicating that men who have sex with men (MSM) with CSA history are almost twice as likely to engage in recent unprotected anal intercourse and 1.5 times more likely to be HIV-positive as compared to MSM without such a history [92]. Studies of HIV-positive women have also been the subject of a meta-analysis, which found that recent PTSD is five times more common and IPV more than twice as common than in HIV-negative women in the general population [93].

A systematic review of studies of HIV-positive men and women indicated an increased risk for PTSD and poorer adherence to antiretroviral regimens in these populations [94]. Strikingly, in a cross-sectional study of HIV-positive biological and transgender women, those who answered affirmatively to a single screening question regarding exposure to abuse or violence in the past month had over four times the odds of antiretroviral failure (defined as having a detectable viral load or ≥75 copies/mm) as compared to women with negative trauma screening [95]. The recursive interactions between trauma, PTSD, substance use disorder, and HIV risk [96] have led more recently to a syndemic conceptualization of the intersecting epidemics of trauma and HIV infection calling for a TIC approach [97], as well as delivery of trauma-specific therapies [98] and trauma-informed risk reduction interventions [99–101].

Mirroring results from the ACE Study, which found a dose-response relationship between ACE score and health risk behaviors [102], a survey with representative samples in three US states (North Carolina, Washington, and Wisconsin) found that sexual orientation was no longer associated with health risk behaviors after adjusting for the increased prevalence of ACEs in sexual minority individuals compared to heterosexuals [103]. Similarly, a large, nationally representative survey found that the increased risk of exposure to early life adversity explained between 10% and 20% of the increased prevalence of tobacco, alcohol and drug use, and psychiatric symptoms among LGB youth versus heterosexual comparisons [104]. Besides family-based childhood adversities, school-based and neighborhood-based abuse and violence have an impact on health risk behaviors as well. A survey of 9th through 12th grade students in Massachusetts and Vermont compared reports of threat or injury with a weapon or deliberately damaged or stolen property while at school among LGBQ and heterosexual youth during the previous year. LGBQ youth reporting high levels of victimization endorsed more health risk behaviors, while health risk behaviors of LGBQ youth who reported low levels of victimization were similar to their heterosexual peers [105]. Another study linked suicidality and relational and electronic bullying reported by sexual minority youth to the rate of neighborhood-level assaultive hate crimes directed at LGBT individuals [106, 107]. Consistent with the increased health risk behaviors reported by LGB and LGBQ youth exposed to violence, a survey of adults recruited at a crowdsourcing internet jobsite showed that maltreatment by adults and peer bullying explained the disparate rates of lifetime physician-diagnosed physical health conditions among sexual minority individuals compared to heterosexuals [108].

In summary, studies reviewed in this section demonstrate that LGBT individuals exhibit a substantially elevated risk of exposure to trauma and that this exposure is highly consequential to physical and mental health outcomes. Additionally, blunted HPA axis reactivity –one of the mechanisms linking trauma exposure to health outcomes– has been observed in sexual minority individuals exposed to environments punctuated by high structural stigma, which may also underlie the association between structural stigma and early death due to cardiovascular causes [109]. This finding argues for considering structural stigma as a context that not only enables individual exposure to violence and abuse, but possibly amplifies neurobiological changes underlying the deleterious impact of trauma on health.

Together, epidemiological, preclinical, and clinical research makes a compelling case for addressing LGBT healthcare needs and well-being at both individual and population health levels through trauma-informed policies and practices. Those policies and practices should be the target of systematic evaluation and empirical investigation in the future. In the meantime, the studies reviewed comprise a solid theoretical foundation for the design and development of trauma-informed prevention, early intervention, and treatment efforts to address the glaring health disparities affecting LGBT populations.

Evidence of the Effectiveness of TIC

Although TIC formulations have evolved since the 1980s, empirical testing of professed benefits remains limited to date. One of the most ambitious efforts in this direction was the Women, Co-occurring Disorders, and Violence Study (WCDVS), a quasi-experimental nine-site longitudinal study that compared the effectiveness of usual care to comprehensive, integrated, trauma-informed services for women with co-occurring substance use and mental health disorders and a history of physical and/or sexual abuse [110]. Primary endpoints in the WCDVS study were alcohol and drug use, general psychological distress symptoms, and posttraumatic symptoms; secondary outcomes included service costs. Importantly, consumers of mental health services, survivors of trauma, and women in recovery were involved in the design, delivery, evaluation, and governance of the study [111]. In addition to providing trauma-informed services, the nine sites provided one of the following trauma-specific services: TREM [11], Seeking Safety [112], Addiction and Trauma Recovery Model (ATRIUM) [113], and/or the Triad Group model [114].

Six- and 12-month follow-up results painted a mixed picture, in part because improvement was observed in both the intervention and the usual care group [115, 116]. At 6 months, patients receiving the intervention experienced significant improvement in substance use outcomes and posttraumatic symptoms, and nearly significant improvement in psychological distress symptoms as compared to usual care [115]. In a similar comparison at 12 months, there was no significant reduction in addiction symptom severity, but the intervention was associated with statistically significant improvements in both psychological distress and posttraumatic symptoms [116]. In the words of the researchers: "Any multi-site study of this magnitude and complexity, governed by committee, is replete with both creative solutions and hard-won compromises to its methodological challenges. The result is a study with

conspicuous strengths and weaknesses" [111]. Considering the similar costs of operating comprehensive, trauma-informed compared with routine services and the potential gains for patients receiving trauma-informed care, the authors concluded that treatment intervention services were cost-effective [117]. In other words, available evidence indicates that there is no reason not to implement trauma-informed and trauma-specific systems.

The reduction or elimination of seclusion and restraint in a wide variety of healthcare settings and populations is congruent with TIC and has received ongoing empirical attention, chiefly in emergency or inpatient psychiatric wards [118–123]. The promise of this practice is illustrated by a randomized controlled trial of an intervention based on the Six Core Strategies TIC model [124] at a psychiatric hospital in Finland involving male patients with schizophrenia who had a history of violent behavior. Before the intervention, the high-security wards used seclusion as the primary coercive method, sometimes preceded by restraints and injectable medication. Four out of the 13 wards served the most treatment-resistant men with schizophrenia (one ward in the control and one ward in the intervention condition). Among other elements, the intervention featured individual crisis plans drawn from a questionnaire of traumatic experiences and violent behavior and a list of common triggers, warning signs, and calming activities. Study outcomes included duration of seclusion-restraint, the number of patient-days with seclusion, restraint, or room observation, and the number of incidents of physical violence against any person, including self-harm. Compared to a 25–19% decrease in seclusion-restraint and observation days in control wards, corresponding decreases of 30–15% were observed in the study wards [125]. Notably, seclusion-restraint time increased in the control wards, from 133 to 150 h per 100 patient-days, while it decreased in the intervention wards from 110 to 56 h [125]. The highly significant statistical differences in study outcomes were achieved without a concomitant increase in patient-to-patient injuries, including self-mutilation [125]. Unfortunately, the authors do not report on other important outcomes, such as associations with duration of hospitalization and symptom severity, which should be investigated in the future. In another study, substantial reductions in seclusion-restraint were observed in child and adolescent psychiatric wards at a state hospital after the Six Core Strategies model was adopted by leadership and staff, although the intervention did not involve a control group [126].

As another example, Project Kealahou is a federally funded program seeking to provide TIC and trauma-specific therapies to female youth exposed to trauma, as well as interagency collaboration among the mental health, education, juvenile justice, and child welfare service sectors in Hawaii [127]. A program evaluation involving 28 youth and

16 caregivers who completed both a baseline and a 6 month follow-up interview, revealed significant improvement in a range of program endpoints, including depression, behavioral problems, emotional problems, and caregiver strain, as well as satisfaction with the program [128].

In summary, these initial studies provide evidence that even a uniform approach to TIC can be beneficial in both healthcare and non-healthcare environments. Studies seeking to determine how approaches can be tailored based on age, setting, sexual orientation/gender identity, etc. are clearly needed.

Knowledge and Practice Gaps in TIC

A trauma-informed approach poses fundamental challenges to certain aspects of human services systems, including the healthcare system, as they are commonly configured in the USA. In its most far-reaching version of TIC, the Sanctuary Model, Bloom challenges the short-term bottom-line focus in for-profit healthcare and calls for commitments to social responsibility and "deep democracy" (i.e., recognizing "the basic ecological fact that everything is interconnected, that all life is a complex and interdependent web" [page 100–101]) in trauma-informed organizations [16]. Even in less comprehensive versions, a trauma-informed approach requires leadership, organizational commitment to change, and investment in the face of limited evidence of effectiveness or efficacy using the gold standard in treatment evaluation, randomized controlled trials. In this instance, it may be beneficial to introduce TIC alongside other social justice and ethical imperatives [129–131].

Development of a trauma-informed workforce is also important to consider. At least in terms of the healthcare workforce, curricular exposure to TIC is limited with few exceptions [132, 133]. Despite increasing inclusion of specific trauma topics (e.g., IPV content) in the curriculum of US medical schools [134], gaps in actual clinical performance remain [135]. Among practicing physicians, few primary care providers and pediatricians regularly screen for trauma exposure across the lifespan or feel confident in their skills [136–138]. Data on actual trauma-informed practices in other healthcare professions are also scarce, despite cogent calls for integration of the science related to ACEs into their work [131, 139]. However, the recent publication of several randomized controlled trials of educational interventions that resulted in self-reported or observed improvement in patient-physician communication around ACEs in primary care providers is decidedly encouraging [140–142].

Anecdotal evidence suggests that one barrier to participation in training and/or routinely incorporate TIC practices is a provider's personal history of trauma. An early survey of providers in social service agencies working with children indicated a prevalence of childhood maltreatment of any type (neglect or abuse) of 28.2% for male providers and 36.8% for female providers [143]. In a second survey of professionals responsible for evaluating child sexual abuse allegations, 13% of men and 20% of women reported a history of childhood sexual abuse, and 7.3% of men and 6.9% of the women reported a history of childhood physical abuse [144]. A third survey involved 297 members of the Massachusetts Academy of Family Physicians who appeared to be representative of the Academy's overall membership, at least in terms of demographics (51.2% female) [145]. Reported rates for childhood abuse were 18.1% and 26.5% for any childhood abuse and 24.3% and 42.4% for any lifetime abuse for men and women, respectively [145]. A fourth, large survey of female nurses ($N = 1981$) found that 17.87% reported childhood physical abuse, 17.99% reported childhood sexual abuse and 10.29% reported witnessing IPV between parents or caregivers during childhood [146]. Childhood maltreatment (but not witnessing IPV during childhood) increased the risk for adult IPV in the sample (25% lifetime) [146].

Interestingly, respondents in three of the surveys who disclosed a history of trauma were more likely to believe children's reports of abuse [143], ascertain abuse in case vignettes [144], or feel confident in their ability to screen patients for a history of childhood abuse [145]. However, the possibility of secondary or vicarious traumatization, particularly for providers who have a personal history of trauma, is an important consideration. If healthcare systems were more trauma-informed, healthcare workers themselves might be less likely to experience both primary traumatization and retraumatization; this is a fertile area for future study. A recent meta-analysis identified a personal trauma history as one of the risk factors for secondary traumatic stress [147].

A study of physicians referred for remediation after making professional boundary violations revealed that 29% of respondents were positive for the minimization/denial subscale of the Childhood Trauma Questionnaire, which indicates a likely underreporting of childhood maltreatment [148]. However, there are no published Childhood Trauma Questionnaire data obtained from nonreferred physicians to serve as a benchmark. Thus, the possibility remains that a significant minority of physicians and other healthcare providers who disavow their histories of childhood adversities may be less likely to engage in trauma-informed practices. This is a tenable question that could be addressed by future research. Future research should also focus on the contrasting hypothesis: Are healthcare providers with avowed histories of trauma that have worked through the psychological sequelae of their trauma particularly competent in TIC practices? Anecdotal experience show that such individuals seek jobs caring for others who have experienced adversity as a means to "give back" and empowerment.

TIC, Resilience, and the Limitations of Resilience

Even if TIC can be adopted faithfully in contexts far removed from the historical and sociopolitical context in which TIC first emerged in the USA, the preeminence of *individual* empowerment, strengths, and resilience in TIC is intricately linked to the values of an individualistic culture. In this type of culture, "societies exist to promote the well-being of individuals" and "individuals are seen as separate from one another," in contrast to collectivistic societies, where "Individuals are seen as fundamentally connected and related through relationships and group memberships"(page 311) [149]. It therefore remains to be seen if this individualistic feature can be adopted in collectivistic cultures. Social psychology has shown that the individualistic-collectivistic distinction is associated with cross-cultural differences in a range of mental processes and behaviors, ranging from the meaning of suffering [150] to the pursuit of individual goals [151] and the extent to which people view themselves as agents acting independently [152]. Most contemporary formulations of resilience revolve around neurobiological or psychological qualities of an individual [153], although there are recent exceptions to this trend proposing a community view of resilience focusing on robust health systems, social connectedness, psychological health, and vulnerable populations [154]. The concerns about a more culturally responsive view of resilience have been reviewed by Buse and colleagues, who consider the impact of culture on expression of emotions, somatization, locus of control, self-enhancement, dissociation, family and community support, and healing rituals or ceremonies [155].

Conclusions

Since its inception in the early 1980s, TIC has evolved from a therapeutic approach for disadvantaged women with mental illness and co-occurring substance misuse to a veritable social movement. During this evolution, the original focus of TIC on healthcare has expanded into other human service arenas, and now includes proposals to transform organizational policies and procedures in addition to the practices of individual service providers. In giving voice to the lived experience of people who have experienced trauma, TIC emphasizes the importance of respect, dignity, and collaborative patient-clinician relationships. These values are congruent with two broad-based approaches to service provision – patient-centered care and cultural competence – that enjoy increasing buy-in from stakeholders at all levels, including consumers and communities. While empirical evidence for the added value of adopting a universal, trauma-informed approach to care is being gathered, this congruence of TIC with other approaches and a strong focus on social justice and equity will likely facilitate widespread uptake and dissemination.

In summary, this chapter reviewed the literature to build a case for the relevance of trauma-informed approaches to the provision of services for LGBT and gender nonconforming or genderqueer individuals across the lifespan and in numerous sectors, including school, child welfare, justice, and healthcare. Burdened by both high rates of trauma exposure and health disparities, these populations can benefit from programs and practices that embed TIC principles in their design, implementation, and evaluation.

References

1. Hopper EK, Bassuk EL, Olivet J. Shelter from the storm: trauma-informed care in homelessness services settings. Open Health Serv Policy J. 2010;3:80–100.
2. Administration. SAaMHS. SAMHSA's concept of trauma and guidance for a trauma-informed approach. Rockville: Substance Abuse and Mental Health Services Administration; 2014.
3. Administration. SAaMHS. Trauma-informed care in behavioral health services. Rockville: Substance Abuse and Mental Health Services Administration (US); 2014.
4. Goodman LA, Dutton MA, Harris M. Episodically homeless women with serious mental illness: prevalence of physical and sexual assault. Am J Orthopsychiatry. 1995;65:468.
5. Goodman LA, Dutton MA, Harris M. The relationship between violence dimensions and symptom severity among homeless, mentally ill women. J Trauma Stress. 1997;10:51–70.
6. Harris M, Anglin J. Trauma recovery and empowerment: a clinician's guide for working with women in groups. New York: Simon and Schuster; 1998.
7. Herman JL. Complex PTSD: a syndrome in survivors of prolonged and repeated trauma. J Trauma Stress. 1992;5:377–91.
8. Courtois CA. Healing the incest wound: adult survivors in therapy. New York: WW Norton & Company; 1996.
9. Janoff-Bulman R, Frieze IH. A theoretical perspective for understanding reactions to victimization. J Soc Issues. 1983;39:1–17.
10. Rosenberg SD, Mueser KT, Friedman MJ, et al. Developing effective treatments for posttraumatic disorders among people with severe mental illness. Psychiatr Serv. 2001;52:1453–61.
11. Fallot RD, Harris M. The trauma recovery and empowerment model (TREM): conceptual and practical issues in a group intervention for women. Community Ment Health J. 2002;38:475–85.
12. Harris M, Fallot RD. Envisioning a trauma-informed service system: a vital paradigm shift. New Dir Ment Health Serv. 2001;2001:3–22.
13. Jacobson A, Koehler JE, Jones-Brown C. The failure of routine assessment to detect histories of assault experienced by psychiatric patients. Psychiatr Serv. 1987;38:386–9.
14. Bloom SL. Creating sanctuary: healing from systematic abuses of power. Ther Communities-London-Assoc Ther Communiities. 2000;21:67–92.

15. Bloom SL, Bennington-Davis M, Farragher B, et al. Multiple opportunities for creating sanctuary. Psychiatry Q. 2003; 74:173–90.

16. Bloom SL, Farragher BJ. Restoring sanctuary: a new operating system for trauma-informed systems of care. Oxford: Oxford university press; 2013.

17. Rivard JC, McCorkle D, Duncan ME, et al. Implementing a trauma recovery framework for youths in residential treatment. Child Adolesc Soc Work J. 2004;21:529–50.

18. Rivard JC, Bloom SL, McCorkle D, et al. Preliminary results of a study examining the implementation and effects of a trauma recovery framework for youths in residential treatment. Ther Community Int J Ther and Supportive Organ. 2005;26:83–96.

19. Borckardt JJ, Madan A, Grubaugh AL, et al. Systematic investigation of initiatives to reduce seclusion and restraint in a state psychiatric hospital. Psychiatr Serv. 2011;62(5):477–83.

20. Bloom SL. The sanctuary model: developing generic inpatient programs for the treatment of psychological trauma. In: Williams M, Sommer JF, editors. Handbook of post-traumatic therapy, a practical guide to intervention, treatment, and research. New York: Greenwood Publishing; 1994. p. 474–49.

21. Raja S, Hasnain M, Hoersch M, et al. Trauma informed care in medicine: current knowledge and future research directions. Fam Community Health. 2015;38:216–26.

22. Stewart M. Patient-centered medicine: transforming the clinical method. London: Radcliffe Publishing; 2014.

23. Tervalon M, Murray-Garcia J. Cultural humility versus cultural competence: a critical distinction in defining physician training outcomes in multicultural education. J Health Care Poor Underserved. 1998;9:117–25.

24. Walls ML, Gonzalez J, Gladney T, et al. Unconscious biases: racial microaggressions in American Indian health care. J Am Board Fam Med. 2015;28:231–9.

25. Balsam KF, Molina Y, Beadnell B, et al. Measuring multiple minority stress: the LGBT people of color microaggressions scale. Cultur Divers Ethnic Minor Psychol. 2011;17:163–74.

26. Sue DW, Capodilupo CM, Torino GC, et al. Racial microaggressions in everyday life: implications for clinical practice. Am Psychol. 2007;62:271–86.

27. Jackson JL, Kroenke K. Difficult patient encounters in the ambulatory clinic: clinical predictors and outcomes. Arch Intern Med. 1999;159:1069–75.

28. Campbell JA, Walker RJ, Egede LE. Associations between adverse childhood experiences, high-risk behaviors, and morbidity in adulthood. Am J Prev Med. 2015;50(3):344–52.

29. Montalvo-Ortiz JL, Gelernter J, Hudziak J, et al. RDoC and translational perspectives on the genetics of trauma-related psychiatric disorders. Am J Med Genet B Neuropsychiatr Genet. 2016;171:81–91.

30. Price LH, Kao H-T, Burgers DE, et al. Telomeres and early-life stress: an overview. Biol Psychiatry. 2013;73:15–23.

31. Frodl T, O'Keane V. How does the brain deal with cumulative stress? A review with focus on developmental stress, HPA axis function and hippocampal structure in humans. Neurobiol Dis. 2013;52:24–37.

32. Nusslock R, Miller GE. Early-life adversity and physical and emotional health across the lifespan: a neuroimmune network hypothesis. Biol Psychiatry. 2015;80(1):23–32.

33. Lim L, Radua J, Rubia K. Gray matter abnormalities in childhood maltreatment: a voxel-wise meta-analysis. Am J Psychiatry. 2014;171:854–63.

34. Odgers CL, Jaffee SR. Routine versus catastrophic influences on the developing child. Annu Rev Public Health. 2013;34:29.

35. Shonkoff JP, Boyce WT, McEwen BS. Neuroscience, molecular biology, and the childhood roots of health disparities: building a new framework for health promotion and disease prevention. JAMA. 2009;301:2252–9.

36. McEwen BS. Brain on stress: how the social environment gets under the skin. Proc Natl Acad Sci. 2012;109:17180–5.

37. Evans A, Coccoma P. Trauma-informed care: how neuroscience influences practice. New York: Routledge; 2014.

38. Frewen P, Lanius R. Healing the traumatized self: consciousness, neuroscience, treatment (Norton series on interpersonal neurobiology). New York: WW Norton & Company; 2015.

39. Shin LM, Liberzon I. The neurocircuitry of fear, stress, and anxiety disorders. Neuropsychopharmacology. 2010;35:169–91.

40. Dannlowski U, Kugel H, Huber F, et al. Childhood maltreatment is associated with an automatic negative emotion processing bias in the amygdala. Hum Brain Mapp. 2013;34:2899–909.

41. Strout TD. Perspectives on the experience of being physically restrained: an integrative review of the qualitative literature. Int J Ment Health Nurs. 2010;19:416–27.

42. Leeners B, Stiller R, Block E, et al. Effect of childhood sexual abuse on gynecologic care as an adult. Psychosomatics. 2007;48:385–93.

43. Leeners B, Stiller R, Block E, et al. Consequences of childhood sexual abuse experiences on dental care. J Psychosom Res. 2007;62:581–8.

44. Swahnberg K, Davidsson-Simmons J, Hearn J, et al. Men's experiences of emotional, physical, and sexual abuse and abuse in health care: a cross-sectional study of a Swedish random male population sample. Scand J Public Health. 2011.

45. Gridley S. The gold–hope tang, MD 2015 humanism in medicine essay contest: third place: gauze and guns. Acad Med. 2015,90.1356–7.

46. Maranets I, Kain ZN. Preoperative anxiety and intraoperative anesthetic requirements. Anesth Analg. 1999;89:1346.

47. Whitlock EL, Rodebaugh TL, Hassett AL, et al. Psychological sequelae of surgery in a prospective cohort of patients from three intraoperative awareness prevention trials. Anesth Analg. 2015;120:87–95.

48. Lovestrand D, Phipps S, Lovestrand S. Posttraumatic stress disorder and anesthesia emergence. AANA J. 2013;81:199–203.

49. Maren S, Phan KL, Liberzon I. The contextual brain: implications for fear conditioning, extinction and psychopathology. Nat Rev Neurosci. 2013;14:417–28.

50. Åhs F, Frick A, Furmark T, et al. Human serotonin transporter availability predicts fear conditioning. Int J Psychophysiol. 2014;98(3):515–9.

51. Giustino TF, Maren S. The role of the medial prefrontal cortex in the conditioning and extinction of fear. Front Behav Neurosci. 2015;9:298. doi:10.3389/fnbeh.2015.00298. PMID: 26617500.

52. Pratchett LC, Yehuda R. Foundations of posttraumatic stress disorder: does early life trauma lead to adult posttraumatic stress disorder? Dev Psychopathol. 2011;23:477–91.

53. Lopresto D, Schipper P, Homberg JR. Neural circuits and mechanisms involved in fear generalization: implications for the pathophysiology and treatment of posttraumatic stress disorder. Neurosci Biobehav Rev. 2016;60:31–42.

54. LeDoux JE. Coming to terms with fear. Proc Natl Acad Sci. 2014;111:2871–8.

55. Wessa M, Flor H. Failure of extinction of fear responses in posttraumatic stress disorder: evidence from second-order conditioning. Am J Psychiatry. 2007;164:1684–92.

56. O'Doherty DCM, Chitty KM, Saddiqui S, et al. A systematic review and meta-analysis of magnetic resonance imaging

measurement of structural volumes in posttraumatic stress disorder. Psychiatry Res Neuroimaging. 2015;232:1–33.

57. VanElzakker MB, Dahlgren MK, Davis FC, et al. From Pavlov to PTSD: the extinction of conditioned fear in rodents, humans, and anxiety disorders. Neurobiol Learn Mem. 2014;113:3–18.

58. Maren S, Holmes A. Stress and fear extinction. Neuropsychopharmacology. 2016;41:58–79.

59. McLaughlin KA, Sheridan MA, Gold AL, et al. Maltreatment exposure, brain structure, and fear conditioning in children and adolescents. Neuropsychopharmacology. 2015;41(8):1956–64.

60. Callaghan BL, Sullivan RM, Howell B, et al. The international society for developmental psychobiology Sackler symposium: early adversity and the maturation of emotion circuits—a cross-species analysis. Dev Psychobiol. 2014;56:1635–50.

61. Ko SJ, Ford JD, Kassam-Adams N, et al. Creating trauma-informed systems: child welfare, education, first responders, health care, juvenile justice. Prof Psychol. 2008;39:396.

62. Sullivan KM, Murray KJ, Ake GS. Trauma-informed care for children in the child welfare system an initial evaluation of a trauma-informed parenting workshop. Child Maltreat. 2015.

63. Bartlett JD, Barto B, Griffin JL, et al. Trauma-informed care in the Massachusetts child trauma project. Child Maltreat. 2015.

64. Holmes C, Levy M, Smith A, et al. A model for creating a supportive trauma-informed culture for children in preschool settings. J Child Fam Stud. 2015;24:1650–9.

65. Briere J, Agee E, Dietrich A. Cumulative trauma and current posttraumatic stress disorder status in general population and inmate samples. Psychol Trauma. 2016;8(4):439–46.

66. Tripodi SJ, Pettus-Davis C. Histories of childhood victimization and subsequent mental health problems, substance use, and sexual victimization for a sample of incarcerated women in the US. Int J Law Psychiatry. 2013;36:30–40.

67. Dierkhising CB, Ko SJ, Woods-Jaeger B, Briggs EC, Lee R, Pynoos RS. Trauma histories among justice-involved youth: findings from the National Child Traumatic Stress Network. Eur J Psychotraumatol. 2013;4 doi:10.3402/ejpt.v4i0.20274. PMID: 23869252.

68. Haugebrook S, Zgoba KM, Maschi T, et al. Trauma, stress, health, and mental health issues among ethnically diverse older adult prisoners. J Correct Health Care. 2010;16:220–9.

69. Joubert D, Archambault K, Brown G. Cycle of coercion: experiences of maltreatment and disciplinary measures in Canadian inmates. Int J Prison Health. 2014;10:79–93.

70. Miller NA, Najavits LM. Creating trauma-informed correctional care: a balance of goals and environment. Eur J Psychotraumatol. 2012;3 doi:10.3402/ejpt.v3i0.17246. PMID: 22893828.

71. Wallace BC, Conner LC, Dass-Brailsford P. Integrated trauma treatment in correctional health care and community-based treatment upon reentry integrated trauma treatment in correctional health care and community-based treatment upon reentry. J Correct Health Care. 2011.

72. Covington SS, Burke C, Keaton S, et al. Evaluation of a trauma-informed and gender-responsive intervention for women in drug treatment. J Psychoactive Drugs. 2008;40:387–98.

73. King EA. Outcomes of trauma-informed interventions for incarcerated women a review. Int J Offender Ther Comp Criminol. 2015.

74. Friedman MS, Marshal MP, Guadamuz TE, et al. A meta-analysis of disparities in childhood sexual abuse, parental physical abuse, and peer victimization among sexual minority and sexual nonminority individuals. Am J Public Health. 2011;101:1481–94.

75. Andersen JP, Blosnich J. Disparities in adverse childhood experiences among sexual minority and heterosexual adults:

results from a multi-state probability-based sample. PLoS One. 2013;8:e54691.

76. Felitti VJ, Anda RF, Nordenberg D, et al. Relationship of childhood abuse and household dysfunction to many of the leading causes of death in adults: the adverse childhood experiences (ACE) study. Am J Prev Med. 1998;14:245–58.

77. Schneeberger AR, Dietl MF, Muenzenmaier KH, et al. Stressful childhood experiences and health outcomes in sexual minority populations: a systematic review. Soc Psychiatry Psychiatr Epidemiol. 2014;49:1427–45.

78. Roberts AL, Austin SB, Corliss HL, et al. Pervasive trauma exposure among US sexual orientation minority adults and risk of posttraumatic stress disorder. Am J Public Health. 2010;100:2433–41.

79. Roberts AL, Rosario M, Corliss HL, et al. Elevated risk of posttraumatic stress in sexual minority youths: mediation by childhood abuse and gender nonconformity. Am J Public Health. 2012;102:1587–93.

80. Finneran C, Stephenson R. Intimate partner violence among men who have sex with men a systematic review. Trauma Violence Abuse. 2013;14:168–85.

81. Badenes-Ribera L, Bonilla-Campos A, Frias-Navarro D, et al. Intimate partner violence in self-identified lesbians a systematic review of its prevalence and correlates. Trauma Violence Abuse. 2015.

82. Rothman EF, Exner D, Baughman AL. The prevalence of sexual assault against people who identify as gay, lesbian, or bisexual in the United States: a systematic review. Trauma Violence Abuse. 2011.

83. Dank M, Lachman P, Zweig JM, et al. Dating violence experiences of lesbian, gay, bisexual, and transgender youth. J Youth Adolesc. 2014;43:846–57.

84. Meyer IH. Minority stress and mental health in gay men. J Health Soc Behav. 1995;36:38–56.

85. Meyer IH. Prejudice, social stress, and mental health in lesbian, gay, and bisexual populations: conceptual issues and research evidence. Psychol Bull. 2003;129:674.

86. Hatzenbuehler ML, Bellatorre A, Lee Y, et al. Structural stigma and all-cause mortality in sexual minority populations. Soc Sci Med. 2014;103:33–41.

87. Hatzenbuehler ML. How does sexual minority stigma "get under the skin"? A psychological mediation framework. Psychol Bull. 2009;135:707.

88. Hatzenbuehler ML, McLaughlin KA. Structural stigma and hypothalamic–pituitary–adrenocortical axis reactivity in lesbian, gay, and bisexual young adults. Ann Behav Med. 2014;47:39–47.

89. Dimock PT. Adult males sexually abused as children characteristics and implications for treatment. J Interpers Violence. 1988;3:203–21.

90. Zierler S, Feingold L, Laufer D, et al. Adult survivors of childhood sexual abuse and subsequent risk of HIV infection. Am J Public Health. 1991;81:572–5.

91. Bartholow BN, Doll LS, Joy D, et al. Emotional, behavioral, and HIV risks associated with sexual abuse among adult homosexual and bisexual men. Child Abuse Negl. 1994;18:745–61.

92. Lloyd S, Operario D. HIV risk among men who have sex with men who have experienced childhood sexual abuse: systematic review and meta-analysis. AIDS Educ Prev. 2012;24:228.

93. Machtinger E, Wilson T, Haberer JE, et al. Psychological trauma and PTSD in HIV-positive women: a meta-analysis. AIDS Behav. 2012;16:2091–100.

94. Spies G, Afifi TO, Archibald SL, et al. Mental health outcomes in HIV and childhood maltreatment: a systematic review. Syst Rev. 2012;1:1.

95. Machtinger E, Haberer J, Wilson T, et al. Recent trauma is associated with antiretroviral failure and HIV transmission risk behavior among HIV-positive women and female-identified transgenders. AIDS Behav. 2012;16:2160–70.

96. Brief DJ, Bollinger A, Vielhauer M, et al. Understanding the interface of HIV, trauma, post-traumatic stress disorder, and substance use and its implications for health outcomes. AIDS Care. 2004;16:97–120.

97. Brezing C, Ferrara M, Freudenreich O. The syndemic illness of HIV and trauma: implications for a trauma-informed model of care. Psychosomatics. 2015;56:107–18.

98. Seedat S. Interventions to improve psychological functioning and health outcomes of HIV-infected individuals with a history of trauma or PTSD. Curr HIV/AIDS Rep. 2012;9:344–50.

99. Williams JK, Glover DA, Wyatt GE, et al. A sexual risk and stress reduction intervention designed for HIV-positive bisexual African American men with childhood sexual abuse histories. Am J Public Health. 2013;103:1476–84.

100. Williams JK, Wyatt GE, Rivkin I, et al. Risk reduction for HIV-positive African American and Latino men with histories of childhood sexual abuse. Arch Sex Behav. 2008;37:763–72.

101. Sikkema KJ, Wilson PA, Hansen NB, et al. Effects of a coping intervention on transmission risk behavior among people living with HIV/AIDS and a history of childhood sexual abuse. JAIDS. 2008;47:506–13.

102. Dube SR, Felitti VJ, Dong M, et al. The impact of adverse childhood experiences on health problems: evidence from four birth cohorts dating back to 1900. Prev Med. 2003;37:268–77.

103. Austin A, Herrick H, Proescholdbell S. Adverse childhood experiences related to poor adult health among lesbian, gay, and bisexual individuals. Am J Public Health. 2016;106(2):314–20. doi:10.2105/AJPH.2015.302904. PMID: 26691127.

104. McLaughlin KA, Hatzenbuehler ML, Xuan Z, et al. Disproportionate exposure to early-life adversity and sexual orientation disparities in psychiatric morbidity. Child Abuse Negl. 2012;36:645–55.

105. Bontempo DE, d'Augelli AR. Effects of at-school victimization and sexual orientation on lesbian, gay, or bisexual youths' health risk behavior. J Adolesc Health. 2002;30:364–74.

106. Duncan DT, Hatzenbuehler ML. Lesbian, gay, bisexual, and transgender hate crimes and suicidality among a population-based sample of sexual-minority adolescents in Boston. Am J Public Health. 2014;104:272–8.

107. Hatzenbuehler ML, Duncan D, Johnson R. Neighborhood-level lgbt hate crimes and bullying among sexual minority youths: a geospatial analysis. Violence Vict. 2015;30:663–75.

108. Andersen JP, Zou C, Blosnich J. Multiple early victimization experiences as a pathway to explain physical health disparities among sexual minority and heterosexual individuals. Soc Sci Med. 2015;133:111–9.

109. Nijm J, Jonasson L. Inflammation and cortisol response in coronary artery disease. Ann Med. 2009;41:224–33.

110. Huntington N, Moses DJ, Veysey BM. Developing and implementing a comprehensive approach to serving women with co-occurring disorders and histories of trauma. J Community Psychol. 2005;33:395–410.

111. McHugo GJ, Kammerer N, Jackson EW, et al. Women, co-occurring disorders, and violence study: evaluation design and study population. J Subst Abuse Treat. 2005;28:91–107.

112. Najavits LM, Weiss RD, Liese BS. Group cognitive-behavioral therapy for women with PTSD and substance use disorder. J Subst Abuse Treat. 1996;13:13–22.

113. Miller D, Guidry L. Addictions and trauma recovery: healing the body, mind and spirit. New York: WW Norton & Co; 2001.

114. Clark C, Fearday F. Triad Women's project group facilitator manual and workbook. Tampa: University of South Florida; 2001.

115. Cocozza JJ, Jackson EW, Hennigan K, et al. Outcomes for women with co-occurring disorders and trauma: program-level effects. J Subst Abuse Treat. 2005;28:109–19.

116. Morrissey JP, Jackson EW, Ellis AR, et al. Twelve-month outcomes of trauma-informed interventions for women with co-occurring disorders. Psychiatr Serv. 2014;56(10):1213–22.

117. Domino M, Morrissey JP, Nadlicki-Patterson T, et al. Service costs for women with co-occurring disorders and trauma. J Subst Abuse Treat. 2005;28:135–43.

118. Substance Abuse and Mental Health Services Administration. The business case for preventing and reducing restraint and seclusion use. HHS Publication No(SMA), 11-4632. Rockville: Substance Abuse and Mental Health Services Administration; 2011.

119. Goetz SB, Taylor-Trujillo A. A change in culture violence prevention in an acute behavioral health setting. J Am Psychiatr Nurses Assoc. 2012;18:96–103.

120. Barton SA, Johnson MR, Price LV. Achieving restraint-free on an inpatient behavioral health unit. J Psychosoc Nurs Ment Health Serv. 2009;47:34–40.

121. Donat DC. An analysis of successful efforts to reduce the use of seclusion and restraint at a public psychiatric hospital. Psychiatr Serv. 2003;54(8):1119–23.

122. Sullivan AM, Bezmen J, Barron CT, et al. Reducing restraints: alternatives to restraints on an inpatient psychiatric service—utilizing safe and effective methods to evaluate and treat the violent patient. Psychiatry Q. 2005;76:51–65.

123. Cole R. Reducing restraint use in a trauma center emergency room. Nurs Clin N Am. 2014;49:371–81.

124. Huckshorn KA, CAP I, Director N. Six core strategies to reduce the use of seclusion and restraint planning tool. National Association of State Mental Health Program Directors. Available at: http://www.wafca.org. Accessed 7 Feb 2016 1.2010, 2005.

125. Putkonen A, Kuivalainen S, Louheranta O, et al. Cluster-randomized controlled trial of reducing seclusion and restraint in secured care of men with schizophrenia. Psychiatr Serv. 2013;64(9):850–5.

126. Azeem MW, Aujla A, Rammerth M, et al. Effectiveness of six core strategies based on trauma informed care in reducing seclusions and restraints at a child and adolescent psychiatric hospital. J Child Adolesc Psychiatr Nurs. 2011;24:11–5.

127. Slavin LA, Suarez E. Insights in public health: project Kealahou—forging a new pathway for girls in Hawai'i's public mental health system. Hawai'i J Med Public Health. 2013;72:325.

128. Suarez E, Jackson DS, Slavin LA, et al. Project Kealahou: improving Hawai'i's system of Care for At-Risk Girls and Young Women through gender-responsive, trauma-informed care. Hawai'i J Med Public Health. 2014;73:387.

129. Services SAaMH. SAMHSA's National Center on trauma-informed care: changing communities, changing lives. Rockville: Substance Abuse and Mental Health Services Administration; 2012.

130. Machtinger EL, Cuca YP, Khanna N, et al. From treatment to healing: the promise of trauma-informed primary care. Womens Health Issues. 2015;25:193–7.

131. Waite R, Gerrity P, Arango R. Assessment for and response to adverse childhood experiences. J Psychosoc Nurs Ment Health Serv. 2010;48:51–61.

132. Raja S, Rajagopalan CF, Kruthoff M, et al. Teaching dental students to interact with survivors of traumatic events: development of a two-day module. J Dent Educ. 2015;79:47–55.

133. Layne CM, Ippen CG, Strand V, et al. The core curriculum on childhood trauma: a tool for training a trauma-informed workforce. Psychol Trauma. 2011;3:243.

134. Hamberger LK. Preparing the next generation of physicians medical school and residency-based intimate partner violence curriculum and evaluation. Trauma Violence Abuse. 2007;8:214–25.

135. Connor PD, Nouer SS, Mackey SN, et al. Intimate partner violence education for medical students: toward a comprehensive curriculum revision. South Med J. 2012;105:211–5.

136. Rodriguez MA, Bauer HM, McLoughlin E, et al. Screening and intervention for intimate partner abuse: practices and attitudes of primary care physicians. JAMA. 1999;282:468–74.

137. Weinreb L, Savageau JA, Candib LM, et al. Screening for childhood trauma in adult primary care patients: a cross-sectional survey. Prim Care Companion J Clin Psychiatry. 2010;12(6). pii: PCC.10m00950. doi: 10.4088/PCC.10m00950blu. PMID: 21494339.

138. Kerker BD, Storfer-Isser A, Szilagyi M, et al. Do pediatricians ask about adverse childhood experiences in pediatric primary care? Acad Pediatr. 2015;16(2):154–60.

139. Larkin H, Felitti VJ, Anda RF. Social work and adverse childhood experiences research: implications for practice and health policy. Soc Work Public Health. 2014;29:1–16.

140. Helitzer DL, LaNoue M, Wilson B, et al. A randomized controlled trial of communication training with primary care providers to improve patient-centeredness and health risk communication. Patient Educ Couns. 2011;82:21–9.

141. Green BL, Saunders PA, Power E, et al. Trauma-informed medical care: a CME communication training for primary care providers. Fam Med. 2015;47:7.

142. Dubowitz H, Lane WG, Semiatin JN, et al. The safe environment for every kid model: impact on pediatric primary care professionals. Pediatrics. 2011;127:e962–e70.

143. Howe AC, Herzberger S, Tennen H. The influence of personal history of abuse and gender on clinicians' judgments of child abuse. J Fam Violence. 1988;3:105–19.

144. Nuttall R, Jackson H. Personal history of childhood abuse among clinicians. Child Abuse Negl. 1994;18:455–72.

145. Candib LM, Savageau JA, Weinreb LF, et al. Inquiring into our past: when the doctor is a survivor of abuse. Fam Med. 2012;44 (6):416–24.

146. Bracken MI, Messing JT, Campbell JC, et al. Intimate partner violence and abuse among female nurses and nursing personnel: prevalence and risk factors. Issues Ment Health Nurs. 2010;31:137–48.

147. Hensel JM, Ruiz C, Finney C, et al. Meta-analysis of risk factors for secondary traumatic stress in therapeutic work with trauma victims. J Trauma Stress. 2015;28:83–91.

148. MacDonald K, Sciolla AF, Folsom D, et al. Individual risk factors for physician boundary violations: the role of attachment style, childhood trauma and maladaptive beliefs. Gen Hosp Psychiatry. 2015;37:489–96.

149. Oyserman D, Lee SWS. Does culture influence what and how we think? Effects of priming individualism and collectivism. Psychol Bull. 2008;134:311–42.

150. Sullivan D, Landau MJ, Kay AC, et al. Collectivism and the meaning of suffering. J Pers Soc Psychol. 2012;103:1023.

151. Elliot AJ, Chirkov VI, Kim Y, et al. A cross-cultural analysis of avoidance (relative to approach) personal goals. Psychol Sci. 2001;12:505–10.

152. Kashima Y, Yamaguchi S, Kim U, et al. Culture, gender, and self: a perspective from individualism-collectivism research. J Pers Soc Psychol. 1995;69:925.

153. Southwick SM, Charney DS. The science of resilience: implications for the prevention and treatment of depression. Science. 2012;338:79–82.

154. Wulff K, Donato D, Lurie N. What is health resilience and how can We build it? Annu Rev Public Health. 2015;36:361–74.

155. Buse NA, Bernacchio C, Burker EJ. Cultural variation in resilience as a response to traumatic experience. J Rehabil. 2013;79:15.

Screening and Assessment of Trauma in Clinical Populations

15

Brian Hurley, Kenny Lin, Suni Niranjan Jani, and Kevin Kapila

Introduction

Given the frequency of trauma in LGBT populations, there are clinical and public health imperatives for routine screening for and subsequent assessment of traumatic experiences and trauma-related symptoms in healthcare settings. Trauma screening and assessments are best performed in a trauma-informed context, where clinicians start by developing trust and rapport with a patient, build on an individual's strengths and encourage utilization of supportive resources, and follow principles of awareness, safety, and autonomy. Such an environment is particularly important when working with individuals who identify as LGBT not only because of the high rates of trauma among LGBT communities, but simply disclosing one's sexual orientation and/or gender identity can be traumatic in an unfriendly environment. Optimizing care to LGBT communities requires healthcare providers to be educated about how sexual and/or gender minority statuses impact both the overall health status and the healthcare

experience of their patients. Clinicians can play a crucial role in facilitating healthy coping and adaptation in LGBT patients who have experienced trauma.

This chapter will begin by outlining the rationale for contextualizing trauma assessment based on sexual orientation and gender identity. We will then describe a stepwise approach to assessment for trauma, including screening, subsequent assessment, and diagnosis of trauma-related sequelae. Next, we will discuss how to contextualize trauma assessment in LGBT populations and conclude by describing the assessment of posttraumatic growth and resilience.

Contextualizing Trauma Assessment Based on Sexual Orientation and Gender Identity

LGBT communities frequently experience social and cultural hardships on the basis of sexual orientation, gender identity, and/or gender expression that range widely from infrequent instances of bias, to chronic everyday discrimination, to overt violence. These experiences are also informed by an individual's age, race/ethnicity, socioeconomic status, and stage of development. Effective healthcare providers appreciate these complexities and educate themselves on how to evaluate and treat LGBT individuals whose medical or psychiatric presentations may or may not be related to their sexual orientation or gender identity minority status. For example, if a patient discloses that they have a long-term same-sex partner during a routine primary care visit, it is important to not automatically stereotype and start asking if the patient has HIV, is sexually promiscuous, uses drugs, has an open relationship, or is a victim of trauma. However, what should healthcare providers do when an LGBT patient discloses trauma? What nuances in history and presentation should be explored in these patient populations? These questions highlight the importance of contextualizing trauma assessment based upon sexual orientation and gender identity.

B. Hurley, MD, MBA, DFASAM (✉)
Los Angeles County Department of Mental Health, Robert Wood Johnson Foundation Clinical Scholar, David Geffen School of Medicine of the University of California, 10780 Santa Monica Blvd., Suite 105, Los Angeles, CA 90025, USA
e-mail: bhurley@ucla.edu

K. Lin, MD
Massachusetts General Hospital, Child and Adolescent Psychiatry Department, Boston, MA, USA
e-mail: kalin@partners.org

S.N. Jani, MD, MPH
Massachusetts General Hospital/McLean Hospital, Harvard Medical School, Child and Adolescent Psychiatry Department, Yawkey Center for Outpatient Care 6A, Boston, MA, USA
e-mail: sjani@mgh.harvard.edu

K. Kapila, MD
Fenway Health, Fenway South End, 142 Berkeley St., Boston, MA 02216, USA
e-mail: kkapila@fenwayhealth.org

© Springer International Publishing AG 2017
K.L. Eckstrand, J. Potter (eds.), *Trauma, Resilience, and Health Promotion in LGBT Patients*,
DOI 10.1007/978-3-319-54509-7_15

Assessment for Trauma

Effective assessment of trauma begins with screening for a past history of traumatic experiences and the presence of symptomatic sequelae. Further assessment for the presence of a trauma-related psychiatric diagnosis is indicated for those with positive screens, and further assessment for other trauma-associated psychiatric sequelae is indicated for individuals who are found to have a trauma-related psychiatric diagnosis.

Screening for Trauma

Screening for trauma is appropriate for primary care, behavioral health settings, emergency rooms, and in tertiary care settings, as patients with a history of traumatic experiences may present in any of these settings. A variety of screening tools may be used, though not all have been validated in LGBT populations (see Table 15.1; see Chap. 18 for discussion of assessment instrument limitations for LGBT patients). The Primary Care PTSD Screen (PC-PTSD-5) is a five-item screen validated in the primary care setting and has additional clinical utility in behavioral health, emergency department, and other clinical settings where a focused and quick screen is indicated [1]. In additional to the PC-PTSD-5, the Short Form of the PTSD Checklist [2], Short Screening Scale for PTSD [3], and Startle, Physiological Arousal, Anger and Numbness (SPAN) Inventory [4] have been validated in primary care settings. An additional screening tool for use when evaluating injured children and their parents, the Screening Tool for Early Predictors of PTSD (STEPP) [5], has been validated in emergency rooms and urgent care settings.

Transition from Screening to Assessment

Prior to proceeding from screening to a detailed assessment, clinicians should ensure that sufficient rapport, trust, and comfort have been established to permit further inquiry into specific aspects of a patient's trauma history [6]. This preparatory conversation provides key information to predict how an individual is likely to tolerate a more detailed

Table 15.1 Trauma screening and assessment instruments

	Tool	Key features	Limitations
Screening tool	Primary Care PTSD Screen for DSM-5 (PC-PTSD-5)	5 items Clinician administered Validated in primary care settings	Cutoff scores were validated in predominantly male veterans Not validated in LGBT-specific populations
	Short Form of the PTSD Checklist	2- or 6-item versions Clinician administered Validated in primary care settings	2-item form has poor specificity Not validated in LGBT-specific populations
	Short Screening Scale for PTSD	7 items Self-administered Validated in primary care settings	Validated for DSM-IV (not DSM-5) Not validated in LGBT-specific populations
	Startle, Physiological Arousal, Anger and Numbness (SPAN)	4 items Self-administered Useful for screening following recent trauma experiences	Validated for DSM-IV (not DSM-5) Not validated in LGBT-specific populations
	Screening Tool for Early Predictors of PTSD (STEPP)	12 items Clinician administered Validated in acute care settings For children and their parents	A triage tool, not a diagnostic measure Validated for DSM-IV (not DSM-5) Not validated in LGBT-specific populations
Assessment tools	PTSD Checklist	17 items Self-administered Validated in primary care settings	Validated for DSM-IV (not DSM-5) High symptom crossover with other psychiatric conditions Not validated in LGBT-specific populations
	PTSD Symptom Scale – Interview for DSM-5	17 items Clinician-administered semi-structured interview Validated in behavioral health settings	20 min to administer Not validated in LGBT-specific populations
	Clinician-Administered Posttraumatic Stress Disorder (PTSD) Scale (CAPS)	30 items Clinician-administered interview Validated in behavioral health settings	45–60 min to administerNot validated in LGBT-specific populations
	LGBT POC (People of Color) Microaggressions Scale	17 items Self-administered Validated in LGBT populations of color	Not a diagnostic tool for DSM-5 conditions Unknown if generalizable to all LGBT populations of color
	The BTQ (Brief Trauma Questionnaire)	10 items Self-administered Assesses history of traumatic events, including items relevant to LGBT populations	Validated for DSM-IV (not DSM-5) Does not include symptoms Not validated in LGBT-specific populations
	ACE (Adverse Childhood Events)	Items in 14 domains Researcher-administered Includes events relevant to LGBT populations	Over 60 min to administer Used for research; not yet a validated clinical tool

discussion. Useful initial questions include "What strengths did (or do) you use to get through or endure your trauma?" or "How did you survive?" [7].

Trauma-informed assessment is guided by the principles of awareness of trauma, safety for the patient, prominence of patient choice and empowerment, and emphasizes strength-based, patient-centered strategies. The socioecological model of trauma includes examining individual and inter-personal factors that shape a person's response to trauma, but also considers community and organizational, societal, cultural, and historical factors that shape the manner in which societal definitions of trauma evolve in response to cultural shifts [8].

Detailed Assessment of Trauma Symptoms

The Diagnostic Statistical Manual of Mental Disorders (DSM-5) [9] defines trauma systems according to four domains: intrusive symptoms, negative alterations in mood and/or cognition, avoidance of trauma-related stimuli, and heightened arousal and reactivity. Given that these domains extend across the cognitive, mood, and anxiety elements of the human experience, a wide range of immediate and delayed reactions have been described in the literature in response to trauma [6].

A variety of assessment tools have been validated for patients with trauma symptoms (see Table 15.1). These instruments include the Clinician-Administered Posttraumatic Stress Disorder (PTSD) Scale (CAPS) [10], the PTSD Symptom Scale – Interview for DSM-5 (PSSI-5) [11], the PTSD Checklist [12], and the Impact of Events Scale [13]. As with the aforementioned screening tools, some but not all of these assessment instruments have been studied in LGBT populations.

Diagnosis of Trauma-Associated Sequelae

The DSM-5 includes two trauma-specific diagnoses: Acute Stress Disorder and Posttraumatic Stress Disorder. The diagnostic criteria for trauma-related diagnoses are discussed in detail in Chap. 1. The DSM-5 also includes additional trauma diagnoses, such as specific trauma-related disorder and unspecified trauma-related disorder, which are broader descriptive diagnostic terms for trauma-related mental illnesses that do not fully meet criteria for either PTSD or ASD.

In clinical practice, a structured psychiatric or psychological interview is generally sufficient to confirm or exclude the diagnosis of PTSD or ASD. In primary care and other settings where full psychiatric or psychological assessments are not routinely feasible, the PTSD Checklist [12] has been

shown to be effective in supporting the diagnosis of PTSD and is feasible to administer and interpret in these settings [14].

In addition to trauma-specific diagnoses, individuals with a history of traumatic experiences have higher rates of other depression and anxiety disorders, substance use disorders, and eating disorders [15]. Further, individuals with severe mental illness may be more vulnerable to trauma [16]. Therefore, screening for and subsequently assessing for the presence of other psychiatric conditions is clinically indicated for individuals with a history of traumatic experiences.

Contextualizing Screening and Assessment of Trauma in LGBT Populations

Rationale for Contextualizing

The impact of stressful life experiences must be considered when screening and assessing for trauma. As discussed in Chap. 1, there has been significant debate in the diagnostic conceptualization of what constitutes a traumatic event. While the DSM-5 defines a traumatic event as "exposure to actual or threatened death, serious injury, or sexual violence," it is well-recognized that nontraumatic events that are not life-threatening but are still emotionally or physically stressful may lead to subsequent psychological distress [17]. For example, exposure to childhood emotional abuse or neglect – which clearly does not threaten life or physical integrity as defined above – is associated with the development of psychiatric illness [18].

For individuals who identify as LGBT or gender nonconforming, an emerging body of research consistently demonstrates associations between minority stress experiences, many of which do not meet the specific criteria for trauma, and adverse health outcomes. High rates of bullying in LGBT and gender nonconforming youth can lead to substance use, depressive symptoms, and PTSD [19, 20]. Further, structural stigma via lack of nondiscrimination policies is associated with greater depression, anxiety, and PTSD among LGB adults [21]. Contextualizing screening for the unique forms of trauma and stress experienced by LGBT individuals is thus critical to identifying the presence of, and risk for, psychiatric distress.

How Is the Assessment of LGBT Patients Similar and Different from Assessment of Their Heterosexual/Cisgender Counterparts?

Regardless of sexual orientation or gender identity, the same standard of care applies when it comes to building an alliance, performing a thorough psychiatric evaluation, and delivering appropriate medical care. Frequently, an interviewer may not discover that a patient identifies as LGBT until sufficient rapport has been established or the patient is convinced that it is relevant to disclose this information. One of the foundations of trauma work is to build a strong therapeutic alliance with the patient as a first step, and this principle is particularly important for LGBT patients.

While there are several similarities in screening and assessing trauma across diverse sexual orientations and gender identities, numerous differences exist. LGBT individuals can experience internal minority stressors, including internalized homo/bi/transphobia and rejection sensitivity, and may conceal their identities. External minority stressors that don't meet the diagnostic criteria for trauma such as sexual and gender minority-related bullying, harassment, and discrimination, frequently remain unassessed via standard screening and assessment instruments. These nuances are particularly important at certain stages in development, such as childhood and adolescence, when the differential vulnerability to stress may have a long-lasting impact on an LGBT individual's mental, physical, and behavioral health. Additionally, the "microtraumas" of daily marginalization and discrimination may have differential effects for LGB individuals who are also members of a stigmatized ethnic or racial minority group experiencing race or ethnicity-related discrimination [22]. Table 15.2 lists questions that can be used in the clinical setting for discussing LGBT-related trauma and stress.

What Specialized Screening and Assessment Considerations Are Relevant for LGBT People of Color?

As discussed in Chap. 10, some LGB individuals may have a difficult time finding support within the LGB community due to racial or ethnic stigmatization factors, including immigration status, acculturation status, language barriers, family of origin, and socioeconomic class. However, counter to evidence that some LGB ethnic and racial minorities have poorer outcomes compared to those with racial and ethnic privilege, some individuals with dual minority status have been shown to have *lower* rates of mental health problems. As suggested in the APA guidelines, a double minority status could provide skills in "negotiating one stigmatized aspect of identity," which "assists the individual in dealing with and protecting the individual from other forms of stigmatization" [23].

The impact of the intersection between racial and LGBT identities can become more complicated if the patient is also an immigrant or forced migrant, as migrant individuals experience unique vulnerabilities (see Chap. 11). For example, family support may be limited if family members are physically living in other countries; alternatively, families of origin are frequently a source of emotional, verbal, physical, and sexual abuse [24]. Repeated and chronic abuse can contribute to psychological barriers that prevent migrant individuals from seeking help, particularly when law

Table 15.2 Questions for assessing trauma, stress, and resilience

Clinical questions discussing minority stress
In what environments are you out about your sexual orientation/gender identity status? In what settings are you not out?
How comfortable are you with others knowing about your sexual orientation/gender identity status? At home? At work?
What, if any, discrimination or unfair events have happened to you as a result of your sexual orientation, gender identity, or gender expression?
How worried are you that others might treat you differently or discriminate against you as a result of your sexual orientation/gender identity?
In what ways, if any, are you bothered or concerned by your sexual orientation/gender identity?
Do you ever feel, or have you ever felt, depressed, anxious, sad, or stressed about your sexual orientation/gender identity?
Do you ever feel you have to say or do things you don't want to in order to fit in with other LGBT individuals?
In what ways, if any, do you feel you struggle with your sexual orientation/gender identity?
Clinical questions discussing resilience
How have your feelings regarding your sexual orientation/gender identity changed over time?
Who are the supportive individuals in your life? How supported do you feel by these people regarding your sexual orientation/gender identity?
How supportive is your family regarding your sexual orientation/gender identity?
Describe your social support network; how comfortable are you with this network?
When you have a stressful life experience, how do you handle it?
When you are in a situation that makes you feel unsafe, how do you handle it?
How do you cope with depression, anxiety, or other challenging emotions?
What ways, if any, do you feel you could be more supported regarding your sexual orientation/gender identity?

enforcement and other officials in countries of origin participated in the abuse.

The LGBT POC (People of Color) Microaggressions Scale can be used to quantify and study stressors specific to LGBT individuals who are also racial or ethnic minorities [25]. The self-report consists of 18 questions divided into three subscales of (a) racism in LGBT communities, (b) heterosexism/transphobia in racial/ethnic minority communities, and (c) racism in dating and close relationships. These authors found that higher microaggression experiences were found in men compared to women, lesbian women and gay men compared to bisexual women and men, and Asian Americans more than African Americans or Latinos. Whereas follow-up studies are needed to determine if higher scores on this specific scale correlate to poorer outcomes, previous studies have revealed the repeating theme that LGBT ethnic minorities often have worse physical and health outcomes (e.g., more smoking or more depression).

What Specialized Screening and Assessment Considerations Are Relevant for LGBT Youth?

As discussed in Chap. 6, children and adolescents who are LGBT or are questioning their sexual orientation, gender identity, or gender expression are at greater risk for certain types of trauma and stress. Over one-third of LGB youth have been bullied on school property as well as electronically, nearly 30% have been in a physical fight, 10% have been threatened with a weapon, and almost one in five LGB individuals have been forced to have sexual intercourse [26]. Few studies exist on the experiences of transgender youth; however, gender nonconforming youth experience higher rates of discrimination and victimization [19]. Unsurprisingly, LGB students are more likely to avoid school due to safety concerns, nearly half have considered suicide, and are more likely to use tobacco, alcohol, and other substances [26]. The behavioral changes identified above may precede an individual's coming out, so universal screening for bullying and violence is recommended for all youth [27].

Screening for childhood abuse and mistreatment can be performed by calculating an individual's ACE (Adverse Childhood Experiences) Score. This is determined through answering 10 questions about potential adverse childhood experiences that can lead to poorer physical health outcomes in adulthood [28]. For the most part, the 10 questions asked are broadly applicable; however, they may not capture SOGI-specific experiences, and thus could potentially give LGBT patients an artificially lower score. For example, the ACE questionnaire omits questions such as "Were you ever discriminated against due to your sexual orientation or gender identity?" Furthermore, question 7 asks specifically about a mother or a stepmother, which automatically excludes two male parents. Thus, even though the ACE study is a valuable tool that helps to explain how trauma (both life threatening and not) can affect future physical health outcomes, it is not clear that it holds the same specificity or sensitivity for LGBT individuals compared to heterosexual and cisgender people.

For LGB youth who have disclosed their sexual orientation and/or gender identity, additional instruments have been developed to assess for trauma and stress. One recently developed instrument, the Sexual Minority Adolescent Stress Inventory [29], includes measures on disclosure of sexual orientation, internalized stigma, family/peer/school interactions, and racial/ethnic intersectionality. Another measure, the Parental Support for Sexual Orientation Scale [30], examines parental support for youth identifying with a sexual orientation minority or are in a same-sex romantic relationship.

What Specialized Screening and Assessment Considerations Are Relevant for LGBT Adults?

Even when reluctant to interact with the healthcare system due to a past history of trauma, LGBT individuals with life-threatening or chronic medical illnesses will at some point present for care. Such presentations can be challenging in many ways. Since the US Supreme Court ruling in 2015, same-sex marriages are legal across the United States [31]. However, that does not end the discrimination and bias that some LGBT couples continue to face in the healthcare system, particularly when they are not legally married. As discussed in Chap. 8, life partners can help in decision-making, provide comfort for the patient, mobilize social supports, and will also need support themselves from providers. When the partner is not recognized or acknowledged, patient care can be adversely impacted. Partners might not receive medical updates or be acknowledged as the next of kin in capacity evaluations. Social services could also potentially be denied, as during disposition to certain programs or nursing homes. Furthermore, for LGB individuals who lose their partner, family support may be limited or nonexistent due to ostracization for being in a gay and lesbian relationship. In such cases, the surviving partner may become even more isolated, placing them at risk for complicated grief or depression.

Unfortunately, validated instruments assessing stress and trauma for LGBT older adults are not available at this time. However, it is recommended that clinicians be able to discuss trauma and stress with LGBT elders across the four domains of successful LGBT aging: physical, mental, emotional, and social health [32].

Assessment of Posttraumatic Growth and Resilience

Most sexual minority identity research has yet to systematically study growth experiences associated with childhood and/or minority stress [33–37]. To date, the literature has focused chiefly on adverse psychological and social outcomes without assessing posttraumatic growth and resilience [33, 37]. However, sexual orientation stress can mediate growth and resilience by stimulating stigma-related coping that confers psychological benefits and overall positive effects on mental health [38]. Indeed, Berger et al. [39] reported that 63% of lesbian and gay participants reported growth associated with the sexual identity development process. Additionally, qualitative research on sexual minority identity development has provided substantial evidence that sexual identity disclosure to others is associated with both losses and gains, and ultimately produces resilience [40, 41], to the extent that some researchers have applied the term "Coming Out Growth" to this process [42]. Figure 15.1 highlights select factors that have been associated with positive health effects among LGBT individuals.

Discussing growth and resilience is a critical component of assessing for trauma, as it can identify an individual's strengths as well as opportunities for clinical intervention or referral to additional resources [42]. Table 15.2 lists several questions that can be used clinically to assess for coping and resilience among LGBT individuals. Indeed, simply discussing coping and resilience with patients can elicit the resilience of LGBT patients they encounter during the process of trauma screening and assessment. Further, while individuals may identify certain aspects of coping and resilience, these can be strengthened clinically through several techniques discussed elsewhere in this text. Some of these factors, such as emotional coping and self-acceptance, can be enhanced through motivational interviewing and use of a trauma-informed approach to care (see Chaps. 17 and 15, respectively). Others, such as social support, can be bolstered by connecting individuals (and their family members, if open to participating) with supportive resources in the community (see Chap. 20).

Conclusion

Deciding where and how to screen for stressful and traumatic experiences is a topic of increasing discussion in clinical practice. While assessment and diagnosis may be nuanced, the myriad negative sequelae of traumatic experiences necessitate early identification and management to optimize the health of individuals who have experienced trauma. Numerous screening and assessment tools

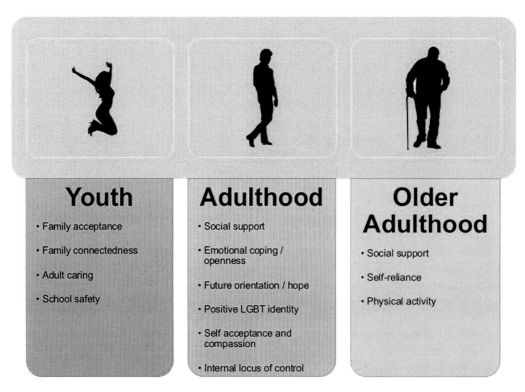

Fig. 15.1 Resilience factors among LGBT individuals

have been developed, although these instruments must be contextualized based on sexual orientation and gender identity. Using the strategies described in this chapter, clinicians can not only develop proficiency in screening and assessing for stress and trauma inclusive of LGBT individuals, they can also begin to promote posttraumatic growth and resilience.

Key Clinical Recommendations

- LGBT populations are at elevated risk for traumatic experiences.
- The assessment of trauma in LGBT individuals should be contextualized to LGBT populations.
- There are tradeoffs when choosing tools for trauma screening and assessment; clinicians should be able to tailor common assessment instruments to evaluate LGBT-specific traumatic and stressful experiences.
- Trauma-informed assessment is guided by the principles of awareness of trauma, patient safety, prominence of patient choice and empowerment, and emphasis on strength-based strategies.
- Healthcare providers should approach LGBT individuals with openness, humility, and a genuine curiosity to understand.
- Resilience can be fostered through use of motivational interviewing and employing trauma-informed principles to elicit openness, hope, and optimism.

References

1. Prins A, et al. The primary care PTSD screen for DSM-5 (PC-PTSD-5): development and evaluation within a veteran primary care sample. J Gen Intern Med. 2016;31:1–6.
2. Lang AJ, Stein MB. An abbreviated PTSD checklist for use as a screening instrument in primary care. Behav Res Ther. 2005;43(5):585–94.
3. Kimerling R, et al. Brief report: utility of a short screening scale for DSM-IV PTSD in primary care. J Gen Intern Med. 2006;21(1):65–7.
4. Sijbrandij M, et al. Early prognostic screening for posttraumatic stress disorder with the Davidson trauma scale and the SPAN. Depress Anxiety. 2008;25(12):1038–45.
5. Winston FK, et al. Screening for risk of persistent posttraumatic stress in injured children and their parents. JAMA. 2003;290(5):643–9.
6. Briere JN, Scott C. Principles of trauma therapy: a guide to symptoms, evaluation, and treatment. Thousand Oaks: Sage Publications; 2014.
7. Bassuk EL, Melnick S, Browne A. Responding to the needs of low-income and homeless women who are survivors of family violence. J Am Med Womens Assoc. 1998;53:57–64.
8. Substance Abuse and Mental Health Services Administration. Trauma-informed care in behavioral health services. Treatment improvement protocol (TIP) series 57. HHS publication no. (SMA) 13–4801. Rockville: Substance Abuse and Mental Health Services Administration; 2014.
9. American Psychiatric Association. Diagnostic and statistical manual of mental disorders (DSM-5®). Washington, DC: American Psychiatric Publishing; 2013.
10. Blake D, et al. A clinician rating scale for assessing current and lifetime PTSD: the CAPS-1. Behav Ther. 1990;13:187–8.
11. Foa EB, et al. Psychometric properties of the posttraumatic stress disorder symptom scale interview for DSM–5 (PSSI–5). Psychol Assess. 2015;28:1159–65.
12. Weathers F, et al. The PTSD checklist for DSM-5 (PCL-5). 2013 [2016 Aug 24]. Available from: www.ptsd.va.gov.
13. Creamer M, Bell R, Failla S. Psychometric properties of the impact of event scale—revised. Behav Res Ther. 2003;41(12):1489–96.
14. Spoont MR, et al. Does this patient have posttraumatic stress disorder?: Rational clinical examination systematic review. JAMA. 2015;314(5):501–10.
15. Brady KT, et al. Comorbidity of psychiatric disorders and posttraumatic stress disorder. J Clin Psychiatry. 2000;61:22–32.
16. Grubaugh AL, et al. Trauma exposure and posttraumatic stress disorder in adults with severe mental illness: a critical review. Clin Psychol Rev. 2011;31(6):883–99.
17. Carlson EB, Dalenberg CJ. A conceptual framework for the impact of traumatic experiences. Trauma Violence Abuse. 2000;1(1):4–28.
18. Schalinski I, et al. Type and timing of adverse childhood experiences differentially affect severity of PTSD, dissociative and depressive symptoms in adult inpatients. BMC Psychiatry. 2016;16(1):295.
19. Roberts AL, et al. Childhood gender nonconformity: a risk indicator for childhood abuse and posttraumatic stress in youth. Pediatrics. 2012;129(3):410–7.
20. Association, A.P. Guidelines for psychological practice with lesbian, gay, and bisexual clients. Am Psychol. 2012;67(1):10–42.
21. Hatzenbuehler ML, Keyes KM, Hasin DS. State-level policies and psychiatric morbidity in lesbian, gay, and bisexual populations. Am J Public Health. 2009;99(12):2275–81.
22. Alessi EJ, Meyer IH, Martin JI. PTSD and sexual orientation: an examination of criterion A1 and non-criterion A1 events. Psychol Trauma. 2013;5(2):149.
23. American Psychological Association. Guidelines for psychological practice with lesbian, gay, and bisexual clients. Am Psychol. 2012;67(1):10–42.
24. Shiloh A, Aloha J. Mental health challenges of LGBT forced migrants. Forced Migr Rev. 2013;42:9.
25. Balsam KF, et al. Measuring multiple minority stress: the LGBT people of color microaggressions scale. Cultur Divers Ethnic Minor Psychol. 2011;17(2):163.
26. Kann L. Sexual identity, sex of sexual contacts, and health-related behaviors among students in grades 9–12—United States and selected sites, 2015. MMWR Surveill Summ. 2016;65:1–202.
27. Committee on Injury, V., and Poison Prevention. Policy statement-role of the pediatrician in youth violence prevention. Pediatrics. 2009;124(1):393–402.
28. Felitti VJ, et al. Relationship of childhood abuse and household dysfunction to many of the leading causes of death in adults: the adverse childhood experiences (ACE) study. Am J Prev Med. 1998;14(4):245–58.
29. Goldbach JT. Measuring stress among diverse adolescents. In development. https://projectreporter.nih.gov/project_info_descrip tion.cfm?aid=8931800&icde=32046403&ddparam=&ddvalue=&ddsub=&cr=1&csb=default&cs=ASC.
30. Mohr JJ, Fassinger RE. Self-acceptance and self-disclosure of sexual orientation in lesbian, gay, and bisexual adults: an attachment perspective. J Couns Psychol. 2003;50(4):482.

31. Obergefell v. Hodges, in S. Ct. Supreme Court; 2015. p. 2071.

32. Van Wagenen A, Driskell J, Bradford J. "I'm still raring to go": successful aging among lesbian, gay, bisexual, and transgender older adults. J Aging Stud. 2013;27(1):1–14.

33. Bonet L, Wells BE, Parsons JT. A positive look at a difficult time: a strength based examination of coming out for lesbian and bisexual women. J LBGT Health Res. 2007;3(1):7–14.

34. Lasser J, Tharinger D. Visibility management in school and beyond: a qualitative study of gay, lesbian, bisexual youth. J Adolesc. 2003;26(2):233–44.

35. Moradi B, et al. Counseling psychology research on sexual (orientation) minority issues: conceptual and methodological challenges and opportunities. J Couns Psychol. 2009;56(1):5.

36. Savin-Williams RC. Then and now: recruitment, definition, diversity, and positive attributes of same-sex populations. Dev Psychol. 2008;44(1):135.

37. Riggle ED, et al. The positive aspects of being a lesbian or gay man. Prof Psychol. 2008;39(2):210.

38. Wang K, Rendina HJ, Pachankis JE. Looking on the bright side of stigma: how stress-related growth facilitates adaptive coping among gay and bisexual men. J Gay Lesbian Ment Health. 2016;20(4):363–75.

39. Berger RM. Passing: impact on the quality of same-sex couple relationships. Soc Work. 1990;35(4):328–32.

40. LaSala MC. Gay male couples: the importance of coming out and being out to parents. J Homosex. 2000;39(2):47–71.

41. Savin-Williams RC. Mom, Dad. I'm Gay: how families negotiate coming out. Washington, DC: American Psychological Association; 2001.

42. Vaughan MD, Waehler CA. Coming out growth: conceptualizing and measuring stress-related growth associated with coming out to others as a sexual minority. J Adult Dev. 2010;17(2):94–109.

Sarah M. Peitzmeier and Jennifer Potter

Introduction

Chapter 4 reviewed the impact of trauma on the health of LGBT individuals. In this chapter, we will discuss how understanding trauma may be particularly relevant when conducting a physical exam with an LGBT patient. The laying of hands on the body to examine a patient has been a central part of medical practice for thousands of years and happens in most medical encounters [1]. While physical touch has the potential to be therapeutic and the exam may contribute to diagnosis and healing, it also carries the potential to harm. This is of particular concern for patients with a trauma history, where a history of physical, emotional, sexual, institutional, and healthcare-related traumas can make the physical exam more emotionally or physically challenging. Independent from trauma history, LGBT patients may find physical exams traumatizing if they seem incongruent with their gender identity (such as transgender women receiving a prostate exam). The experience of the physical exam can thus have negative consequences and, in a worst-case scenario, can trigger acute reactions such as dissociation or panic attacks. We review practical techniques of good clinical practice and positive patient-provider interaction that can make physical exams more empowering and prevent

such adverse reactions; we also discuss how to manage these reactions when they do occur. Most of the literature on performing a trauma-informed physical exam concerns pelvic exams for individuals with natal female reproductive anatomy; where possible we also present evidence about other types of exams and guiding principles that can be generalized to many different exam procedures.

Performing a Trauma-Informed Physical Exam That Is LGBT-Inclusive

See Table 16.1 for some guiding principles for performing a trauma-informed physical exam that is LGBT-inclusive.

Screen for Trauma

Screening for trauma is critical in the medical setting (see Chap. 14 for more details on how to build a trauma-informed practice). Even when a patient screens negative, the clinician can never be completely sure of the patient's trauma history, since not all patients who have experienced trauma recall the event or perceive events that are consistent with clinical definitions of trauma to be "traumatic." Others may make a conscious decision not to disclose. Therefore, it is important to avoid following one set of procedures for physical exams with patients who screen positive for trauma, and a completely separate set of procedures for those who screen negative. One should always act in a way that conforms to basic principles of trauma-informed care, though extra precautions to avoid retraumatization due to the exam can be taken with those who screen positive (see section "Additional Considerations for Patients Who Have Experienced Trauma").

S.M. Peitzmeier, MSPH (✉)
Johns Hopkins Bloomberg School of Public Health, Department of Population, Family and Reproductive Health, 615 N. Wolfe St, Baltimore, MD 21205, USA

The Fenway Institute, 1340 Boylston St, Boston, MA 02215, USA
e-mail: speitzme@jhsph.edu

J. Potter, MD (✉)
Associate Professor of Medicine and Advisory Dean and Director, William B. Castle Society, Harvard Medical School

Director, Women's Health Center, Beth Israel Deaconess Medical Center

Director, Women's Health Program, Fenway Health Center

Director, Women's Health Research, The Fenway Institute, Boston, MA, USA
e-mail: jpotter@bidmc.harvard.edu

© Springer International Publishing AG 2017
K.L. Eckstrand, J. Potter (eds.), *Trauma, Resilience, and Health Promotion in LGBT Patients*,
DOI 10.1007/978-3-319-54509-7_16

Table 16.1 Guiding principles

1. Ensure that the *locus of control* remains with the patient – i.e., that the patient feels they have voluntarily consented to the exam and feels empowered to stop the exam, communicate with you, or ask for modifications at any time
2. Engage in *shared decision making* regarding what screening the patient opts to do, especially in the face of uncertain evidence or conflicting guidelines
3. *Explain* the procedure to the extent preferred, using the patient's preferred terminology for body parts
4. Discuss what *modifications to the exam* can be made to promote patient comfort
5. *Acknowledge* the patient's trauma history and *validate* any negative consequences they feel resulting from the trauma

Consider if You Actually Need to Perform the Exam

Although most patients will not be traumatized by a physical exam, any exam has some potential to be traumatizing. This is especially true if the exam requires the patient to become particularly vulnerable (as during a breast, pelvic, prostate, or rectal exam) or if the patient has a history of trauma of any kind. Posttraumatic distress can be triggered even years after the index traumatic event by strong emotions (e.g., feeling helpless, out of control, trapped, or unprotected), physical discomfort, and/or any sensation that is reminiscent of the original trauma. Because all aspects of the physical exam have the potential to cause such harm, it is important to avoid asking patients to submit to exams that are not clearly warranted – especially those aspects of an exam that cause the greatest vulnerability.

Review the evidence in your specialty for what aspects of the physical exam are supported by reliable and consistent evidence, and which are not. For instance, the American College of Physicians conducted a systematic review and in 2014 concluded that there is no evidence to suggest that routine screening with bimanual examination (BME)[1] for asymptomatic, average-risk, nonpregnant women reduces morbidity or mortality as long as cervical cancer screening guidelines are followed [2], with some calling BMEs "more of a ritual than an evidence-based practice" [3]. Nevertheless, many gynecologists continue to regularly perform this exam on asymptomatic patients [4, 5]. Similarly, testicular exams are no longer recommended to screen for testicular cancer in asymptomatic adolescent or adult individuals with natal male anatomy [6]. In another example, the US Preventive Services Task Force (USPSTF) ruled in 2009 that there is insufficient evidence to suggest any benefit to clinical breast exams above and beyond mammography as a screening procedure for breast cancer, and also recommends against teaching breast self-exams [7], as does the American Cancer Society [8].

If you are in the middle of a visit and are not sure whether a particular screening exam is indicated, let the patient know

you need to obtain consultation to determine the most up-to-date medical recommendations, and step out of the room to confer with a knowledgeable colleague in the moment. If such guidance is not immediately available, set an intention with the patient to complete the discussion at their next visit rather than proceeding with the exam, particularly if the exam has a higher potential to be traumatizing (e.g., breast, pelvic, prostate, or rectal exams).

Completely unnecessary exams must be avoided. For instance, asking to see trans patients' body parts merely out of curiosity about anatomical changes or surgical results is unprofessional and a form of harassment. In a qualitative study we conducted, one patient recounted a story of a surgeon who, while preparing to perform a breast augmentation for a trans woman, asked to see her vagina because he was curious about what it looked like [9]. This sort of curiosity is never appropriate.

Consider if There May Be Alternative Procedures to Recommend to or Offer the Patient

Increasingly, alternatives exist to physical exams that are backed by evidence and may be preferred by some patients. For instance, self-collected swabs for gonorrhea and chlamydia testing, including vaginal, anal, and throat samples, are actually superior to physician-collected samples in their sensitivity and specificity [10]. While some patients will prefer to have a provider collect the sample, others will appreciate having the option to perform sample collection themselves.

Make No Assumptions About Patients' Preferences and Discuss the Benefits, Potential Harms, and Limitations of the Examination, Particularly with Regard To Data Pertaining to LGBT Populations

After reviewing the benefits and risks of exams to decide whether they are indicated (see section "Consider If You Actually Need to Perform the Exam"), the clinician should engage in shared decision making with LGBT patients about whether to perform the exam. Involving the patient in this decision helps the locus of control remain with the patient

---

[1] A bimanual examination is when the clinician places two fingers inside the vagina and the other hand on top of the abdomen in order to palpate internal pelvic structures such as the cervix, uterus, and ovaries.

and helps ensure that they fully understand and consent to the exam.

This discussion should include a review of data (or lack thereof) pertaining to benefits and risks in specific LGBT communities, especially transgender patients, for whom high-quality evidence is frequently limited. For instance, no studies have specifically evaluated the benefits and harms of clinical breast exams, mammography, testicular or prostate exams, and Pap tests of the neovagina among postsurgical trans women. In the absence of definitive data, expert consensus recommendations are available to guide care [11–13]. For example, the University of California San Francisco (UCSF) Center of Excellence for Transgender Health recommends against performing Pap tests of the neovagina in trans women because its walls are typically composed of keratinized skin or urethral/colon mucosa and recommends screening mammograms for trans women 50 or older with more than 5 years of estrogen and progesterone use and additional risk factors (family history, BMI > 35) [14]. While recommended exams should be promoted, patients should nevertheless be made aware of the quality of the evidence that underlies such consensus recommendations.

This discussion should also review potential harms of the exam, which include the possibility that it may cause emotional distress and/or physical discomfort. After validating the patient's concerns, discuss modifications that can be made to the exam to make it more acceptable to the patient (see section "Before Proceeding with the Exam, Discuss Whether the Patient Desires Any Modifications to the Exam to Reduce the Potential for Retraumatization"). If an exam is clearly indicated, it is the clinician's job to help the patient feel comfortable enough to adhere to the recommended guidelines as closely as possible. However, this should never be accomplished at the expense of true informed consent. In our qualitative work with transgender men, several reported being told they could not obtain hormones if they did not first agree to have a cervical Pap [15]. This echoes the outdated practice of withholding birth control if the patient has not had a Pap test [16], another coercive and medically unsupported practice.

In addition, clinicians should avoid assuming that either discussing the physical exam in advance or performing the exam will necessarily cause psychological harm, and should refrain from broaching the topic of an exam with exaggerated caution. Some LGBT patients may have extra sensitivities or concerns about an exam while others may not. Simply ask about a patient's prior experience with similar exams, and find out which aspects went well and which could be improved in the future.

Before Proceeding with the Exam, Discuss Whether the Patient Desires Any Modifications to the Exam to Reduce the Potential for Retraumatization

Explain to the patient what they can expect in terms of length of time the exam will take and what sensations or discomfort they may experience. To the extent preferred, explain the mechanics of the exam (e.g., offering to show a speculum before a Pap test if they would like to know the details). These conversations should take place while the patient is still clothed and in a location where the patient is empowered to participate in such a conversation [17].

Discuss potential modifications to the exam to increase individual comfort. In a qualitative study of transgender men's preferences with regard to cervical cancer screening, patients reported a wide range of comfort with the exam and many found modifications helpful [15] including:

1. Self-insertion of the speculum
2. Use of a pediatric speculum
3. Use of lubricant and/or topical lidocaine to ease speculum insertion
4. Having a trusted support person accompany them as a chaperone
5. Positioning alternatives
6. Use of antianxiety medications

Allowing the patient to make modifications to reduce physical and/or emotional discomfort with the exam shifts the locus of control toward the patient and makes retraumatization less likely. Alternative positioning diagrams and descriptions are available elsewhere [18]. Different patients will have different preferences, so asking the patient "What we can do to make this exam easier for you?" and briefly providing some options to open up the discussion is important. Regardless of trauma history, modifications can make the exam more tolerable for any patient.

It is extremely important that the locus of control with respect to both proceeding with an exam and stopping the exam at any point resides at all times with the patient. Review with the patient that it will always be their choice whether and when to proceed with an exam and that they retain the right to change their minds at any time and stop the exam. If choosing to proceed, agree in advance on the signal the patient will use to indicate that they want to stop the exam and be sure to respect that signal immediately.

Always Obtain Assent Before You Physically Touch or Examine a Patient

Prior to performing any aspect of a physical exam it is important to explain to the patient what you plan to do and obtain assent. For example, one might say, "Now that we've completed your history, I'd like to check your blood pressure and listen to your heart and lungs… Is that OK?" Once a patient has assented, it is important to continue to provide verbal notice before touching the patient; for example, one might say, "Now you'll feel the stethoscope touching the right side of your back." When performing a particularly sensitive exam that involves touching vulnerable parts of the body (e.g., the genitals), provide a warning before each maneuver ("Now I'm going to separate the outer folds"… "Now you'll feel a little pressure as I insert the speculum"). These warnings help patients prepare themselves so the touch does not come as a surprise and cause a startle response. It may be helpful to students just learning these techniques to perform the exam as if the patient cannot see what is going on, as in this case explaining every action prior to doing it comes very naturally. As many members of the treatment team (e.g., medical assistants, nurses, etc.) may have occasion to touch patients in the course of providing care, it is important to teach all team members these trauma-informed exam techniques and to observe their performance to make sure they achieve the desired level of competence.

Non-gendered or less-gendered terminology can be particularly important to use with transgender patients who experience body dysphoria unless they indicate a preference for traditional clinical terms, e.g., using "folds" instead of "labia" when performing pelvic exams with transgender men. Language with sexual ("I'm going to come into you now") or violent connotations (such as "blades" of the speculum) should be avoided. See Potter et al. [15] for alternative language suggestions.

Particular sensitivity is required in situations in which extra caregivers, such as translators, American Sign Language (ASL) interpreters, personal care attendants, etc., are present in the exam room. In these cases, you should discuss how the patient wants or needs the exam to be conducted (e.g., with the translator in the room but standing behind a curtain, using hand signals agreed upon in advance and the ASL interpreter stepping outside the room, etc.) before proceeding [17]. These steps are particularly important when caring for patients with a known trauma history and for transgender patients, who may be more likely to experience additional people in the room as voyeurs.

During the Exam, Be particularly Mindful of Your Tone and Reactions

The patient may feel most vulnerable during the actual exam itself due to physical positioning or touch and thus may be most sensitive to triggers at this time. Speak and move calmly and slowly, as these actions will help both you and the patient remain calm during what can be a stressful situation for both parties. Avoid expressing surprise or making any remarks during the exam about the patient's body that are not relevant to the performance of the exam. For instance, some trans patients may have anatomical changes as the result of hormones or surgery, while others may not. In a qualitative study of trans men's experiences with cancer screening, one participant reported feeling disturbed when a clinician commented during an exam of his postmastectomy chest, "I bet you were happy when those were gone!" While the clinician may have been trying to build rapport by validating the patient's decision to have gender-affirming chest surgery, the comment was medically unnecessary, made the patient feel like an object of scrutiny, and drew attention to a part of their body that had been the focus of considerable dysphoria in the past. Body piercings or tattoos should also not be commented on unless medically relevant.

Additional Considerations for Patients Who Have Experienced Trauma

While the above steps apply to all patients, additional steps may be necessary for patients with a history of trauma who are having a difficult time approaching the exam.

Validate the Patient

Normalize that many people have an impulse to avoid exams in the wake of trauma. Emphasize the importance of locus of control and of accomplishing needed exams as a key ingredient to self-care.

For patients who have experienced violence and abuse, self-care may seem like a foreign concept, exhausting to contemplate or pointless to consider. Gently remind such patients that everyone deserves to be cared for, we all have the power to take care of ourselves, and caring for one's body is an important aspect of healing from trauma and abuse.

Be Patient and Focus on Building a Relationship

In our qualitative work with transgender men and cervical cancer screening, an established, trusting relationship with the provider was a key facilitator to screening: many patients were unwilling to receive a cervical Pap test with a new provider, but were willing to do so once trust was established. Supportive and gentle encouragement by a provider repeatedly over multiple visits can enhance a patients' intrinsic motivation to undergo a needed procedure, despite initial reluctance.

Brainstorm Additional Ways to Support the Patient

When working with patients who have experienced trauma, it is particularly important to discuss adaptations to the exam that can be used to optimize comfort. These adaptations are analogous to the accommodations you would make for any patient who has additional needs that must be addressed in order to perform a thorough exam (e.g., a patient with an above-the-knee amputation who is unable to place both lower extremities in footrests for a pelvic exam and requires collaborative problem solving to achieve a comfortable and feasible position in which the exam can be performed successfully). Such time spent up front can be pivotal in establishing an environment in which the patient eventually feels sufficiently safe to proceed with the exam. It is often useful to devote an entire visit to this discussion to allow enough time to discuss concerns and preferences, and to not rush the patient. In our qualitative work, transmasculine patients who were reluctant to undergo cervical cancer screening often expressed the desire for a consult visit where they would be able to talk to the provider about what the procedure would entail and how to manage challenges that might occur during the exam, such as emotional and/or physical discomfort. This approach further allows for patients to prepare themselves for a subsequent exam and to feel more in control of the process.

Discuss potentially pursuing a team-based approach to accomplishing the exam, such as involving a therapist in helping the patient learn techniques to manage discomfort and/or inviting a supporter of the patient's choosing to attend the exam. If participation of an office assistant or chaperone is anticipated, an explanation of the reason for that person's attendance is crucial. Some patients may feel more uncomfortable undergoing certain exams in the presence of chaperones as they can feel like a voyeur [15]; therefore, whenever possible, the patient should be given the choice of whether to have one.

For some patients, premedication with a short-acting anxiolytic medication (e.g., benzodiazepine) may also be helpful. Keep in mind that such medicines may cause dissociation during the exam or even amnesia, which may be alarming to patients who have experienced trauma [19]. When using such medicines, it is therefore a good idea to discuss these side effects with patients prior to their administration. Again, inviting a person the patient trusts to witness the encounter if medication is used can create a space that feels more safe [15].

Patients who have experienced trauma in the past may be more likely to experience physical pain due to factors such as anxiety leading to involuntary pelvic floor muscle contraction and/or spasm, which can also impede insertion of specula or digits in the case of pelvic and rectal exams.

Strategies to reduce pain include application of topical lidocaine gel for vaginal or rectal exams, topical nitroglycerin for rectal exams, and oral anesthetic spray for pharyngeal swabs. Postmenopausal women and transgender men on testosterone may also benefit from a 5-day course of estrogen or suppository prior to a pelvic exam to reduce atrophy-mediated discomfort upon speculum insertion. Transgender men may have some sensitivities around using estrogen cream, so the discussion should be broached thoughtfully, emphasizing that the effects are highly localized and short term.

Be Prepared to Handle Dissociation or Distress During the Exam

If a patient seems to be experiencing mild distress during the exam, even if they have not signaled or asked for you to stop, ask the patient if they would like you to do so. Some patients will prefer to continue and get the exam over with despite some distress (particularly if the only distressing aspect is physical pain and not emotional distress), while others will appreciate the opening to ask you to stop. If a patient is having more severe distress or dissociates during the exam (e.g., eyes become glazed, stares off into space, seems to no longer be engaged in the present, begins to cry, or has a flashback), stop the exam immediately. Have the patient sit up fully covered, and utilize grounding techniques. These are techniques designed to bring the patient back to the present:

- Verbally reorient the patient using safety statements ("I am Dr. XX"... "You are safe right now"... "You are in the present, not the past"... "You are at ___ and the date is ___").
- Ask the patient to keep their eyes open and look around the room. Ask the patient to describe the exam room in detail using all of their senses (e.g., objects, sounds, textures, colors, smells, shapes, numbers, temperature).
- Reconnect the patient with their body by asking them to grip the table as hard as they can with their hands, wiggle their toes in their socks, or place their feet on the floor and literally feel the ground supporting them.
- Once the patient is reengaged in the present, and preferably when they are once again fully clothed, talk about what happened, reassure the patient that such reactions are common and make sense after a person has experienced trauma. Reassure the patient that they did not "fail" in some way, that you are not upset that they were not able to complete the exam at this visit, and that you are invested in continuing to work together to make sure they receive the best possible care.

Debrief After the Exam and Make Sure the Patient Has a Plan for Self-Care After Leaving the Office

For patients who experience distress during the physical exam, always conclude the encounter by assisting the patient in reconstituting and developing a self-care plan for after they leave the office. This plan might include:

- Connecting with a therapist, friends, family, or pet
- Picturing themselves in a safe and soothing place (e.g., the beach, mountains, or a favorite room)
- Repeating a coping statement ("I can handle this"... "This will pass"), poem, or prayer
- Self-soothing by setting an intention to give themselves a safe treat (e.g., nice dinner, warm bath, listening to favorite music, etc.)
  - If they feel their gender identity was undermined by the exam (e.g. some transmasculine patients report feeling their identity feels challenged or destabilized after undergoing a Pap test), they may want to make a plan for affirming their gender in positive ways (e.g. one patient in our qualitative study reported going shopping for men's clothing and asking his friends to text him and call him "handsome" after his Pap test).

Make sure the patient has a follow-up appointment scheduled before they leave the office. If possible, give the patient a transitional object to take home – such as a business card with your name and contact information on it – to help them stay tangibly connected.

Case Example

The patient is a 55-year-old woman who is brought in to your office by a female friend. She does not make eye contact with you as you attempt to make introductions but answers all of your questions, and you learn that she goes by "Mary," identifies as a lesbian, and uses the pronouns "she/her"/"hers." When you ask what brings her in today, she hesitates initially and then says after encouragement from her friend: "I've been having bleeding down there." With supportive prompting, you learn that she underwent menopause at around age 50 but has been having erratic, sometimes heavy vaginal bleeding for the past 6 months. She admits that because of a history of childhood sexual abuse, she has always hated having her vagina penetrated with any object, including tampons, fingers or toys during sex, or the device doctors use during a pelvic exam. In fact, her last

attempt to have a Pap test more than 15 years ago was unsuccessful because she developed extreme pain on insertion of the speculum. After that experience, she made a decision to avoid medical care altogether "unless it's an absolute emergency."

Discussion Questions

- What exams are warranted in this case?
  - Visual inspection of entire perineum, speculum exam of vaginal vault and cervix with cervical Pap test, and bimanual palpation.
- How will you prepare the patient for the exam given her reluctance?
  - Explain time frame for the exam: 3–5 min
  - See example introductory language below for points you may want to consider discussing.
- What strategies can you use to adapt the exam to optimize comfort?
- If an exam cannot be performed due to patient preference, what else can be done to evaluate her chief complaint?

Example Introductory Language to the Physical Exam

Having explained the general principles to follow, here we provide example language adapted from a script developed for our work providing cervical Paps to transgender men [20]. The provider uses gender-neutral language and open-ended questions to explain the exam to the extent preferred by the patient, check in about past experiences with the Pap, offer a number of modifications, and allow space to discuss, validate, and address patient concerns. This script can be adapted for other types of exams.

- In a moment, I'll step out to let you get ready for the examination. Before I do that, I wanted to make sure that you understand the examination. What terms would you prefer I use or avoid when discussing your body?
- The Pap test looks for cells from the cervix that appear to be abnormal and might be a sign of a cancer developing so that we can monitor closely or treat any abnormal cells found in order to prevent cancer. The cervix is an internal organ located at the end of the frontal canal [or patient's preferred term for vagina]. During the exam, I use a tool called a speculum to widen the [patient's preferred term for vagina] so I can insert a small spatula and then a brush that collect cells from the inside and outside of the cervix.

The process usually takes about 5 min. We send the cells to a lab for further testing and get the results back in about 2–3 weeks.

- [When appropriate, e.g., for patients aged 30–65]: Because we know that infection with the HPV virus can trigger cells to start growing abnormally and possibly turn into cancer, the lab will also test the samples we collect today for HPV.
- If any of the tests we do today are abnormal, we will help you arrange further testing or treatment.
- Have you had a Pap test before? [If yes] What aspects of the procedure were difficult or that you would like to do differently this time? [Discuss with patient; offer modifications that address their specific concerns].
- Traditionally, when a pelvic and Pap test are done, the patient lies on their back on the exam table with their feet in these footrests, but you can choose a different position if you wish. Some people prefer to have their feet flat on the end of the table; other people lie with the soles of their feet together and their legs out in a frog-like position. Some people prefer to have the top of the exam table raised up a bit so that they can see what is going on during the examination. How would you like to be positioned for the examination?
- Some people also find that they have discomfort when the speculum is inserted and that it helps them to insert the speculum themselves with my guidance. Is this something that you would like to do or try?
- Sometimes people want another person, perhaps a friend or another medical professional, in the room during the exam. Who, if anyone, would you like in the room to be with you while you are having the examination?
  OR: Usually when I perform this exam, I have a medical assistant in the room with me who helps hand me the tools I need. How would you feel if he/she/they were in the room during your exam?
- Before we do the exam, would you like to see the speculum and the swabs and brushes that we use?
- Would you like me to talk you through what I'm doing as the exam goes along or would you prefer that I remain silent?
- Finally, I want you to know that you are in control of the examination. If at any point, you would like me to pause or stop the examination for any reason, just let me know. You can tell me to stop or simply hold up your hand, and I'll check in with you about what you want to do. How does that sound?
- What other questions do you have before the exam?
- Great, I'll leave now and give you a few minutes to change. Please take off your pants and underpants, put on this gown, and sit on the end of the table with this sheet over your lap.

Performing a Physical Exam in the Immediate Posttrauma Setting

Clinicians may be called upon to perform a physical exam immediately after a patient has experienced trauma, including physical or sexual child abuse, elder abuse, intimate partner violence, or hate crimes. These can be some of the most difficult exams for a person who has a history of trauma, and there are special considerations for LGBT survivors. As a case example, we focus in this section on how to make sexual assault forensic exams (SAFEs) trans-inclusive. We do not attempt to provide a comprehensive tutorial for performing a SAFE exam, but instead focus on aspects of the exam that require special consideration in transgender patients. The principles discussed here extend to other LGBT populations, types of trauma, and types of physical exams immediately after a traumatic event.

The goal of a SAFE is to provide medical care, including treatment of injuries, postexposure prophylaxis of sexually transmitted infections, and emergency contraception as relevant, and to document evidence that can be used if the patient decides to report to law enforcement. SAFEs are usually conducted by sexual assault nurse examiners due to the specialized nature of evidence collection, but clinicians working in an emergency department or primary care setting also may need to provide acute care to someone following an assault [21].

Special Considerations: Data, Disparities, and Context

Members of LGBT populations experience sexual violence at rates comparable to or higher than their heterosexual, cisgender counterparts (see Chap. 18). Best estimates suggest that some 50% of transgender people have been sexually assaulted [22].

Trans survivors of sexual violence often report that anti-trans bias was a key factor that motivated the assault. In a 2005 survey by FORGE, 42% of survivors reported that their assault was motivated at least in part by their gender [23], while in a study of transgender people in Virginia, 71% of transfeminine survivors and 40% of transmasculine survivors felt they had been targeted due to their gender [24]. Hate and bias-motivated crimes generally result in greater psychological trauma than non-bias crimes as the person's sense of themselves, their identity, and their community is also under attack [25]. Thus, transgender survivors of sexual violence are more likely to have to cope with the fact that their identity was under attack than would cisgender survivors. Transgender survivors of color also have to grapple with the sense that they were targeted because of their intersectional racial and gender identities; a review of anti-trans hate crimes in Los Angeles found that many perpetrators expressed both racialized and anti-LGBT slurs [26]. In addition to more complex emotional scars, assaults motivated by animus toward transgender individuals often leave more complex physical scars as well, as hate crimes motivated by anti-LGBT bias tend to be more violent than hate crimes against racial or religious groups [27], and injuries may be more likely to include disfigurement to the face, chest, genitals, or other gendered body parts [28]. The nature of the attack may be otherwise tied to gender, as when one transgender woman was beaten using her own high heels [26]. In order to fully support transgender patients, clinicians should educate themselves about federal hate crime laws, just as they should seek to be informed about the Violence Against Women Act (VAWA) and reporting considerations for cisgender women.

Receiving a full-body exam, including a pelvic exam, immediately after a sexual assault can be traumatic. Further complicating post-assault care, transgender survivors may have to deal with the simultaneous challenge of reentering the healthcare setting where they have also experienced trauma in the past. The National Transgender Discrimination Survey found that 10% of respondents had been sexually assaulted by a healthcare provider, 26% had been physically assaulted by a medical provider, and 19% had been denied medical care because of their identity [29]. These numbers may be higher among transgender people of color [30]. This context may make the physical exam feel overwhelming. Data about to what degree transgender survivors are able to access SAFEs specifically are not available, but disparities in accessing healthcare due to either avoidance or being denied care may carry over to SAFEs as well. Due to the importance of forensic evidence in prosecuting sexual assault, transgender individuals may be more likely to be assaulted, less likely to receive a SAFE, and less likely to receive justice.

Special Considerations: Administrative Issues, Forms, and Interacting with Others Besides the Patient

As with general intake forms, care should be taken to use forms related to the exam that accommodate a range of gender identities and sexual orientations. Despite the best forms, however, a trans person may or may not indicate their identity on intake forms, particularly if they are accompanied by someone who does not know they identify as trans. During an exam, it is important to avoid expressing surprise or alarm if body parts are not concordant with what you expected based on the intake.

As with any SAFE exam, take the initial assault history in private, away from any support person. If the patient requests the presence of a support person during portions of the history and exam, ensure that exam findings are not shared with the support person without the patient's knowledge and consent. Keep in mind that any person accompanying the patient – regardless of the gender of this companion – might actually be the person who abused the patient. Also, do not disclose to the support person that the patient is trans unless the patient explicitly gives permission to do so.

An important part of the SAFE involves marking a body diagram for where the patient has injuries. Use a gender-neutral diagram such as the one in Fig. 16.1. If your organization or state requires the use of gendered body maps or forms, or such forms are necessary to best document injuries from the assault, then explain to the patient why you are required to use such forms, and explain that this is not done to disrespect their gender identity. These explanations can minimize distress caused by forms that are not inclusive.

If consultation with or referral to an outside provider is necessary for follow-up, the patient may be anxious about having to meet with a new provider and once again disclose that they are transgender. Where possible, identify providers in your area in advance who have experience working with transgender patients, so you can assure the patient that the providers will be both welcoming and knowledgeable. Offer to assist the patient in informing the consultant of the patient's gender identity in advance, if the patient would find this introduction helpful.

Special Considerations: Clinical Considerations for Trans Patients

Be aware of anatomical changes that trans people may have as a result of hormones or surgery, and common physical findings that results from practices such as chest binding (compressing chest tissue for a flatter appearance) or genital tucking (pushing the testes into the inguinal canal and the penis between the legs). For instance, chest binding can result in scarring, abrasions, rashes, and cuts to the torso [31], while tucking may cause defects or hernias at the external inguinal ring [32]. This background helps the examiner evaluate what may be normal for the patient and what may be related to the assault. However, make no assumptions and nonjudgmentally ask the patient whether abrasions, cuts, and other physical findings are assault-related. For example, rather than assuming that cuts on the chest are from chest binding – or from self-harm practices, which are relatively common in this population [33] – nonjudgmentally ask how long the person has had the cuts [28] and where the cuts come from. Document all injuries

Fig. 16.1 Gender-neutral body diagram for use documenting injuries in post-assault exams

ANATOMICAL DIAGRAMS-SKIN SURFACE ASSESSMENT

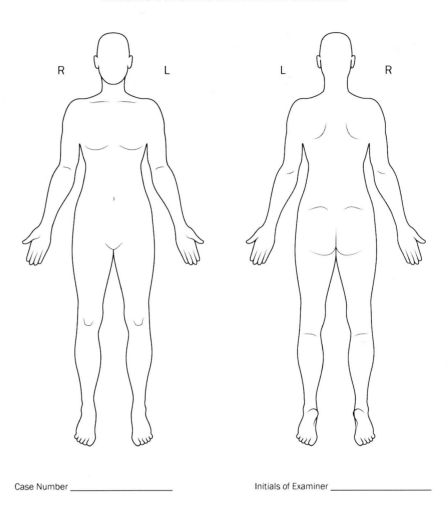

Case Number _____   Initials of Examiner _____

[34], including details such as the location, size, number, color, and depth of injuries. Use imaging studies where clinically appropriate. The role of the clinician is not to judge whether an assault occurred [21] or to use legal terms in the patient record (e.g., "patient alleges") but instead to document in detail the injuries present and information reported by the patient.

Trans men on testosterone experience vaginal atrophy and the vaginal wall becomes less elastic, more fragile, and prone to perforation [35, 36]. For trans women who have had genital reconstruction, the neovagina is also often less elastic than a cisgender woman's vagina [32]. While data are not available, trans individuals may therefore be more likely to experience genital injuries during a sexual assault, which may make acquisition of HIV/STIs more likely. During a pelvic exam, it also means that a pediatric, shorter-billed or narrower speculum may be necessary during the exam to avoid further trauma [28]. For neovaginal exams, consider using an anoscope rather than a vaginal speculum, as the neovagina has an inferior angle and lacks fornices and a cervix.

While numbers are hard to obtain, particularly for transgender individuals, anal penetration is likely more common among sexual assault survivors with natal male anatomy than among cisgender female survivors of sexual assault; in one study of gay and bisexual male survivors, 45.2% were anally penetrated [37]. Particular attention to anorectal trauma may therefore be warranted.

Trans men may not be aware that they can become pregnant as a result of penile-vaginal penetration, even if they are on testosterone and are experiencing amenorrhea [38]. It is the examiner's job to sensitively counsel the patient that pregnancy is a concern in this context if the patient has not had a hysterectomy and is not using birth control. The examiner should explain the options around emergency contraception (EC). Be aware that some patients may be reluctant to take estrogen or even progesterone-containing pills, either because the idea conflicts with their gender identity, or because they are concerned that these hormones will inhibit or conflict with testosterone therapy. There are no known contraindications to giving oral EC to patients on testosterone, though this practice has not been studied in transgender men specifically [38]. Explain that commonly prescribed oral EC methods do not contain estrogen and are either progesterone-only or contain ulipristal acetate. The copper IUD contains no hormones and thus may be a more palatable form of emergency contraception for some patients. There is no need to halt testosterone use in transgender men receiving emergency contraception [28].

For trans women who use silicone injections, physical assault may dislodge silicone deposits, which can be dangerous [28]. As mentioned earlier, assailants may particularly target gendered body parts where silicone injections are commonly used, such as buttocks, breasts, and face; therefore, these areas should be carefully examined and any injuries documented.

Be prepared to arrange specialty consultation if there is damage to the neophallus or neovagina that requires surgical repair beyond your ability. Ideally, make a standing arrangement with a surgeon in your area, so that you do not need to rush to find someone when presented with a patient in a crisis. You may also need to consult with the surgeon who performed the original operation on a particular patient, with the patient's consent [28].

Prosthetics can have evidentiary value and patients should be asked to bring prosthetics in for evidence collection if they were worn during the assault [34]. While generally clothing is taken and submitted as evidence for testing, there may be special sensitivities toward taking prostheses, wigs, and other gender-related items from the patient. First, these can be expensive to replace. Second, leaving the facility without these items can leave a patient emotionally and/or physically vulnerable, particularly if they feel they need to "pass" for safety. If the patient feels strongly that they need to keep a prosthetic, try swabbing or collecting samples from the surface of the item rather than taking the item entirely, if possible. Regardless, counsel the patient on how to access victim compensation funds to replace prostheses that are damaged or submitted as evidence. If possible, have extra wigs or prostheses available for the patient to take with them, and makeup available for trans women to use before leaving if desired. Most facilities that perform SAFEs have underwear and clothing available for patients after a SAFE, and having these additional items can be important in facilitating evidence collection and promoting the patient's mental health and safety after the exam [28].

Special Considerations: Patient-Provider Interaction

Clinicians should take special care to explain what they want to do and why they want to do it before each step of the exam, giving the patient the opportunity to ask questions or deny a specific procedure before proceeding. While providing a detailed explanation is important for any patient, experiences of being treated as a medical or anatomical curiosity and mistrust of healthcare system in general make this practice particularly critical for transgender clients. Specific aspects of a SAFE may be particularly important to explain to trans patients; for example, having body parts photographed can be important from a legal perspective, but may make a patient feel that they are being subjected to unnecessary scrutiny unless properly prepared as to why this step is necessary.

Before the patient leaves the acute care setting, it is important to help the patient make a safety plan that considers trans-specific issues. These include bringing crucial documents, medication, or other items related to gender transition with them if they decide to leave an abusive relationship and how to locate LGBT-competent survivor support organizations. An example of a comprehensive safety planning tool for trans clients can be found at http://forge-forward.org/wp-content/docs/safety-planning-tool.pdf. It is also crucial for clinicians to assess for suicidal ideation, which is common among trans individuals [39, 40], and may be triggered by an acute experience of assault or abuse.

Clinicians and organizations should develop partnerships with trans-competent community organizations, advocacy services, and providers, so that transgender patients can be smoothly referred to established and trustworthy services for medical and/or psychosocial follow-up. Building professional relationships ahead of time permits clinicians to conduct "warm handoffs" by helping patients connect with services while still in the office, thereby increasing the likelihood of engagement in follow-up care compared to simply providing patients with contact information and sending them home.

Conclusion

The physical exam is an important part of most medical encounters. Principles such as being thoughtful about whether an exam is medically necessary, engaging in shared decision making as to when the exam should be performed, understanding sensitivities that may be more common in LGBT patients, explaining the exam and discussing patient concerns, being open to making modifications to the exam to increase physical and emotional comfort, and being prepared to identify and address distress during the exam can make the physical exam both trauma-informed and LGBT-competent.

Acknowledgments We would like to thank Dr. Maddie Deutsch for editing this chapter and Katja Tetzlaff for creating the illustration. We would also like to thank Dr. Jocelyn Anderson, Dr. Tim Cavanaugh, Dr. Ami Multani, Dr. Henry Ng, Dr. Lori Panther, Dr. Sari Reisner, and Dr. Faiza Yasin for their contributions.

References

1. Bruhn JG. The doctor's touch: tactile communication in the doctor-patient relationship. South Med J. 1978;71(12):1469–73.

2. Bloomfield HE, Olson A, Greer N, Cantor A, MacDonald R, Rutks I, et al. Screening pelvic examinations in asymptomatic, average-risk adult women: an evidence report for a clinical practice guideline from the American College of Physicians. Ann Intern Med. 2014;161(1):46–53.

3. Sawaya GF, Jacoby V. Screening pelvic examinations: right, wrong, or rite? Ann Intern Med. 2014;161(1):78–9.

4. Henderson JT, Harper CC, Gutin S, Saraiya M, Chapman J, Sawaya GF. Routine bimanual pelvic examinations: practices and beliefs of US obstetrician-gynecologists. Am J Obstet Gynecol. 2013;208 (2):109.e1–7.

5. Burns RB, Potter JE, Ricciotti HA, Reynolds EE. Screening pelvic examinations in adult women: grand rounds discussion from the Beth Israel Deaconess Medical Center. Ann Intern Med. 2015;163 (7):537–47.

6. United States Preventive Services Task Force. Screening for testicular cancer: US preventive services task force reaffirmation recommendation statement. Ann Intern Med. 2011;154(7):483.

7. United States Preventive Services Task Force. Screening for breast cancer: US preventive services task force recommendation statement. Ann Intern Med. 2009;151(10):716.

8. American Cancer Society. American Cancer Society recommendations for early breast cancer detection in women without breast symptoms. http://www.cancer.org/cancer/breastcancer/moreinformation/breastcancerearlydetection/breast-cancer-early-detection-acs-recs2015. 19 Nov 2015.

9. Potter J, Peitzmeier S, Reisner S, Bernstein I. If you have it, check it: Overcoming barriers to cervical cancer screening with patients on the female-to-male transgender spectrum. http://www.lgbthealtheducation.org/training/on-demand-webinars/2014.

10. Schachter J, Chernesky MA, Willis DE, Fine PM, Martin DH, Fuller D, et al. Vaginal swabs are the specimens of choice when screening for Chlamydia trachomatis and Neisseria gonorrhoeae: results from a multicenter evaluation of the APTIMA assays for both infections. Sex Transm Dis. 2005;32(12):725–8.

11. Center of Excellence for Transgender Health. Primary care protocols for transgender patient care. http://transhealth.ucsf.edu/trans?page=protocol-00-002011. 22 Jan 2016.

12. Hembree WC, Cohen-Kettenis P, Delemarre-van de Waal HA, Gooren LJ, Meyer III WJ, Spack NP, et al. Endocrine treatment of transsexual persons: an Endocrine Society clinical practice guideline. J Clin Endocrinol Metabol. 2009;94(9):3132–54.

13. Coleman E, Bockting W, Botzer M, Cohen-Kettenis P, DeCuypere G, Feldman J, et al. Standards of care for the health of transsexual, transgender, and gender-nonconforming people, version 7. Int J Transgend. 2012;13(4):165–232.

14. Center of Excellence for Transgender Health. General prevention and screening. http://transhealth.ucsf.edu/trans?page=protocol-screening. 29 Nov 2015.

15. Potter J, Peitzmeier SM, Bernstein I, Reisner SL, Alizaga NM, Agénor M, et al. Cervical cancer screening for patients on the female-to-male spectrum: a narrative review and guide for clinicians. J Gen Intern Med. 2015;30(12):1857–64.

16. Stewart FH, Harper CC, Ellertson CE, Grimes DA, Sawaya GF, Trussell J. Clinical breast and pelvic examination requirements for hormonal contraception: current practice vs evidence. JAMA. 2001;285(17):2232–9.

17. Bates CK, Carroll N, Potter J. The challenging pelvic examination. J Gen Intern Med. 2011;26(6):651–7.

18. Simpson KM, Lankasky K. Table manners and beyond: the gynecological exam for women with developmental disabilities and other functional limitations. 2001. http://lurie.brandeis.edu/pdfs/TableMannersandBeyond.pdf.

19. Badura AS, Reiter RC, Altmaier EM, Rhomberg A, Elas D. Dissociation, somatization, substance abuse, and coping in women with chronic pelvic pain. Obstet Gynecol. 1997;90(3):405–10.

20. Reisner S, Pardee DJ, Deutsch M, Peitzmeier S, Potter J, editors. Preventive sexual health screening in female-to-male trans masculine (TM) adult patients. Oakland: National Transgender Health Summit; 2015.

21. Linden JA. Care of the adult patient after sexual assault. N Engl J Med. 2011;365(9):834–41.

22. Stotzer RL. Violence against transgender people: a review of United States data. Aggress Violent Behav. 2009;14(3):170–9.

23. Forge. Transgender sexual violence project. Milwaukee: Forge; 2005.

24. Xavier J, Honnold JA, Bradford JB. The health, health-related needs, and lifecourse experiences of transgender Virginians. Richmond: Virginia Department of Health; 2007.

25. Herek GM, Gillis JR, Cogan JC, Glunt EK. Hate crime victimization among lesbian, gay, and bisexual adults prevalence, psychological correlates, and methodological issues. J Interpers Violence. 1997;12(2):195–215.

26. Stotzer RL. Gender identity and hate crimes: violence against transgender people in Los Angeles County. Sex Res Soc Policy. 2008;5(1):43–52.

27. Dunbar E. Race, gender, and sexual orientation in hate crime victimization: identity politics or identity risk? Violence Vict. 2006;21(3):323–37.

28. Day K, Stiles E, Munson M, Cook-Daniels L. Forensic exams with transgender sexual assault survivors. 2014. http://forge-forward.org/event/forensic-exams/

29. Grant JM, Mottet L, Tanis JE, Harrison J, Herman J, Keisling M. Injustice at every turn: a report of the National Transgender Discrimination Survey. Washington, DC: National Center for Transgender Equality; 2011.

30. Bradford J, Reisner SL, Honnold JA, Xavier J. Experiences of transgender-related discrimination and implications for health: results from the Virginia transgender health initiative study. Am J Public Health. 2013;103(10):1820–9.

31. Acevedo K, Corbet A, Gardner I, Peitzmeier SM, Weinand J. Chest binding among transgender and gender non-conforming adults: health impact and recommendations for healthy binding. Under review. 2015.

32. Feldman JL, Goldberg JM. Transgender primary medical care. Int J Transgend. 2006;9(3–4):3–34.

33. House AS, Van Horn E, Coppeans C, Stepleman LM. Interpersonal trauma and discriminatory events as predictors of suicidal and nonsuicidal self-injury in gay, lesbian, bisexual, and transgender persons. Traumatology. 2011;17(2):75.

34. US Department of Justice Office of Violence Against Women. A national protocol for sexual assault medical forensic examinations adults/adolescents. US Department of Justice, Office of Justice Programs, National Criminal Justice Reference Service, Publications; 2004. Retrieved from https://www.ncjrs.gov/App/publications/Abstract.aspx.

35. van Trotsenburg MA. Gynecological aspects of transgender healthcare. Int J Transgend. 2009;11(4):238–46.

36. O'Hanlan KA, Dibble SL, Young-Spint M. Total laparoscopic hysterectomy for female-to-male transsexuals. Obstet Gynecol. 2007;110(5):1096–101.

37. Hickson FC, Davies PM, Hunt AJ, Weatherburn P, McManus TJ, Coxon AP. Gay men as victims of nonconsensual sex. Arch Sex Behav. 1994;23(3):281–94.

38. Erickson-Schroth L. Trans bodies, trans selves: a resource for the transgender community. New York: Oxford University Press; 2014.

39. Haas AP, Eliason M, Mays VM, Mathy RM, Cochran SD, D'Augelli AR, et al. Suicide and suicide risk in lesbian, gay, bisexual, and transgender populations: review and recommendations. J Homosex. 2010;58(1):10–51.

40. Nuttbrock L, Hwahng S, Bockting W, Rosenblum A, Mason M, Macri M, et al. Psychiatric impact of gender-related abuse across the life course of male-to-female transgender persons. J Sex Res. 2010;47(1):12–23.

Motivational Interviewing for LGBT Patients

17

Blake E. Johnson and Matthew J. Mimiaga

Over the past century, there has been a remarkable shift in the leading causes of death in the United States. In 1900, infectious diseases including influenza and pneumonia, tuberculosis, and gastrointestinal infections were among the most common causes of death [1]. With advances in healthcare in the twentieth century, the burden of mortality caused by infectious diseases waned. The leading causes of death today have shifted to cancers, heart disease, diabetes, HIV/AIDS, and obesity – all of which are strongly linked to lifestyles and health behaviors. Contemporary theories of disease distribution link biomedical and lifestyle perspectives to understand patterns of disease occurrence as being influenced by a patient's genetic background, their environment, and their behaviors [2]. While many illnesses and afflictions that drive individuals to seek the advice of a healthcare professional are biomedical in origin, many may be preventable or their progression mitigated through behavior change.

For many patients, a visit to a healthcare professional is seen as an encounter in which they are asked questions about their health and the reason for their visit, undergo a targeted physical examination, and are then recommended an appropriate treatment that is often pharmaceutical in nature. While some visits with practitioners may look like this, others may be more conversational in nature, with a healthcare provider giving advice and counsel related to a patient's health and behavior. The process of visiting a provider can be incredibly stressful for LGBT-identified patients, who have life experiences and unique health challenges with which many

health providers are unfamiliar and poorly equipped to handle. Many LGBT individuals have felt a societal pressure to conform to specific behaviors throughout their life, perhaps to be less "gay," to act "normal," or to "blend in" with a desired community [3–5]. Behavior change is tricky to accomplish and must be facilitated in a manner that is intrinsically tied to the individual's participation and consent, particularly with individuals whose autonomy has been diminished personally, socially, and institutionally.

The classic example in behavior change theory is related to patients with high alcohol consumption and liver disease [6]. While treatment options may be available to address progression to liver disease and subsequent complications, talking with such patients about changing their chosen drinking patterns to improve their health is also an integral aspect of care. As another example, consider an HIV-positive patient with suboptimal adherence to their antiretroviral therapy (ART). A prescriber might opt to shift the patient to an easier treatment regimen with fewer pills, but there is also an opportunity for the provider to help the patient address behavioral barriers that are contributing to their adherence difficulties. Behavior change thus plays an important part in modern healthcare; however, some methods of facilitating this change are more effective than others.

Conversations with patients about behaviors that impact their health are common occurrences for all types of medical professionals who provide direct patient care. The importance of these conversations is clear; however, the manner in which these dialogues are structured so as to both respect the patient's autonomy and be most effective at changing unhealthy behaviors is less apparent. In this chapter, we discuss the utility of motivational interviewing (MI), a type of counseling that emphasizes a patient's own intrinsic motivations to change a behavior with a focus on a specific goal [7]. At its core, behavior change does not happen by a provider *telling* a patient how to behave [8], e.g., telling a patient to curtail their number of sexual partners to reduce their risk for HIV and sexually transmitted infections (STIs)

B.E. Johnson, ScM (✉)
UNC School of Medicine, The University of North Carolina at Chapel Hill, 321 S. Columbia St, Chapel Hill, NC 27516, USA
e-mail: blake_johnson@med.unc.edu

M.J. Mimiaga, ScD, MPH
Epidemiology and Behavioral & Social Health Sciences, Institute for Community Health Promotion, Brown University, Providence, RI, USA

© Springer International Publishing AG 2017
K.L. Eckstrand, J. Potter (eds.), *Trauma, Resilience, and Health Promotion in LGBT Patients*,
DOI 10.1007/978-3-319-54509-7_17

will most likely not result in effective behavior change. Rather, MI relies on building an internal motivation within the patient to change behaviors that the patient realizes are having a negative impact on an aspect of their life and health that they want to improve (Fig. 17.1).

The patient-centric, nonjudgmental, and nonconfrontational nature of MI is a flexible and empathetic approach to working with patients who identify as LGBT. The supportive tone of MI is particularly well suited to the LGBT community in that it promotes behavior change and resilience without condescension or overt direction, which may turn LGBT patients away from affecting a positive change in their health behaviors. For an LGBT person with a history of trauma, be it physical, sexual, emotional, cultural, or institutional, MI works well to return the locus of control to the individual, who may otherwise feel that their ability to control events and situations in their life has been lost [9, 10]. Beyond this, MI allows providers to better understand their patient's perspectives and become more effective resources for their patients. This chapter presents the basic principles of MI, provides tips and techniques to effectively integrate these principles into everyday interactions with patients, and discusses how MI techniques can be inclusive of LGBT populations.

Origins of Motivation Interviewing in Theories of Behavior Change

William Miller, a psychologist at the University of New Mexico, developed motivational interviewing techniques during the late 1970s and early 1980s in an effort to change behaviors of individuals with alcohol addiction [6]. Stephen Rollnick then described the application of MI to clinical practice in 1995 [11]. Miller and Rollnick argue that behavior change can be communicated in three distinct styles: following, directing, and guiding.

Following

In the communication style of following, the key skill is listening and understanding. A patient-provider interaction in which the provider relies on the following to effect a change in behavior puts the emphasis on the patient's vocalizations about their behaviors and trusting that the patient will set the pace and goals that are appropriate to effect a change in their own behavior. This allows the patient to take the lead in their decisions to make a change in their own behavior and embodies the locus of control within the patient.

Directing

A directing style of communicating behavior change resembles the more traditional type of behavior change practiced in healthcare, in which providers attempt to influence an individual's behaviors directly [12]. In essence, providers who utilize a directing style of communicating behavior change tell their patient what to do, without much explanation or reason. While many patients have come to expect this of their providers, the top-down nature of directing often creates a barrier between patient and provider, ultimately failing to facilitate behavior changes [13]. For example, consider the following encounter between a family medicine physician and Anthony, a 52-year-old gay man being seen for a chronic cough. Anthony has been smoking tobacco for 35 years (Fig. 17.2).

PROVIDER: How has your cough been since the last time I saw you?
ANTHONY: Well, it hasn't improved much and it's keeping me awake at night. I can't seem to figure out why it won't go away.
PROVIDER: Have you quit smoking like I asked you to the last time you visited?

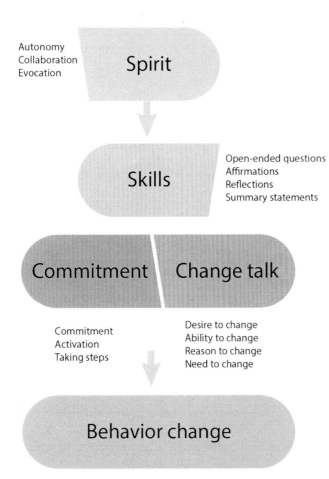

Fig. 17.1 Components of motivational interviewing

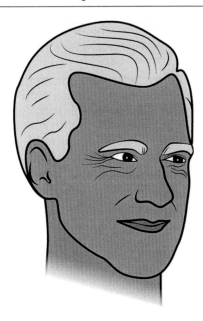

Fig. 17.2 Anthony is a 52-year-old gay man being seen for a chronic cough

ANTHONY: No….well smoking helps me stay awake at work, and since I haven't been sleeping that well because of the cough, I've been having some trouble quitting. Also, I smoke most when I'm out at the bar with friends, and that's the only time I have with my gay friends given my work schedule.

PROVIDER: Well, my recommendation is that you need to quit smoking. I can put you in touch with a smoking cessation counselor, but you really need to focus on quitting.

Here, the provider solely utilizes a directing style and comes off as gruff and uninterested in the details surrounding the patient's struggle to quit smoking. The top-down directing style, albeit useful to emphasize importance when used sparingly, is not effective when used as the sole communication style.

Guiding

Of the three styles of communicating behavior change, MI is most embodied in guiding. In essence, a practitioner can use a guiding style to serve as a resource and help an individual realize, set, and achieve their goals. Using principles of guiding, a practitioner provides their expertise to set up options and alternatives to help a patient, rather than communicating about one set path that a patient must follow, as seen in the directing style above.

While providers can, and should, skillfully integrate following, directing, and guiding communication styles into all

conversations with patients, MI is rooted in a guiding style of communication in which a provider focuses on helping the individual move past feelings of ambivalence to build their internal motivation to effect behavior change. As we will discuss in the remainder of the chapter, MI is nonjudgmental, nonconfrontational, and nonadversarial, making it a well-suited framework to guide conversations between providers and their LGBT-identified patients. In the context of resilience and health promotion, shifting to a guiding communication style is a simple way to support patients in everyday conversations by engaging the patient in their own healthcare. Further, while providers may not have training in discussing topics of sexual orientation, gender identity, or sexual behavior, the process of MI can support the provider's own growth by virtue of listening to the patient's experience, their chosen language to talk about themselves and their lives, and the diversity of motivations for which people initiate – and change – behaviors.

Fundamentals of Motivational Interviewing

A core goal of MI is to build the patient's internal motivations to change a specific behavior. Stated simply, this involves guiding the patient to think about their life experiences and concerns, and to examine the consequences that specific behaviors and decisions have on their aspirations and goals. As discussed with the three core communication styles of behavior change earlier in this chapter, a provider *guides* their patient to thinking about behavior change by leading patients to explore the effect a behavior change would make in their life, i.e., building the patient's internal motivation for behavior change. In this vein, Miller and Rollnick describe the fundamental spirit of MI to be collaborative, evocative, and honoring of patient autonomy [7].

In MI the provider and patient are equal in power and make decisions *collaboratively* to help the patient enact change. To do this, a provider must often *evoke* a patient's own internal motivations to affect a health behavior change, usually by guiding the patient to make the connection between their goals or concerns and the behavior change. To facilitate this, MI is always conducted with the utmost respect for patient autonomy. While a provider can advise, instruct, or encourage a behavior change within a patient, MI recognizes that it is the patient who must ultimately decide what to do and whether or not they will actually make an agreed-upon behavior change. Further, MI can be strategically used to enhance an individual's self-efficacy in engaging in a particular behavior. If a behavior change or an action plan suggested by a provider seems overwhelming for a patient, a provider can use MI to break that plan or behavior change into smaller steps. By empowering a patient to accomplish each of these smaller steps, a provider can enhance the confidence an individual has in their ability to get through their struggle to achieving healthy behavior change.

While seemingly simple, complexities arise in motivation interviewing. *Ambivalence* in an individual is the first core complexity. Consider the following interaction, noting the use of contrasting conjunctions (but, however, although, though, etc.) to express ambivalence. Here a provider is meeting with Sarah, a transwoman who was diagnosed with HIV 20 years ago, before she began transitioning (Fig. 17.3). Sarah's viral load has been consistently undetectable but has recently started to rise.

PROVIDER: By taking your HIV medications every day as scheduled, you can keep your viral load down. That would help keep you healthy, and it will also protect your partner from acquiring HIV. Improved adherence to HIV medications helps keep everyone in a relationship healthy.

SARAH: Yes, I do know all of this and I want to keep my partners healthy. *But* when I don't take my HIV meds, I'm less bloated and I feel more alert and awake. And my viral load has always been low, even when I've missed some doses, and I make my partners wear condoms.

Here, the patient is ambivalent about the idea of changing her behavior regarding how she takes her HIV medications. On the one hand, she feels okay – perhaps even better – when she skips doses; on the other, she doesn't want her partners to contract HIV from her and feels she currently tries to minimize this risk by having her partners wear condoms. While many providers may perceive patient ambivalence as impossible to navigate, ambivalence is best understood as a natural response to being encouraged to change. For example, no matter how many times a dentist explains the benefits of flossing, a patient might be resistant to make flossing part of their daily routine because of time constraints during the

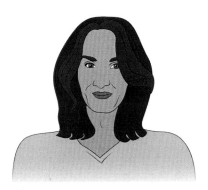

Fig. 17.3 Sarah is a transwoman who was diagnosed with HIV 20 years ago before she began transitioning

morning rush or their gums feeling sore after flossing. Thus, patients may understand that a health behavior is appropriate for them, but because of certain constraints or limitations, they are ambivalent about making a change in their behaviors or lifestyle [14]. By coming forward and suggesting a change in behavior, a provider may provoke an opposing or ambivalent response. To avoid this outcome, the provider should use MI techniques to get the patient to articulate the arguments in support of behavior change rather than vocalize a counterargument to behavior change. To navigate these conversations, MI relies on four guiding principles, easily remembered using the acronym RULE, first described by Miller and Rollnick in 1992 [11, 15].

R: Resist the Righting Reflex

In the previous example demonstrating a patient's ambivalence to improve their HIV medication adherence, a provider's suggestion for a behavior change was met with ambivalence and would likely result in a failed attempt at health behavior change if the provider continues in a directing communication style. It makes sense that clinicians often instinctually attempt to correct what they perceive is an unhealthy behavior, in an effort to protect a patient's health. However, the reflex to "right" a patient is frequently determined based on what the provider perceives to be of the utmost importance – optimizing health. This reflex can come through in a directing style, establishing an uneven power dynamic in the patient-provider interaction. To effectively utilize MI, providers must check their reflex to right and instead allow a patient to vocalize their motivations and understanding of what behaviors they may need to change. This technique will help providers navigate through a patient's ambivalence, and helps to avoid the patient vocalizing any ambivalence they may have, as an individual tends to attach to or believe what they hear themselves say [7].

U: Understand the Motivations of Your Patient

MI can be adapted for individuals from all backgrounds, and techniques can be adjusted to account for different levels of client readiness to change their behaviors. A key aspect to helping guide a patient to a health behavior change is to understand their perspectives, motivations, and thoughts about their behaviors, as well as their goals and concerns related to changing those behaviors. When ample time is available, providers can explore a patient's current situation in depth to understand the patient's motivations. However, patient-provider interactions are often constrained to 20-min visits, and providers may therefore be limited in their ability to fully examine all of a patient's motivations. In situations with limited time, it is helpful to focus on understanding a patient's motivations for change and discussing how they might make a change in an incremental fashion in an effort to establish a foundation for additional discussions in the future.

L: Listen to Your Patient

Perhaps the most important aspect of MI is listening to the patient. Effective listening is a difficult skill to master, particularly as many providers are seen as having the answers to concerns that patients may come with to a visit. As MI relies on understanding perspectives within the patient, the "answers" more often than not originate within the patient rather than the provider. Listening techniques, including reflective listening, are discussed in the next part of this chapter.

E: Empower, Engage, and Encourage Your Patient

There is a clear body of evidence suggesting that patients who are engaged in their own healthcare experience better outcomes than patients who are disinterested or disengaged in their treatment plans and overall healthcare [16–19]. The fourth guiding principle of MI centers on empowering a patient to make a behavior change in their lives.

Let's revisit the conversation with Sarah, this time approaching her challenges with taking her HIV medications using RULE, the four guiding principles of MI.

PROVIDER: Can you tell me about how taking your HIV medication has been since the last time I saw you? [R, U]

SARAH: It's been more a challenge in the last few months – I've been taking my meds for so many years and I'm tired of them.

PROVIDER: When you say that you're tired of your meds, what do you mean? [R, U, L]

SARAH: Well, the routine of taking my meds every day has never bothered me. More recently, I have been thinking that over the past 20 years I haven't felt sick and my counts have always been low, even when I've missed a few doses here and there. Maybe it's not the drugs that are keeping me healthy – maybe it's something else. The drugs just make me feel bloated and I don't feel attractive some days.

PROVIDER: So you don't feel like the drugs are what are keeping you healthy? Why might you want to keep taking your medications on schedule? [U]

SARAH: Yeah…and being bloated makes me want to skip my medications. The rational part of me knows that I should be better at taking my meds to keep my counts low and I want to be healthy for both me and my partner.

PROVIDER: I'm glad to hear that keeping your counts low is a priority for you, but that feeling bloated may distract on that goal. Let's focus on keeping you healthy, and also try tweaking when you take your meds to try and minimize the times that you feel bloated. How important is it to you to focus on keeping your counts low? [E]

SARAH: It's really important to me – especially if we could do something to help with the bloating and my feelings about my body image when I take my meds.

Here, the provider skillfully avoids prompting Sarah to vocalize her ambivalence by using the RULE principles. Rather than talking to Sarah with a directing style that prompts Sarah to express her ambivalence, the provider guides Sarah and hones in on her goals to stay healthy, while also considering her concerns. Simply focusing on going through each of the RULE principles is key technique to skillfully navigate through a patient's ambivalence. In the next portion of this chapter we will discuss more techniques that can be used to incorporate MI into healthcare practice, particularly for LGBT patients.

Incorporating Motivational Interviewing into Patient-Provider Interactions

Motivational interviewing builds on key skills that providers may use in everyday practice, focusing on the *guiding* communication style and the core principles of RULE. Here we detail the three skills of MI: asking, informing, and listening.

Asking

There are a number of considerations that must be taken into account when asking questions in the context of MI. Asking is particularly useful in getting to understand your patient, so as to direct conversation and guide patients toward thinking about behavior change with respect to their unique perspectives and goals.

Open vs. Closed Questions

In time-limited settings such as healthcare clinics, closed-ended questions can be helpful in ascertaining the most relevant information in a patient encounter. However, this leaves little room for the patient to respond and elaborate. Consider the following closed questions:

"On a typical night, how many drinks do you have?"

"When you have sex, what percentage of the time are you using a condom?"

"How many times a week do you exercise?"

"Are you depressed or anxious?"

"Have you missed any doses of your HIV medications in the last month?"

While these questions may seem informative, they each have an expected, limited response. For example, if a patient responds to the second question above saying they use a condom 75% of the time, this does not provide any insight into the gender of their sexual partners, the type of sexual activities in which they are engaging (oral, anal, vaginal, etc.), their positioning during sexual activities (top, bottom, versatile, etc.), or any other information that may be crucial to understanding a patient's sexual risk. These types of questions may appear to be efficient in their direct nature, but they often require a number of follow-up questions. By transitioning to questions that are more open in format, providers can ascertain more information and cultivate a conversational rapport with their patient, allowing the patient to provide more information that they feel is relevant in each of their answers. Consider the following open versions of the five questions posed above:

"What role does alcohol play in your life?"

"How do condoms fit into your sex life?"

"In what ways do you incorporate exercise into your life?"

"What does depression feel like to you?"

"How has taking your HIV medications this past month been?"

Shifting to asking open questions allows the patient to share a story, rather than a simple answer, and provides an opportunity for patients to elaborate on their perspectives. This plays into RULE, specifically into understanding your patient's perspectives [U], and is one technique that can be used to successfully incorporate MI into a 20-min consultation. The manner in which a provider asks follow-up questions is also important. Open-ended follow-up questions are particularly useful and emphasize a pattern of asking-listening-asking. Here, the provider guides the conversation to focus on the patient's internal motivations and to progressively gain more and more insight into the patient's perspectives.

Agenda Setting

Another reason to begin an interaction with open questions is to allow the patient to bring specificity to the conversation on their own accord. In contrast, if the provider focuses on a topic that they think is important – for example, discussing body image with a patient who identifies as lesbian who has high blood pressure and an above-average BMI – this may prematurely focus the conversation, boxing the patient-provider interaction into a conversation about the patient's body, when the patient may also have other things they would like to discuss. Rather, the provider should allow the patient to discuss things broadly, and then set an agenda with follow-up questions in an effort to allow a conversation to touch multiple aspects of behavior change. This may include the patient's concerns with body image, but also can include other aspects of the patient's life that she may feel are relevant to discuss with a provider. By beginning with a patient's concerns, rather than the provider's, the patient will be more likely to be receptive to suggestions. With agenda setting, a provider can outline a few different aspects of a specific behavior that they want to discuss with the patient during a single visit, based on their patient's background discussed at the beginning of the consultation. This agenda can be set to incorporate both the topics that a patient brings up in the first few minutes of open questioning in a patient-provider interaction and also the items that a provider wants to discuss with a patient, without being overly directing. This reduces the pressure on both provider and patient and is likely to make the patient more receptive to suggestions from the provider.

Consider the following interaction with Stephen, a gay man in his mid-20s who is in the emergency room after passing out during a workout. Stephen works out at least eight times a week and presents anxious and irritable, with abnormally high creatinine kinase levels, suggesting that Stephen is overexerting himself with an unhealthy gym use.

PROVIDER: Can you tell me about your gym use, including what motivates you to go to the gym and how you fit going to the gym into your daily life?

STEPHEN: You're the fiftieth person today to ask me these questions – seriously, I'm fine, I am just exhausted from work and friends. I work out a lot to burn stress off and to keep my body tight – really just trying to look and feel good for the summer in P-town, you know, Provincetown, Massachusetts – gay beach destination.

PROVIDER: I completely understand, and I just want to help get a better picture of your gym use, to help me understand how you came to the ER today and how using the gym fits into your everyday life. If you like, we can talk about your gym habits – when you go, how often you go, what you do when you're at the gym, what motivates you to go to the gym so often. I'd then like to talk about some techniques to help you keep you from over-training and some changes you can make to improve your health. Would this be an okay order for our conversation? Or are there perhaps other things that you would like to bring up in our conversation?

Here, the provider uses agenda setting to outline an interaction with a patient, which is particularly useful considering Stephen's mood. The provider sets a tone for a dialogue about behavior change, set in the context of understanding Stephen's motivations for his gym use. Agenda setting can also be useful when a provider is offering a number of potential options or solutions for a patient to take going forth, and is laden with asking the patient for consent to continue a conversation. The provider can present a list of these options to the patient, allowing the patient to choose a handful of options to discuss together, thus engaging the patient in setting the course of the conversation and creating a positive rapport for change dialog.

Key Techniques to Asking the Right Questions

1. "What next?" questions

   "What next?" questions serve a variety of purposes in gauging where a patient is on their journey to behavior change. Primarily, these types of questions ask an individual what the next step for them will be, and help to establish the *how* when building internal motivations for a change in behavior. For example:

   > "With everything we just talked about in mind, what will you do next?"

   > "So what do you think about your adherence to your HIV medication now?"

   "What will you do next with regard to your smoking?"

   These questions serve a "check-in" function in assessing the patient's commitment to change and can be followed up with further planning questions or may indicate the need to backtrack and reassess the patient's perspectives and goals before proceeding further.

2. "What if?" questions

   "What if?" questions pose hypothetical situations that can be used to foster motivation in patients who may be less inclined to make a change in their behavior and present a friendly way to envision change, particularly in situations where the patient is more ambivalent. Potential hypotheticals include:

   > "Suppose you were able to use condoms more frequently with your outside partners: what might some of the benefits be for you and your primary partner?"

   > "If your relationship with your parents were stronger, how would your life be different?"

   > "What do you think your life will be like in 10 years if you don't make any change in your substance use?"

3. Scales to assess motivations [1–10]

   For a patient who you feel is less motivated to change a behavior, scales can be a useful tool to help gauge their motivations and to brainstorm what might help them become more confident in their ability to change. Scales, partnered with hypotheticals and targeted follow-up questions, can be useful for both the provider and the patient to gain insight into a patient's perspective. The Miller and Rollnick set of scales have two sides: one side holds the advantages associated with doing a particular behavior and the expected disadvantage of making a behavior change, while the other side holds the disadvantages experienced with doing a particular behavior and the expected advantages of making a behavior change [7, 11, 15]. Providers can utilize scales to help determine a patient's readiness for behavior change, and a patient's responses can identify potential hurdles for the provider and patient to work through to facilitate effective behavior change. Consider the following interaction between a family medicine physician and Max, a genderqueer teenager, born female, who has been struggling with an eating disorder and their body dysmorphia (Fig. 17.4).

PROVIDER: On a scale of 1–10, how ready would you say you are to use a food diary to help you keep track of what you are eating for each meal, with 1 being "not ready at all" and 10 being "extremely ready."

MAX: I don't know, maybe a 6 or so?

PROVIDER: Okay, why did you say 6 and not a lower number, say a 1?

MAX: Well, I want to be able to make sure I'm eating regularly – I don't want my grades to slip anymore than they already have and thinking about my weight has been really stressful. So I guess I'm ready to try something to help me keep track of how I'm doing with eating.

PROVIDER: If you could have anything in the world to help you, what would it take to get you feeling like a ten, or extremely ready to use the food journal?

MAX: Hmm…maybe if some of my friends knew about my struggles with my weight they could help me out – but I feel like I've already been labeled as the odd one out, you know, since the girls in my class think I'm too

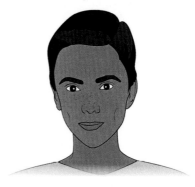

Fig. 17.4 Max is a genderqueer teenager, born female, who has been struggling with an eating disorder and their body dysmorphia

boyish and the boys in my class aren't really comfortable with my masculinity. I don't know if I know how to approach my friends to talk about my diet.

PROVIDER: Do you have one or two friends that are close to you and would support you and help you be more attentive to your diet? I think it's a great idea to help expand your support – and, if you'd like, I have some tools that we can discuss that may help you with talking to your friends about helping you keep track of your eating and may help you boost your social support.

Scales are particularly useful in checking back with the patient after you have made a preliminary plan, typically toward the end of a patient-provider interaction. Here, Max expresses some doubt about how they feel about using a specific strategy to help them with their eating behaviors. By posing hypotheticals and asking Max how they may be able to increase their confidence and readiness to use a specific tool, the provider can better understand what might be holding Max back and adjust their recommendations accordingly.

4. Listen!

Above all, when asking questions, be sure to listen to your patient. It's an easy trap to do all the talking as a provider, but in MI the primary source of information should always be the patient. We'll delve into listening in the next section.

Listening

Listening provides the opportunity to develop an understanding of a patient's perspectives and the foundation for developing a strong rapport between the provider and the patient. Listening serves many purposes in the context of MI, but above all, good listening alone indicates that a provider is taking the time to invest in a patient, and patients can be extremely perceptive of this subtlety. Listening is a key aspect of the *following* style of communicating behavior change, and holds particular importance at the beginning of a visit, when a provider can gather detailed information about the reasons for the patient's visit and motivations for and against a potential behavior change. Additionally, listening is of utmost importance after asking questions and when patients express concern, confusion, or have some other emotional response during the course of a patient-provider interaction. It is important to note that the act of asking a question does not constitute listening; do not fall into the trap of asking a question without listening to the answer.

In particular, providers should listen for "change talk," honing in on a patient's language that is directly related to behavior change [7, 20]. Change talk can be broadly broken into seven categories, easily remembered using the acronym D-A-R-N C-A-T:

1. *Desire* statements express an individual's preferences for change or lack thereof.
2. *Ability* statements express an individual's perception of their ability to accomplish something, which, in part, signifies their motivation to accomplish something. Regardless of an individual's ability, if they are not motivated they may perceive their ability to change their behavior to be lacking or nonexistent.
3. *Reason* statements express why an individual wants to make a change or why they want things to remain the same.
4. *Need* statements express the feeling of necessity to make a change.
5. *Commitment* statements can vary in degree from considering making a change to promising or expressing will to making a change.
6. *Activation* statements express an individual's readiness for change.
7. *Taking steps* statements express actual actions an individual has taken toward making a change in their lives, and tend to be expressed more commonly at repeat visits with a patient, when they occur.

Each of the DARN CAT categories of change talk may express a patient's favor for change, or may favor the sustaining existing behaviors (see examples of change talk in Table 17.1). If you hear change talk that favors "sustain talk," work on exploring an individual's goals and concerns, guiding them to change talk that favors behavior change. Consider the following interaction between a therapist and Cindy, a 45-year-old lesbian who has recurring suicidal thoughts (Fig. 17.5). Notice how the therapist asks questions in search of change talk, and Cindy's expression of different types of change talk, categorized by DARN CAT.

PROVIDER: Why would you *want* to work on reducing how often you think about suicide? [*assessing: desire*]

CINDY: It's been taking such a toll on my everyday life. Sometimes I can't even get out of bed because I feel so hopeless, and I don't *want* to lose my job or my friends. These irrational thoughts are getting in the way of my life and I *need* to find a way to get them out of my head. [*stating: desire, reasons, need*]

PROVIDER: It's clear to me that you want to address your thoughts in an effort to focus more on your life and to get back to a feeling of normalcy. If you decided to work

Table 17.1 Examples of statements with each of the seven kinds of change talk (DARN CAT)

Desire	Statements expressing an individual's preference for change Key verbs: *wish, want, like to, desire*… "I want to be better at quitting smoking" "I would like to focus on taking my HIV medications more regularly" "I wish I was able to make my partner happier"
Ability	Statements expressing an individual's perception of their ability to change Key verbs: *can, may be able to, could*… "I can try to change how I communicate with my friends" "I could try and go to the gym more" "I may be able to cut back on my partying"
Reasons	Statements expressing reasons to make a change Key verbs: no specific verbs, but reason statements may be tied into other change talk "My depression is affecting my relationships with my family and friends" "I want to be able to keep my viral load down" "My issues with eating and thinking about food are too consuming"
Need	Statements expressing necessity for a change Key verbs: *need, must, have to*… "I need to make sure my partner can't hurt me anymore" "I have to get better about not drinking too much when I go out" "I should make a change in my life"
Commitment	Statements committing to making a change Key verbs: *am going to, promise, am ready to*… "I am going to quit smoking" "I promise to focus on using condoms to help me stay healthy" "I am ready to improve my adherence"
Activation	Statements expressing will to make a change Key verbs: *will, would, want*… "I will consider cutting out herbal hormones I buy off the internet" "I think that speaking up for myself with my partner will help me be happier" "I would think about setting up calendar alerts to pick up my prescription"
Taking steps	Statements about steps that an individual will take to make a change Key verbs: no specific verbs, but these statements outline plans or attempts "I picked up my prescription for PrEP" "I talked to my partner about negotiating our relationship agreement" "I think if I focus on establishing a daily routine, that will help"

Adapted from Miller and Rollnick [7]

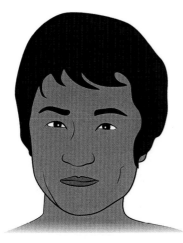

Fig. 17.5 Cindy is a 45-year-old lesbian who has chronic suicidal thoughts

more on these, how do you think you *would* do it? [*assessing: ability*]

CINDY: If I knew, I wouldn't be here talking to you! But, I suppose I *could* try and dig more into the root of my thoughts in my sessions with you. Or maybe I *could* try and build my social support more and get involved with something like community yoga. I don't know… [*stating: ability*]

Here, the provider works to elicit change talk with Cindy, prompting her with specific questions. Together, the first four categories of change talk (desire, ability, reason, and need) convey aspects of motivation for making a change, while the final three categories (commitment, activation, and taking steps) relate to the steps actually necessary for behavior change to occur. In these interactions, listen for change talk, and prompt your patients with questions that are asked with enough specificity to assess their arguments for change or lack thereof. It is important to guide a patient to express the first four categories, but hearing these is not enough to affect a change in behavior, as these expressions merely represent precommitment forms of change talk – that is, expressing a possibility for change. By listening for change talk while going through the RULE principles, a provider can gain a deeper understanding of their patient's background and readiness for change talk and guide the patient toward effective behavior change.

Silence

If you find yourself asking a patient questions and are met with no response or silence, do not fear! Silence is a useful tool in MI. Sitting in silence can allow a patient more time to adjust to the style of the conversation and formulate a response, whereas interrupting the silence may cut off the conversation and shift it to a top-down directing style of communication between the provider and patient. Additionally, if the provider breaks the silence before the patient, this trend is likely to continue throughout the encounter. This creates a one-sided conversation in which the provider must draw answers out of the patient and is less likely to develop the rapport needed to identify change talk and facilitate behavior change.

Reflective Listening and Summarizing

Throughout a patient-provider interaction, it is helpful to reflect on illustrative statements made by the patient, particularly when these statements are related to change talk. To listen reflectively, the provider touches back on previous statements the patient made, demonstrating that they were listening and guiding the conversation to highlight and revisit key topics. This is a type of active listening, which helps the conversation flow, demonstrates a provider's genuine interest in the patient's situation, and serves as a check of the provider's understanding of the patient's perspective. Reflective listening can be used to steer a conversation away from digressive topics and focus instead on statements that are relevant to facilitating behavior change. At the end of an interaction with a patient, and at intermittent points throughout the conversation, the provider should summarize what has been discussed thus far, piecing together the most salient points and allowing the conversation to transition to the next step in the journey toward facilitated behavior change. Reflective summary statements are essential to agenda setting, and can keep a time-limited conversation with a patient on track. Consider the following dialogue between a provider and Andy, a young transman who recently came out (Fig. 17.6). Andy lives in a small rural community and has been struggling with feelings of isolation and depression. Notice how Andy's provider utilizes reflection and summary statements in this excerpt of their interaction.

ANDY: I've just been feeling so lonely recently – coming out was a huge thing for me, and I'm so glad that I am coming into my own identity. But by actually coming out, I've put a huge barrier between me and my classmates who just don't get that I'm a guy. It's so lonely.

PROVIDER: So what I hear is that you're feeling good about being open with your identity, but lonely because you

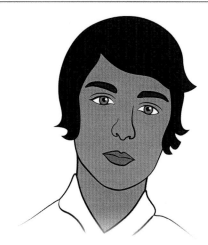

Fig. 17.6 Andy is a young transman who recently came out

sense that some of your peers have put some distance between themselves and you. [*reflection*]

ANDY: Yeah, for sure.

PROVIDER: How has that made you feel? [*open question*]

ANDY: Pretty crappy. I thought that by coming out I would gain at least some support with my friends, but by actually stating it, there's a wedge between us. I don't really want to socialize with anyone or go to school now – everything is just uncomfortable.

PROVIDER: So you're finding yourself retreating and spending more time alone? [*reflection*]

ANDY: Yeah – and I need more support. More friends – a community. I don't want to spend all this time alone, waiting to go to college in a more welcoming environment. I want to get out of my shell.

PROVIDER: Let me recap to make sure that I'm understanding everything you've just told me. Coming out has made you feel more confident about your identity, but you're finding yourself spending more time alone to avoid interacting with classmates and people at school who you feel are a bit more distant than they were before you came out. You're feeling a bit more lonely and want to find more of a community to be yourself in. [*summarizing*]

Here, the provider skillfully reflects on key points that Andy makes. By recalling certain points that Andy makes, the provider indicates that he is actively listening. Beyond this, the provider can use reflection and summary statements to guide a conversation and hone in on change talk that he hears Andy use.

Informing

As a guide, the provider serves as a resource for their patient, providing unbiased information about various options to facilitate behavior change. Informing is a tool that can be used by providers in a variety of clinical circumstances, including sharing information, explaining results or procedures, and providing general advice. Information is critical within the context of MI, and it is important to deliver information in a manner that respects patient autonomy and to avoid transitioning the conversation in a direction that is dominated by the provider.

A key aspect to informing within MI settings is asking the patient for permission to share information with them, whether it is educational material, information about treatment options, information that other patients in similar situations have found useful, or other information that the provider feels necessary to convey. By asking for the patient's permission, the patient maintains a sense of control over the patient-provider interaction, shifting the locus of control to the patient. This ensures that the power dynamic between the provider and the patient remains equal and balanced, and is particularly useful if information is heavy or complicated, as asking for permission helps material feel more digestible. Consider the following interaction between a primary care provider and Meg, a 27-year-old transwoman who occasionally attends pumping parties, where she injects nonsurgical silicone in a medically unsupervised environment (Fig. 17.7). Notice how her provider uses informing selectively, and with permission.

MEG: So at these parties, I go into a backroom and there's a man back there that tells me to lie down on a table. He'd use a needle to inject a couple of cups of silicone into my butt and my hips – really help me get that hourglass figure, you know? My insurance won't cover it, and it's the only choice I have to feel more like me. It's worth the pain – he never uses any numbing – and it's way cheaper than I would pay if I went to a plastic surgeon – no way that I could afford that.

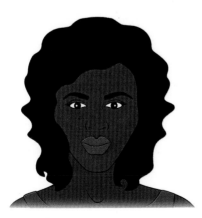

Fig. 17.7 Meg is a 27-year-old transwoman who occasionally attends pumping parties, where she injects nonsurgical silicone in a medically unsupervised environment

PROVIDER: There are a couple of concerns that I have about these pumping parties, would it be alright if I told you about them and then we can talk about some things that other patients of mind have done in the past?

MEG: Okay...

PROVIDER: I understand the appeal of these parties for sure – your body can feel more feminine and look more like what you want it to look like at a lower cost. But over time, these implants will most likely start to shift, and can cause infections and visible deformities on your skin since they're not being placed by a trained medical professional. While they may feel good now in the short-term, in the long-term, you'll save more money by getting them done in a professional setting. If you would like, I can show you some information and pictures of correctly placed silicone and what it should look like over time.

MEG: Hmm...I didn't realize that there was such a risk – I figured that they would keep looking good. But I know I can't afford these treatments, and they do help me feel better about myself now.

PROVIDER: Some of the other transwomen that I work with have had this conflict as well – they want the procedure to feel more at home in their bodies, but they can't afford the procedure or their insurance won't cover it. If you'd like, I can set you up with a health navigator who can talk to you about your insurance options and what doctors we work with who may be able to work with you to get you the care that you need in a safe and affordable way. Would you like me to set up that appointment with the health navigator?

Asking permission is laden throughout this excerpt, in which the provider carefully provides information in a manner that is not overwhelming to the patient. While providers are often seen as the voice of guidance by many patients, it is important that providers using informing in the context of MI maintain a sense of conversation by continually engaging the patient. Additionally, it is imperative that the task of informing does not come off in the *directing* style of communication, and maintains a sense of the provider as a guide. To accomplish this, the provider should endeavor to offer the patient choices that are informed and tailored to that patient's situation, rather than presenting them with only one option. A single option tells the patient what to do, *directing* rather than *guiding* the patient. When presenting options, it is best to present a group of options together, and then discuss the details of choices that interest the patient, rather than singularly presenting an option, explaining it, then explaining a subsequent option, and explaining it. The second method leads to a common trap where the patient will ask you to stop presenting options, choosing the first one presented and opting not to listen to all the options available.

Presenting options is particularly useful in the setting of informing the patient of some options that have worked for other patients, then allowing the patient to explore and grapple with the option that may work best for them.

Balancing Asking, Listening, and Informing

In summary, MI asks the provider to serve as a guide during an interaction with a patient, integrating and balancing the techniques of asking, listening, and informing. The MI process enhances the patient's understanding of their uncertainty surrounding behavior change, guides the patient to resolve their ambivalence by weighing pros and cons, and motivates the patient to accomplish feasible and sustained goals. As we have seen, MI relies on several key skills: the ability to ask open-ended questions, the ability to provide affirmations to the patient, the ability to listen reflectively and verbalize this reflection, and the ability to provide summary statements throughout a patient interaction. MI has a diverse application and can be adapted for individuals at different levels of motivation and readiness for behavior change. While some individuals are completely ready for change and simply need to rely on a provider as a guide to facilitate that change, others may have tried and failed to change their behaviors, and still others may be completely unaware that their behaviors are impacting their lives in unhealthy ways. Regardless, an interaction utilizing MI always begins with assessing where a patient is in the moment and can be seamlessly integrated into routine patient-provider interactions. Although the techniques we have described may feel clunky and unfamiliar at first, with time and practice, they can quickly become second nature.

Applications of Motivational Interviewing in LGBT Health

Motivational interviewing is an effective method for behavior change, and has particular utility for promoting resilience in clinical practice. With respect to LGBT health, MI can be used as a tool to think critically about a population that has unique health needs and a need for informed healthcare providers. Broadly, MI is particularly well suited to patient-provider interactions with LGBT individuals as it can support the individual, promoting resilience within members of populations that have historically been told how they should act or carry out their lives. By utilizing MI to approach interactions with LGBT-identified patients, providers can educate themselves regarding their patients' perspectives, and support patients to make behavior changes in a manner that is affirming and

built on intrinsic motivations, rather than external encouragement and/or overt pressure. By focusing on creating a dialogue between the patient and the provider within MI, the locus of control of behavior change shifts from being provider centric, in a directing style of communication, to being within the individual. This shift is useful and works to build resilience and promote the health of individuals, and is well suited to LGBT-identified individuals with a history of trauma.

As discussed throughout this book, LGBT patients have unique life histories and experiences that influence their behaviors later in life. MI approaches behavior change with a focus on shifting the locus of control to the patient. The affirming nature of MI can build a patient's resilience, and is a key tool in health promotion for LGBT individuals, particularly those with a history of trauma. Further, MI can be used to break seemingly overwhelming behavior changes into smaller steps. In this fashion, a provider can promote the confidence an individual has in their ability to accomplish healthy behavior change, and can develop strategies for behavior change that are more likely to have a meaningful impact.

In this chapter we utilized a number of examples related to health behaviors of LGBT-identified individuals, but the application is broad when you consider traumatic experiences related to childhood trauma, sexual assault, bullying, societal rejection, feelings of isolation or shame, disclosure and coming out, intimate partner violence, self-harm, mental health challenges, and other experiences that are frequently experienced by LGBT individuals. The potential application for MI with LGBT patients is near limitless, and includes the following:

- Sexual risk behaviors (condomless sex, HIV prevention, STI prevention, risky sexual behaviors, sexual assault, engaging in sex work, etc.)
- HIV treatment and prophylaxis (PrEP use/adherence, ART use/adherence, retention in the HIV care continuum, engagement with HIV care providers, etc.)
- Diet and exercise (anabolic steroid use, disordered eating, elevated body mass index among some lesbian populations, etc.)
- Gender-affirming care without medical supervision in the transgender community (herbal preparations or hormones purchased off the Internet, pumping parties, etc.)
- Substance use disorders (smoking, alcohol use, party drugs, etc.)
- Mental health treatments and care (depression, anxiety, feelings of shame or isolation, self-harm, suicidal thoughts, etc.)

In summary, motivational interviewing is a useful tool for a wide range of patients and can be applied to patient-provider interactions in varying degrees. While this chapter focused on LGBT-specific examples, the tools and techniques discussed here – particularly those related to skillful question asking and reflective listening – are useful to promote insightful conversations in any consultation setting. By using the key skills of MI (asking open questions, providing affirmations, listening reflectively, and providing summary statements) and thinking critically about RULE, you can gain an understanding of your patients' motivations and perspectives and guide them toward their goals by facilitating behavior change. Fundamentally, MI promotes resilience in all individuals, regardless of background, empowering them to make changes in their lives that may previously have been unattainable. While each interaction does not need to follow a formal motivational interviewing process, by picking and choosing appropriate counseling techniques, you promote health for patients who identify as LGBT and those who do not and expand your knowledge of patients with backgrounds different from your own or your typical patient base while working to become a better resource for all of your patients.

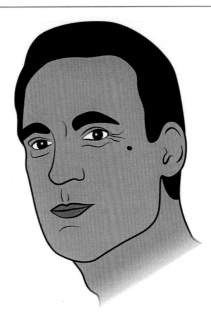

Fig. 17.8 47-year-old White male presenting with a slightly elevated viral load after being on HIV medications for over 20 years

Case Study #1

In the following example, pair up with a colleague to role-play an interaction between a provider and a patient. Halt the dialogue after 10–15 min, and evaluate the interaction using the questions listed below as a guide. Do not read the patient vignette before you decide who will be the patient and who will be the provider. If there are more than two of you working together, those not directly conducting the role play can observe the interaction, practice active listening, and provide feedback after the scenario is complete.

Instructions for Provider (Actor 1)

Introduce yourself to your patient and begin your interaction, obtaining information about what brings them to the visit today and guiding them using key skills in motivational interviewing. You have the following information on your patient: 47-year-old White male, presenting with a slightly elevated viral load after being on HIV medications for over 20 years (Fig. 17.8).

Instructions for Patient (Actor 2)

You are a man who has been living with HIV for over 20 years. You have been on a number of different treatment regimens over the years, many of which have failed. Your current regimen has a lot of side effects, including diarrhea, and you don't like to take the medications on days where you can't afford to have gastrointestinal distress. You've slowly stopped taking your medications, sometimes for weeks at a time. You understand the risks of poor adherence, but you feel okay and don't feel the need to take your meds. You have a partner who is HIV negative, and you are unhappy in your relationship and not motivated to protect your own or your partner's health. At today's meeting, while discussing the fact that your viral load is now slightly elevated, you begin to explain that you've been skipping some of your doses. Challenge your provider, expressing ambivalence about medication adherence: on the one hand, you want to be healthy and should protect your partner, and on the other hand, your medication makes you feel ill and you've already failed other medications so why would this one be different? Attempt to redirect the conversation away from discussion of medication adherence on several occasions to challenge the provider to continue focus on fostering behavior change.

Provider Follow-Up Questions

1. What were your overall impressions of the interaction?
2. How did the types of questions you asked work in the *guiding* style of communicating behavior change?
3. Were you able to listen for different types of change talk and provide reflective summaries on these statements?

4. If your patient had presented with strong ambivalence, or even resistance to change, how would you have approached this interaction?
5. How might you change your approach to this interaction as a provider?

Patient Follow-Up Questions

1. What were your overall impressions of the interaction?
2. What questions were most helpful in eliciting motivation for change?
3. How might the provider improve their interaction to better support behavior change?

Continue practicing with other patients of your own creation, and challenge each other to work through ambivalence, get to understand your patients' perspectives, and foster internal motivations while listening for change talk.

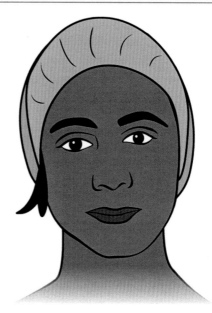

Fig. 17.9 19-year-old Hispanic female complaining of fatigue, feelings of isolation, and a lack of motivation

Case Study #2

In the following example, pair up with a colleague to role-play an interaction between a provider and a patient. Halt the dialogue after 10–15 min, and evaluate the interaction using the questions listed below as a guide. Do not read the patient vignette before you decide who will be the patient and who will be the provider. If there are more than two of you working together, those not directly conducting the role play can observe the interaction, practice active listening, and provide feedback after the scenario is complete.

Instructions for Provider (Actor 1)

Introduce yourself to your patient and begin your interaction, obtaining information about what brings them to the visit today and guiding them using key skills in motivational interviewing. You have the following information on your patient: 19-year-old Hispanic female complaining of fatigue, feelings of isolation, and a lack of motivation to engage in activities she once enjoyed (Fig. 17.9).

Instructions for Patient (Actor 2)

You are teenager who has recently come out as a lesbian. You have been feeling lonely, lacking the motivation to engage in activities you once enjoyed, and are sleepy all the time. You feel anxious about your relationships with your family and friends at school, some of whom haven't been accepting of your coming out. Present to the provider without much motivation to start therapy or treatment for your depression, and slowly introduce some change talk as the provider guides you toward wanting to address your depression. Challenge your provider with ambivalence: on the one hand, you want to feel like your "normal" self again and be open with people about how their lack of support has impacted you and on the other hand, you worry about being rejected by your family and friends and feel that being seeking treatment for depression would just give people something else to make fun of. Attempt to redirect the conversation away from discussion of depression treatment on several occasions to challenge the provider to continue focus on fostering behavior change.

Challenge your provider with ambivalence, but inject change talk slowly. Feel free to resist change, and include diversions to challenge your provider to guide the conversation in the direction of fostering behavior change.

Provider Follow-Up Questions

1. What were your overall impressions of the interaction?
2. How did the types of questions you asked work in the *guiding* style of communicating behavior change?
3. Were you able to listen for different types of change talks and provide reflective summaries on these statements?

4. If your patient had presented with strong ambivalence, or even resistance to change, how would you have approached this interaction?
5. How might you change your approach to this interaction as a provider?

Patient Follow-Up Questions

1. What were your overall impressions of the interaction?
2. What questions were most helpful in eliciting motivation for change?
3. How might the provider improve their interaction to better support behavior change?

Continue practicing with other patients of your own creation, and challenge each other to work through ambivalence, get to understand your patients' perspectives, and foster internal motivations while listening for change talk.

Additional Resources

Many youtube.com videos demonstrate patient-provider interactions using motivational interviewing techniques. Try a Google Search for some examples. Here are a few that we identified as particularly useful:

1. Good and bad examples of MI, Alan Lyme.
   (a) Good example: https://youtu.be/67I6g1I7Zao?list=PL0Iq5_Y7Dui-KRC5Z4ordPG1j7syCsLhq
   (b) Bad example: https://www.youtube.com/watch?v=_VlvanBFkvI
2. Dr. Jonathan Fader demonstrates MI skills: https://www.youtube.com/watch?v=ZxKZaKFzgF8
3. MI: Evoking Commitment to Change: https://www.youtube.com/watch?v=dm-rJJPCuTE&list=PL0Iq5_Y7Dui-KRC5Z4ordPG1j7syCsLhq&index=5
4. Advanced MI: Depression: https://www.youtube.com/watch?v=3rSt4KIaN8I
5. The effective physician: MI Demonstration: https://www.youtube.com/watch?v=URiKA7CKtfc&list=PL0Iq5_Y7Dui-KRC5Z4ordPG1j7syCsLhq&index=10

References

1. Farley TA, Dalal MA, Mostashari F, Frieden TR. Deaths preventable in the US by improvements in use of clinical preventive services. Am J Prev Med. 2010;38(6):600–9.
2. Krieger N. Epidemiology and the people's health: theory and context. New York: Oxford University Press; 2011.
3. Bogart LM, Revenson TA, Whitfield KE, France CR. Introduction to the special section on lesbian, gay, bisexual, and transgender (LGBT) health disparities: where we are and where we're going. Ann Behav Med. 2014;47(1):1–4.
4. Kosciw JG, Palmer NA, Kull RM. Reflecting resiliency: openness about sexual orientation and/or gender identity and its relationship to well-being and educational outcomes for LGBT students. Am J Community Psychol. 2015;55(1–2):167–78.
5. Poteat VP. Peer group socialization of homophobic attitudes and behavior during adolescence. Child Dev. 2007;78(6):1830–42.
6. Miller WR. Motivational interviewing with problem drinkers. Behav Psychother. 1983;11(02):147–72.
7. Miller WR, Rollnick S. Motivational interviewing: helping people change. New York: Guilford press; 2012.
8. Abraham C, Michie S. A taxonomy of behavior change techniques used in interventions. Health Psychol. 2008;27(3):379.
9. Lefcourt HM. Locus of control. In: Robinson JP, Shaver PR, Wrightsman LS, editors. Measures of personality and social psychological attitudes. San Diego: Academic Press; 1991. p. 413–99. xiv, 753.
10. Solomon Z, Mikulincer M, Avitzur E. Coping, locus of control, social support, and combat-related posttraumatic stress disorder: a prospective study. J Pers Soc Psychol. 1988;55(2):279.
11. Rollnick S, Miller WR. What is motivational interviewing? Behav Cogn Psychother. 1995;23(04):325–34.
12. Rogers CR. Client-centered therapy: its current practice, implications and theory. Boston: Houghton Mifflin; 1951.
13. Emmons KM, Rollnick S. Motivational interviewing in healthcare settings: opportunities and limitations. Am J Prev Med. 2001;20(1):68–74.
14. Ajzen I, Fishbein M. Attitude-behavior relations: a theoretical analysis and review of empirical research. Psychol Bull. 1977;84(5):888.
15. Rollnick S, Heather N, Bell A. Negotiating behaviour change in medical settings: the development of brief motivational interviewing. J Ment Health. 1992;1(1):25–37.
16. Hibbard JH, Greene J. What the evidence shows about patient activation: better health outcomes and care experiences; fewer data on costs. Health Aff. 2013;32(2):207–14.
17. Hibbard JH, Cunningham PJ. How engaged are consumers in their health and healthcare, and why does it matter. Res Briefs. 2008;8:1–9.
18. Guadagnoli E, Ward P. Patient participation in decision-making. Soc Sci Med. 1998;47(3):329–39.
19. Greene J, Hibbard JH. Why does patient activation matter? An examination of the relationships between patient activation and health-related outcomes. J Gen Intern Med. 2012;27(5):520–6.
20. DiLillo V, West DS. Incorporating motivational interviewing into counseling for lifestyle change among overweight individuals with type 2 diabetes. Diabetes Spectr. 2011;24(2):80–4.

Promoting Healthy LGBT Interpersonal Relationships

18

Kerith J. Conron, Nathan Brewer, and Heather L. McCauley

Promoting healthy interpersonal relationships – those that, at minimum, are respectful, caring, and free from violence and coercion – is a large social undertaking in which health-care providers can play a critical role. Providers have the capacity to model respectful and caring communication, as well as to establish norms related to interpersonal relationships and help-seeking behaviors. By routinely assessing for intimate partner violence (IPV), providers communicate that IPV, physical and sexual violence, stalking, and psychological aggression, whether by a current or former intimate partner [1], are pervasive problems that merit attention. Once IPV has been identified, providers have an opportunity to provide trauma-informed care and discuss harm reduction strategies with patients who are ready and able to engage with services. The aim of this chapter is to provide guidance on IPV assessment and trauma-informed behavioral health care that considers the ways in which lesbian, gay, bisexual, and transgender (LGBT) patients may be similar to and differ from heterosexual and/or cisgender (nontransgender) patients.

Background

Intimate partner violence (IPV) is a major public health problem in that it is both highly prevalent and a known risk for mortality and morbidity over the life course, with related health conditions including depression, HIV and other sexually transmitted infections, unintended pregnancy, child maltreatment, migraines, asthma, and gastrointestinal problems [2–5]. In the general US population, nearly one in three US women (31.5%) and over one in four men (27.5%) experience physical violence victimization by an intimate partner at some point in their lifetimes [6]. Physical violence includes hitting, biting, strangulating, burning, and the use of weapons. In addition, almost half (47%) of women and men report psychological aggression [6], which includes degrading statements, threats of physical or sexual abuse, and threats to harm loved ones or pets, within an intimate relationship in their lifetimes. The pervasiveness of psychological aggression suggests a universal need to improve communication and conflict resolution skills. Sexual violence, including rape (reported by 8.8% of women and 0.5% of men), attempted rape, and forced sex, as well as the use of alcohol or other means to coerce sexual contact, and including deliberate exposure to sexually transmitted infections, is common among women [6]. Lifetime experiences of stalking such as repeated or unwanted messages through phone or email, spying in person or via devices, and watching or following from a distance by a current or former intimate partner are reported by 9.2% of women and 2.5% of men [6]. Finally, although data are not captured on this expression of IPV, practitioners and advocates widely acknowledge the existence of financial abuse including restricting a person's access to financial resources, forcing them to financially support the partner, or intentionally disrupting their credit.

In about half of relationships in which IPV occurs, perpetration is reported by both partners [7]. This pattern appears to hold across opposite-sex and same-sex relationships [8]. Importantly, providers should note that physical injury is more likely to be reported by female than male victims [7] and that women are more than twice as likely to report rape and other sexual violence within the context of intimate relationships than are male victims [6]. Thus, what is often termed "reciprocal" violence may differ in composition,

K.J. Conron
Blachford-Cooper Research Director and Distinguished Scholar, The Williams Institute, UCLA School of Law and Affiliated Investigator, The Fenway Institute, Fenway Health, Boston, MA, USA

N. Brewer
Simmons College, Boston, MA, USA

H.L. McCauley, ScD (✉)
Human Development and Family Studies, Michigan State University, 3414 Fifth Avenue, CHOB 109, Pittsburgh, PA 15213, USA
e-mail: mccaul49@msu.edu

Table 18.1 Lifetime prevalence of rape, physical violence, and stalking victimization by an intimate partner by sex and sexual orientation identity, National Intimate Partner and Sexual Violence Survey 2010 ($N = 16{,}507$) [10]

	Females			Males		
	Lesbian	Bisexual	Heterosexual	Gay	Bisexual	Heterosexual
	%[a]	%[a]	%[a]	%[a]	%[a]	%[a]
Rape	[b]	22.1	9.1	[b]	[b]	[b]
Physical violence	40.4	56.9	32.3	25.2	37.3	28.7
Stalking	[b]	31.1	10.2	[b]	[b]	2.1

Adapted with permission from the U.S. Centers for Disease Control and Prevention
[a]Weighted proportions
[b]Data are too sparse to provide an estimate

severity, and consequence for each partner, particularly when one is female and the other is male. For instance, reproductive coercion, including sabotage related to contraception and/or condom use to promote pregnancy, is a particular form of gendered sexual violence victimization for which bisexual women with current male partner(s) who utilize family planning clinics are at particular risk [9].

As shown in Table 18.1, rates of IPV among lesbian, gay, and bisexual people are comparable to or exceed those observed among heterosexuals [8, 10–13]. Bisexual women are far more likely to report IPV than are heterosexual women [10–13], particularly in the context of male-female relationships [11]. Given that bisexual women are the largest segment of the LGBT community, particularly among younger cohorts [14], it is critical that providers and health institutions identify bisexual women in "opposite-sex" relationships in order to meet their needs.

Population-based data about IPV experiences among transgender people have not yet been collected, but data from the large National Transgender Discrimination Survey indicate that nearly one in five (19%) of transgender adults has experienced domestic violence by a family member because they are transgender or gender nonconforming [15]. Actual rates of IPV are likely considerably higher, assuming that transgender people also experience IPV for reasons that are unrelated to being transgender.

Rates of IPV are lower than expected for most LGBT subgroups, given that stigma and discrimination increase risk for IPV through elevated rates of child maltreatment [13, 16, 17], depression [17–22], and unemployment and poverty [12, 15, 23–25] – established risks for IPV [26]. IPV may take additional forms among LGBT people, related to their socially marginalized status, and include threats to out a partner's gender or sexual identity [27]. For example, perpetrators may deliberately sabotage fragile relationships with disapproving families of origin to further isolate the partner [28]. Clients in same-sex relationships may also be more susceptible to identity theft or impersonation as abusive tactics.

Stigma and discrimination also limit access to IPV resources, including LGBT-competent medical and behavioral health care and LGBT-inclusive IPV prevention education and treatment, including domestic violence shelters and batterer intervention programs. Experiences of rejection and discrimination in health-care settings are all too common for LGBT people [29] and are associated with medical mistrust and delays in help-seeking [30]. Thus, providers will need to establish trust with LGBT patients and are encouraged to screen routinely for IPV and associated modifiable risk factors, as disclosure may not occur until trust has been established.

Trauma-Informed Violence Screening and Assessment in Primary Care

Strategies for IPV Screening in Primary Care

Screening for IPV in primary care settings is recommended by the Institute of Medicine and supported by leading professional health-care organizations [31–33]. The goal of screening in the clinical setting is to identify patients at risk for IPV and connect them to patient-centered intervention services at the time of a health-care encounter [34]. As patient safety is paramount, screening must be conducted with the patient in a private setting, without partners, friends, or other family members present, any of whom could be abusing the patient. From a patient perspective, qualities of effective screening include trust between the patient and the provider, being routinely asked about IPV [35], and a clinical atmosphere of safety and support [36]. When those qualities are achieved, screening appears to be associated with few adverse effects [37], and patients whose providers ask about their relationships are more likely to be able to identify abusive behaviors and know about the violence recovery resources available to them.

There are several screening approaches that have been tested, although much of what is known about IPV screening and assessment in the clinical setting comes from studies of cisgender heterosexual women primarily (although not exclusively) in reproductive health settings [38]. Consequently, current IPV screening recommendations are specific to these populations. That said, given evidence that LGBT populations experience abuse at similar or higher levels compared to their heterosexual counterparts, strategies to promote conversations with LGBT patients about IPV are warranted. One approach includes having patients complete an IPV screening tool while they are waiting for their clinical visit; results are then reviewed by the clinician, who can engage the patient in further discussion during the encounter. Embedding an IPV screening tool into a set of psychosocial screeners that a patient completes on a computer tablet prior to the clinical encounter is one strategy for collecting and communicating the results of IPV screening data to the provider. This approach, referred to as electronic Patient Reported Outcomes (e-PRO), was initially developed to collect data on behavioral health and HIV-related health status from HIV-positive patients [39] and is being expanded to collect self-report patient data on an array of topics, including IPV, and is being used with broader patient populations.

Another strategy is using the electronic health record to prompt clinicians to screen for IPV, including reminders in progress notes or "smart links" to tools such as IPV resources in the community or additional screening tools (e.g., Danger Assessment Instrument) [40]. While the psychometric properties of common screening tools vary widely by study [41], screening tools with generally strong sensitivity and specificity include the four-item Hurt, Insult, Threaten, and Scream (HITS) instrument [41, 42], and the Ongoing Violence Assessment Tool [43]. The Danger Assessment is another well-validated tool to assess the lethality of an abusive relationship [44, 45] and can be used in the clinical setting, as described under *Behavioral Health* below. These tools, as well as others, can be found at http://www.cdc.gov/violenceprevention/pdf/ipv/ipvandsvscreening.pdf.

Studies assessing the psychometric properties of common IPV screening tools among LGBT populations are scarce. One recent study developed a six-item tool using a mixed methods approach with more than 1,000 gay and bisexual men [46]. In addition to physical and sexual violence, the tool included controlling behaviors and HIV-related IPV and resulted in recording a significantly higher prevalence of IPV compared to the CDC's IPV screening items only [46].

Promising IPV screeners in use at the Fenway Health Center, an urban community health center with expertise in LGBT health, are provided in Table 18.2.

For LGBT patients, disclosing to a clinician that they have experienced abuse in the context of an intimate relationship may be more nuanced than among heterosexual and/or cisgender patients. In some cases, patients may be coming out to their providers for the first time. Sexual identity and behavior also do not perfectly overlap, such that it may be challenging for people who identify as heterosexual yet have same-sex sex partners to discuss abuse

occurring in the context of their relationships. Moreover, similar to cisgender populations, LGBT patients may perceive the behaviors they are experiencing as normative, and therefore may not recognize their experiences as abuse. For all of these reasons, health-care systems and individual providers should strive to create safe spaces for patients by asking about both sexual identity and behavior nonjudgmentally, screening all patients for IPV, and, if making a community referral, discussing the patient's comfort level in disclosing their sexual orientation and gender identity to staff at community-based agencies [47].

IPV Assessment in Primary Care: Universal Education, Routine Inquiry, and Brief Counseling

While IPV screening has been recommended since the 1980s, barriers exist to implementing routine screening in the clinical setting. These perceived barriers by clinicians include limited time, discomfort asking about abuse, and lack of training or confidence regarding how to respond to a positive disclosure [48]. In recent years, leading violence prevention organizations have proposed an approach to providing IPV services in the clinical setting focused on *assessment* rather than screening. With this approach, the goal is not necessarily to achieve disclosure, but to normalize discussions of healthy relationships as an integral aspect of a clinical evaluation. Central to this approach is the perspective that disclosure is not required for providers to practice trauma-informed care and consider that a patient's presentation to the clinic may be connected to events in their intimate relationships [36, 49]. A trauma-informed assessment approach also aligns with research indicating that survivors seek safe environments in which to share their experiences and do not want to feel targeted or judged by their health-care providers [36]. IPV assessment provides an opportunity for primary prevention (for those never exposed), secondary prevention (for individuals with histories of IPV), and intervention for those who are currently experiencing IPV in their relationships [40].

IPV assessment consists of: (1) universal education or anticipatory guidance, (2) routine inquiry, and (3) brief counseling. Futures Without Violence, a national nonprofit organization focused on violence prevention, has developed guidelines to assist providers in conducting IPV assessment in clinical settings (http://www.futureswithoutviolence.org/). Their first curriculum designed for patients of all sexual orientations and gender identities – the Hanging Out or Hooking Up curriculum – has been tested with adolescent and young adults [50]. Using these guidelines and a palm-sized safety card, which discusses healthy and unhealthy relationships, clinicians provide universal education or

Table 18.2 IPV Screeners in use at the Fenway Health Center and suggested additions

Fenway Health IPV Screening

Many patients have health problems due to abuse from a partner. We are giving this questionnaire to all of our patients. Your provider is interested in your answers so that s/he can provide you with the best possible care. Your provider will offer you further resources if you are interested

Please circle your answers and give this form back to your provide. If you prefer not to answer, please check the box below. Thank you

☐ I prefer not to answer these questions

1. In the last year, have you felt isolated, trapped, or like you are walking on eggshells in an intimate relationship?
   ☐ Yes
   ☐ No

2. In the last year, has your partner controlled where you go, who you talk to, or how you spend your money?
   ☐ Yes
   ☐ No

3. In the last year, has someone pressure or forced you to do something sexual that you didn't want to do?
   ☐ Yes
   ☐ No

4. In the last year, has someone hit, kicked, punched, or otherwise hurt?
   ☐ Yes
   ☐ No

Suggested additions

5. What was the gender of the partner or partners who acted this way toward you? (Check all that apply)
   ☐ Man (cisgender, that is not transgender)
   ☐ Woman (cisgender, that is not transgender)
   ☐ Transgender man
   ☐ Transgender woman
   ☐ Genderqueer person (assigned male sex at birth)
   ☐ Genderqueer person (assigned female sex at birth)

6. In the last year, have you controlled where your partner goes, who they talk to, or how they spend their money?
   ☐ Yes
   ☐ No

7. In the last year, have you pressured or forced your partner to do something sexual that they didn't want to do?
   ☐ Yes
   ☐ No

8. In the last year, have you hit, kicked, punched, or otherwise hurt your partner?
   ☐ Yes
   ☐ No

anticipatory guidance as an important first step during all patient encounters. The goal is to have a discussion about healthy relationships with all patients. After briefly initiating the conversation (e.g., "I talk to all of my patients about..."), the provider conducts a routine inquiry. The goal of this phase is for both clinicians and patients to recognize that patients' relationships affect their health. Clinicians may ask questions specific to the context in which a patient is seeking care. For example, when a patient seeks testing for sexually transmitted infections (STI), a savvy clinician will recognize that abusive relationships may impact a patient's ability to negotiate condom use, instead of assuming that the patient does not know how to use a condom or making a judgment about the patient's sexual behavior.

Conversations about healthy relationships should be conducted using affirming, nonjudgmental language. For example, in the case of discussing condom use when seeking STI testing above, a clinician might affirm and reflect, "You're working hard to make decisions to stay healthy, and regularly using condoms is something you recognize would help you achieve that goal. What has made this difficult in the past?" Even in light of affirming, supportive routine questions, some patients may not be ready to disclose abusive experiences. Whether or not a patient discloses or acknowledges abuse, validating an individual's experiences and reactions to those experiences is critical ("Your partner has said very hurtful things to you in the past, and you're struggling with feeling both hurt and still loving your partner"). Further, regardless of disclosure, providers should strive to create a safe environment that supports patients advocating for their health-care needs and preferences (e.g., anonymous STI partner notification). Finally, when patients do disclose, providers should engage in shared decision-making with patients regarding options for continued care referrals for community resources.

The aforementioned approach is supported by mounting scientific evidence. The Hanging Out or Hooking Up guidelines and materials were tested in school-based health centers that serve adolescents ages 14–19 of all sexes and genders. A randomized controlled trial of over 1000 students in eight school-based health centers in California found that youth who received care in intervention clinics were more likely to recognize sexual coercion at 3 month follow-up compared to youth in control clinics. Among those youth who reported IPV victimization at baseline, youth receiving the intervention were more likely than controls to disclose IPV to their providers and less likely to report IPV victimization at 3 month follow-up, which is promising for this brief intervention [51]. A similar approach has also been tested among women seeking care in reproductive health clinics, with evaluation results including reduced pregnancy coercion at follow-up among intervention participants compared to controls [52]. Pilot testing of materials designed specifically for LGBT community members of all ages is currently underway. These materials include a safety card for lesbian, gay, and bisexual patients and one for transgender patients. Safety cards will include information about healthy and unhealthy relationships (e.g., "Do you or your partner threaten to out a partner's gender identity, sexual orientation, HIV status, or immigration status to friends, family, or at work?"), and questions to help patients make the connection between IPV and their health. Moreover, they will include hotline numbers and websites of national resources for LGBT people who have been victimized or perpetrated relationship abuse.

Behavioral Health

Assessment of IPV

Behavioral health assessments with LGBT clients should include a screening for trauma generally, and interpersonal violence specifically. Effective clinical approaches begin with rapport building. It is particularly important to mirror the client's language when describing their identity, their experience of violence, and their resulting symptomatology. Gender and sexual minority clients may be less likely to label their experience as "domestic violence" or "intimate partner violence." This may be due to a variety of reasons, including a lack of LGBT inclusion in prevention education with a resultant lack of cultural references to relationship violence in LGBT communities.

Culturally appropriate IPV education campaigns, as reflected in the public awareness posters and created by TOD@S Collaborative with funding from the Office of Violence Against Women, U.S. Department of Justice, are, unfortunately, rare (Fig. 18.1). TOD@S is an interagency collaboration between the Hispanic Black Gay Coalition, The Network / La Red, Renewal House Shelter, a program of the Unitarian Universalist Urban Ministry and The Violence Recovery Program (VRP) at Fenway Health.

The TOD@S Collaborative website, which provides information about IPV within black and Latin@ LGBT communities, is http://todosinaction.org.

A particularly difficult component of IPV assessment with LGBT clients engaged in behavioral health care is screening for the presence and directionality of controlling behaviors. Screening can require significant questioning regarding relationship dynamics. Clinicians should ask themselves: Who has the ability to make decisions in this relationship? Is one person deferential to another out of fear? If there is physical or psychological violence, what is the *context* of that violence? For instance, did the person enacting the violence react to ongoing psychological abuse? Answering these questions requires solicitation of examples from clients, and probing beyond the initial language used by the respondent. Of particular importance is screening for the presence of coercive control, including the subcomponents of demands, threats, and negative consequences [54]. Individuals experiencing IPV often worry that they are the ones behaving abusively, especially if they have acted in self-defense by perpetrating physical violence. It is imperative that clinicians appropriately contextualize these acts within the greater dynamics of the relationship.

In addition to screening for the presence of violence and the directionality of coercive control, clinicians should assess for the dangerousness and potential lethality of the violence present in the relationship. It is important to probe for information regarding the severity and frequency of violence, as well as changes over time. A widely used tool for assessment of potential lethality (dangerousness) is the Danger Assessment (https://www.dangerassessment.org/)[55]. This assessment screens for known factors associated with homicide from an abusive partner, including threats of homicide, presence of weapons, and past strangulation, among others. Although research on this tool has been limited to heterosexual relationships in which the victim is cisgender and female, it is used with gender and sexual minorities in clinical practice settings.

Treatment of Individuals Following IPV

Treatment of individuals experiencing IPV can be conceptualized in four stages, as described by Judith Herman [56]: (1) ongoing violence, (2) stabilizing trauma symptoms, (3) metabolizing trauma, and (4) integrating trauma. There is often overlap between these stages and they are not meant to be linear. For example, some individuals who have experienced abuse do not leave the person abusing them, and some that do initially leave may eventually return to the relationship.

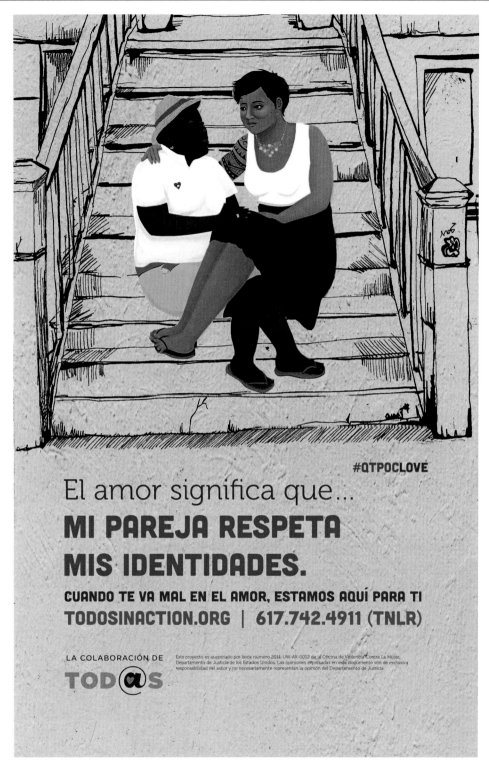

Fig. 18.1 (**a**, **b**) Culturally appropriate IPV Education Campaigns created by TOD@S Collaborative [53] (Used with permission from the TOD@S Collaborative)

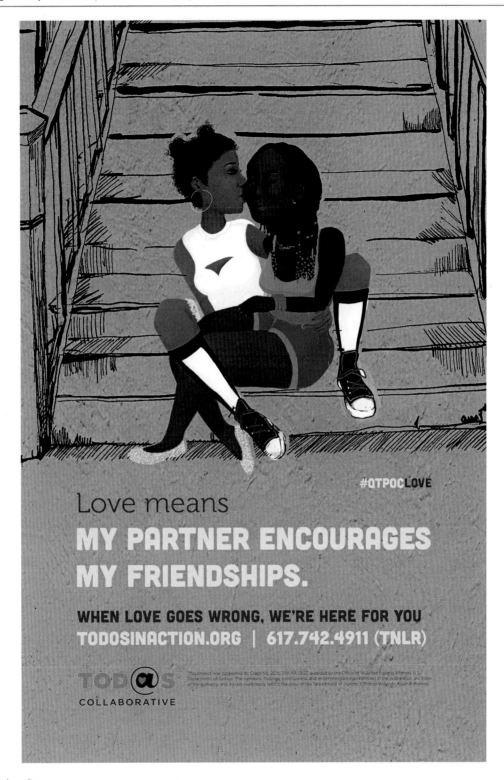

Fig. 18.1 (continued)

Ongoing Violence

When victims are engaged in an ongoing violent relationship, the primary concern should be the safety of the client. The initial danger assessment should be supplemented with repeat assessments over time to identify changes in violent behavior, with a particular focus on potential increases in frequency and severity. It is important to focus on harm reduction rather than being prescriptive or directive in one's approach, and imperative to avoid replicating the kind of power differential that the client is experiencing in their intimate relationship by demanding changes that they are unwilling or unprepared to enact. Particular care should be taken to assess for danger when a client does decide to leave their relationship, as this is a time of increased risk of injury and homicide. A comprehensive safety plan should be developed before an attempt to leave, and should include strategizing ways to limit the risk of harm to the client, as well as loved ones, including children and pets.

Often the safety phase of treatment includes connecting the client to social services, and may include using telephone or web-based platforms to access appropriate care where resources are limited, such as in remote or resource-poor areas [57, 58]. It should be noted that many domestic violence services were created for cisgender women who have male perpetrators. However, some domestic violence shelters are becoming more inclusive, and a few agencies focus on gender and sexual minorities, including The National Coalition of Anti-Violence Programs (http://www.avp.org/), Community United Against Violence (http://www.cuav.org/), Northwest Network of BTLG Survivors of Abuse (http://www.nwnetwork.org/), and The Network/La Red (http://tnlr.org/).

Clients may also rely on family supports during this time of seeking safety; however, this may not be an option for gender and sexual minority clients who are estranged from their families of origin. When possible, including patient-identified supportive individuals in discussions about community-based resources may decrease barriers to utilization of available supports.

Stabilization of Trauma Symptoms

For many clients who have experienced violence in their intimate relationships, mental and physical health symptoms will present during or after leaving the relationship. These symptoms are associated with the three F's: fight, flight, and freeze [59] and can manifest as panic attacks, exaggerated anxiety, irritability, depression, and/or dissociation (e.g., appearing detached, disengaged, or distracted). A major goal of this early stage of care is to assist the client in developing the skills of grounding, allowing patient to stay focused on the present, thereby reducing symptoms of panic and dissociation. Such techniques can include physical sensations (e.g., tracing a nearby object with one's fingers, deep breathing, stretching) or verbal statements (e.g., describing the environment, reciting lyrics to a favorite song). One strategy clinicians can use is to assist the client in cultivating awareness of the connection between environmental triggers and corresponding physiological and psychological symptoms. For example, clinicians can ask patients to describe what it feels like when they experience panic or dissociation, and then work backwards to identify what was occurring in the environment when they started to experience these feelings. Additionally, clients can be

supported in identifying and developing health-promoting coping skills. One way of exploring these coping skills is asking about successes in managing trauma symptoms, that is, "Were there times when you were able to overcome your panic/dissociation/etc.? What do you think helped you to overcome those thoughts and feelings?" As clients begin to develop these skills and feel more grounded, their identity may shift from one of victimhood to one of survivorship.

Stabilization of symptoms may be more difficult for gender and sexual minority clients given high levels of prior and concurrent trauma exposure. Child maltreatment, peer bullying, harassment, and microaggressions (daily insults) are cumulative stressors that are experienced disproportionately by sexual and gender minorities. This insidious trauma or minority stress can create mental health problems and complicate recovery from IPV-related trauma. Clients who are concurrent members of other minority groups (i.e., racial-ethnic minorities, individuals who are foreign-born or those who live with disabilities) may present with higher levels of cumulative trauma for which multiple types of microaggressions may compound the trauma of IPV. It is important for clinicians to be aware that cumulative minority stress, occurring along multiple axes of inequality, may increase the likelihood of internalized stigma (the adoption of negative societal beliefs about one's own group or groups), and risk of poor mental health, in addition to limiting access to resources.

Metabolizing Trauma

For many clients who have begun to develop the necessary grounding techniques to stabilize their functioning, clinical efforts can shift toward metabolizing the trauma. In many cases, this takes the dual form of sadness in response to the loss of their relationship and anger due to the injustice of their experiences; however, it is important to affirm and normalize any emotional or physical reactions individuals may have. Clinicians should be careful to allow space for clients to mourn the loss of their relationships, remembering that clients often love (d) their partners despite the abuse and miss the positive aspects of the terminated relationship. Clinicians should make efforts to validate clients' anger at the injustice of their experience of the IPV. For some clients who successfully metabolize the trauma experience, their identity can shift from that of survivor to one of victor or healer, particularly when their recovery includes helping other survivors. However, specific identity labels may differ from person to person, so it is important for providers to mirror the language created and/or used by their clients.

Integrating Trauma

The final stage of recovery often includes integrating the trauma into the client's larger narrative and identity. Clinical work in this stage may include assisting the client to reconnect with loved ones, including family, and form new relationships. This stage may include asking questions about the experience of trauma, and reconnection may involve the client reconnecting with God or developing a newfound sense of spirituality. For gender and sexual minorities, the integration of trauma can be more complex, as prior experiences of rejection within faith-based settings may complicate the formation of a strong spiritual connection. Clinicians can assist clients in identity exploration, and validate the complexity of thoughts and feelings that arise during this exploration.

The Violence Recovery Program, Fenway Health

Here we will describe the Violence Recovery Program (VRP; http://fenwayhealth.org/care/behavioral-health/vrp/), as it represents a promising clinical practice model for violence prevention and recovery. An integral program of Fenway Health, a multidisciplinary community health center where LGBT people and neighborhood residents receive comprehensive behavioral health and medical care, regardless of ability to pay; the VRP has worked with LGBT survivors of violence for over three decades and provides a wide menu of free services that address anti-LGBT hate violence, domestic violence, sexual assault, and police misconduct.

Direct services are provided in English and Spanish and include individual counseling, group counseling, advocacy, and case management. Counselors and advocates provide trauma-informed services to stabilize acute symptoms of posttraumatic stress, educate clients about the impact of violence, and provide support during the healing process. Survivors are assisted in accessing a range of services and resources, including shelter and housing, public assistance, and social services. Education and assistance is also provided in navigating the criminal justice and legal systems and assisting survivors in filing police reports and obtaining restraining orders; connecting survivors to LGBT-sensitive medical and legal services, and advocating on behalf of survivors with police departments, District Attorneys' offices, the Attorney General's Civil Rights and Victim Compensation divisions, and other victim service agencies. Clients of the VRP may also participate in psycho-educational and support groups that can reduce isolation and improve self-esteem by providing connections to other survivors.

Clients are made aware of the VRP's free services through Fenway Health's medical, behavioral health, and research staff, website, brochures, and other outreach materials, as well as print advertising. The VRP conducts regular outreach to target survivors and specific agencies that are likely to refer victims. This includes outreach to domestic violence agencies, sexual assault programs, legal and criminal justice offices, colleges, and mental health organizations where VRP staff distribute conduct outreach. Prospective clients call the VRP intake line to request an intake, which is scheduled within a few days of the call. Non-VRP providers at Fenway utilize an on-call pager system to request an immediate, in-person introduction by VRP staff to potential clients in the health center.

The VRP also provides trainings on trauma and recovery for LGBT clients and recognizing and treating same-sex domestic violence for a variety of audiences, including but not limited to mental health professionals, law enforcement, legal personnel, students, victim service providers, medical personnel, domestic violence coalitions, and community groups.

Case Study

Avery is a 19-year-old black transgender woman presenting at the clinic with severe headaches (Fig. 18.2). Prior to the exam, the front desk staff warns you that Avery is a difficult client who has been arguing with the staff about being seen despite arriving 15 min late for her appointment. When you open the door to the exam room, Avery straightens up, crosses her arms, and looks angrily at you. Upon questioning, you learn that the front desk staff called out Avery's male birth name (Bryant), which is listed on her insurance card, in the waiting area when it was time to bring her back to the clinical consult room. You

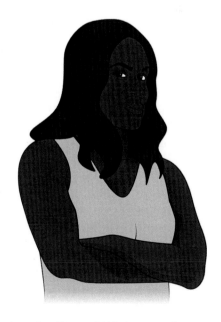

Fig. 18.2 Avery is a 19-year-old black transgender woman presenting at the clinic with severe headaches

also learn that she took three buses to get to her appointment and that the last was running late. You acknowledge the inconvenient location of the clinic and express your appreciation that she got to the appointment, despite the inconvenience. You notice that Avery unfolds her arms. Next, you ask what name and gender pronouns she prefers and then initiate the clinical exam. Upon further questioning, you learn that Avery is taking estrogen at higher levels than was prescribed by another provider and that she is living with a boyfriend who pushes her around when he drinks. She tells you that she is in a rush to complete her transition and is fearful that her employer will learn that she is transgender. As a barista, Avery earns just above minimum wage and is economically dependent on her 42-year-old boyfriend for housing. She states that she does not want to move back home due to conflict with her family about her identity and gender presentation.

Discussion Questions

1. What might be causing Avery's headaches?
2. What can providers do to put patients at ease who expect poor treatment based upon personal and community experience along multiple axes of inequality?
3. How could the topic of where and how to initiate gender affirming care be addressed with Avery?
4. What follow-up questions might a provider ask to better understand Avery's situation with her boyfriend?
5. How can the provider address the topic of healthy/ unhealthy communication within intimate partner relationships even if Avery is reluctant to label or to discuss the abuse that she is experiencing?

Summary Practice Points

1. Patients such as Avery often present with a constellation of social and biological risk factors that may impact physical and mental health. Addressing these risks using a combination of medical, behavioral, and community-based resources may be the most effective approach to promote health and well-being.
2. Providers and patients may have little in common relative to their socioeconomic backgrounds, race-ethnicity, sexual orientation, gender identity, and age. Attentive listening and non-patronizing expressions of concern about the patient may reduce social distance and barriers to effective interpersonal communication.
3. Many transgender patients have had negative experiences with health-care providers and other professionals, and, thus, anticipate rejection. For this reason, patients may be particularly sensitive to being "handed off" to another provider, even when the intention is good (and another provider or clinic has greater

expertise in transgender health). Consequently, transgender patients may prefer to stay with an attentive provider who listens and is willing to obtain information about transgender health rather than being transferred to a new provider or clinic with expertise in transgender health care. It is preferable to ask the patient for her/his/ their preference and to engage them in decision-making regarding their care.

4. Useful questions to ask a patient like Avery to initiate screening include: "Tell me a bit about your relationship with your boyfriend. For how long have you been together? Tell me about your relationship when he is not drinking, what does that look like? How often does he drink? Now, I'd like to ask you a few questions that I ask all my patients."
5. Useful responses to a patient who discloses IPV include: "I am so sorry that this is happening to you. Because many people have this experience, resources are available. I would like to connect you with someone who/program that can offer you some support and information." [Make supported referral.] "Please know that this office is a judgment-free zone. Come and see me any time even if you choose not to make use of the resources that I share with you today."
6. Intimate partner violence is a complicated psychosocial disorder that will require provider persistence and use of external resources to address. The patient may not label abusive behavior as abuse or fully disclose all aspects or the extent of abuse during one visit; however, asking about exposure to IPV on a regular basis signals that the clinic space is a safe one in which to disclose. Providers can say, "I talk to all of my patients about their relationships because our relationships influence our health and how we feel on a day-to-day basis." Moreover, universal education about healthy/unhealthy relationships is beneficial to all patients. Providers can say, "I give out these resources to all of my patients, if you or a friend ever needs it."

References

1. Breiding MJ, et al. Intimate partner violence surveillance: uniform definitions and recommended data elements, version 2.0. Atlanta: National Center for Injury Prevention and Control, Centers for Disease Control and Prevention; 2015.
2. Breiding MJ, Black MC, Ryan GW. Chronic disease and health risk behaviors associated with intimate partner violence-18 U.S. states/ territories, 2005. Ann Epidemiol. 2008;18(7):538–44.
3. Coker AL, et al. Physical health consequences of physical and psychological intimate partner violence. Arch Fam Med. 2000;9 (5):451–7.
4. Campbell JC. Health consequences of intimate partner violence. Lancet. 2002;359(9314):1331–6.

5. Conron KJ, et al. A longitudinal study of maternal depression and child maltreatment in a national sample of families investigated by child protective services. Arch Pediatr Adolesc Med. 2009;163 (10):922–30.
6. Breiding MJ, et al. Prevalence and characteristics of sexual violence, stalking, and intimate partner violence victimization – national intimate partner and sexual violence survey, United States, 2011. MMWR Surveill Summ. 2014;63(8):1–18.
7. Whitaker DJ, et al. Differences in frequency of violence and reported injury between relationships with reciprocal and nonreciprocal intimate partner violence. Am J Public Health. 2007;97(5):941–7.
8. Renner LM, Whitney SD. Examining symmetry in intimate partner violence among young adults using socio-demographic characteristics. J Fam Violence. 2010;25:91–106.
9. McCauley HL, et al. Sexual and reproductive health indicators and intimate partner violence victimization among female family planning clinic patients who have sex with women and men. J Womens Health (Larchmt). 2015;24(8):621–8.
10. Walters ML, Chen J, Breiding MJ. The National Intimate Partner and Sexual Violence Survey (NISVS): 2010 findings on victimization by sexual orientation. Atlanta: National Center for Injury Prevention and Control, Centers for Disease Control and Prevention; 2013.
11. Goldberg NG, Meyer IH. Sexual orientation disparities in history of intimate partner violence: results from the California health interview survey. J Interpers Violence. 2013;28(5):1109–18.
12. Conron KJ, Mimiaga MJ, Landers SJ. A population-based study of sexual orientation identity and gender differences in adult health. Am J Public Health. 2010;100(10):1953–60.
13. Roberts AL, et al. Pervasive trauma exposure among US sexual orientation minority adults and risk of posttraumatic stress disorder. Am J Public Health. 2010;100(12):2433–41.
14. Chandra A, Mosher WD, Copen C. Sexual behavior, sexual attraction, and sexual identity in the United States: data from the 2006–2008 National Survey of Family Growth, in National Health Statistics Reports; no 36. Hyattsville, MD: Centers for Disease Control and Prevention, National Center for Health Statistics; 2011.
15. Grant JM, et al. Injustice at every turn: a report of the National Transgender Discrimination Survey. Washington, DC: National Center for Transgender Equality and National Gay and Lesbian Task Force; 2011.
16. Corliss HL, Cochran SD, Mays VM. Reports of parental maltreatment during childhood in a United States population-based survey of homosexual, bisexual, and heterosexual adults. Child Abuse Negl. 2002;26(11):1165–78.
17. Nuttbrock L, et al. Psychiatric impact of gender-related abuse across the life course of male-to-female transgender persons. J Sex Res. 2010;47(1):12–23.
18. Kann L, et al. Sexual identity, sex of sexual contacts, and health-risk behaviors among students in grades 9–12 – youth risk behavior surveillance, selected sites, United States, 2001–2009. MMWR Surveill Summ. 2011;60(7):1–133.
19. D'Augelli AR, Grossman AH, Starks MT. Parents' awareness of lesbian, gay, and bisexual youths' sexual orientation. J Marriage Fam. 2005;67(2):474–82.
20. Cochran SD, Mays VM, Sullivan JG. Prevalence of mental disorders, psychological distress, and mental health services use among lesbian, gay, and bisexual adults in the United States. J Consult Clin Psychol. 2003;71(1):53–61.
21. Cochran SD, et al. Mental health and substance use disorders among Latino and Asian American lesbian, gay, and bisexual adults. J Consult Clin Psychol. 2007;75(5):785–94.
22. Gilman SE, et al. Risk of psychiatric disorders among individuals reporting same-sex sexual partners in the National Comorbidity Survey. Am J Public Health. 2001;91(6):933–9.
23. Cochran SD, Mays VM. Physical health complaints among lesbians, gay men, and bisexual and homosexually experienced heterosexual individuals: results from the California Quality of Life Survey. Am J Public Health. 2007;97(11):2048–55.
24. Badgett MV, Durso LE, Schneebaum A. New patterns of poverty in the lesbian, gay, and bisexual community. Los Angeles: UCLA, Williams Institute; 2013.
25. Conron KJ, et al. Transgender health in Massachusetts: results from a household probability sample of adults. Am J Public Health. 2012;102:118–22.
26. Centers for Disease Control and Prevention, National Center for Injury Prevention and Control, Division of Violence Prevention. Intimate partner violence: risk and protective factors. 2015 [13 Jan 2016]. https://www.cdc.gov/violenceprevention/intimatepartnerviolence/riskprotectivefactors.html. Last accessed 14 Mar 2017.
27. Freedner N, et al. Dating violence among gay, lesbian, and bisexual adolescents: results from a community survey. J Adolesc Health. 2002;31(6):469–74.
28. Brown TNT, Herman JL. Intimate partner violence and sexual abuse among LGBT people: a review of existing research. Los Angeles: The Williams Institute, UCLA; 2015.
29. Lambda Legal. When health care isn't caring: Lambda Legal's survey of discrimination against LGBT people and people with HIV. New York: Lambda Legal; 2010. www.lambdalegal.org/health-care-report.
30. Cruz TM. Assessing access to care for transgender and gender nonconforming people: a consideration of diversity in combating discrimination. Soc Sci Med. 2014;110:65–73.
31. Nelson HD, Bougatsos C, Blazlna I. Screening women for intimate partner violence: a systematic review to Update the U.S. Preventive Services Task Force recommendation. Ann Int Med. 2012;156 (11):796–808.
32. American College of Obstetricians and Gynecologists. Intimate partner violence. Committee Opinion No. 518. Obstet Gynecol. 2012;119:412–7.
33. National Research Council. Clinical preventive services for women: closing the gaps. Washington, DC: National Academies Press; 2011.
34. Ghandour RM, Campbell JC, Lloyd J. Screening and counseling for intimate partner violence: a vision for the future. J Womens Health. 2014;24(1):57–61.
35. Raissi SE, et al. Implementing an intimate partner violence (IPV) screening protocol in HIV care. AIDS Patient Care and STDs. 2015;29(3):133–41.
36. Chang JC, et al. Asking about intimate partner violence: advice from female survivors to health care providers. Patient Educ Couns. 2005;59(2):141–7.
37. Nelson HD, Bougatsos C, Blazina I. Screening women for intimate partner violence:a systematic review to update the U.S. preventive services task force recommendation. Ann Intern Med. 2012;156:796–808.
38. Bair-Merritt MH, et al. Primary care-based interventions for intimate partner violence: a systematic review. Am J Prev Med. 2014;46(2):188–94.
39. Crane HM, et al. Routine collection of patient-reported outcomes in an HIV clinic setting: the first 100 patients. Curr HIV Res. 2007;5 (1):109–18.
40. Miller E, et al. Integrating intimate partner violence assessment and intervention into healthcare in the United States: a systems approach. J Womens Health. 2015;24(1):92–9.
41. Rabin RF, et al. Intimate partner violence screening tools: a systematic review. Am J Prev Med. 2009;36(5):439–445.e4.
42. Chen P-H, et al. Screening for domestic violence in a predominantly Hispanic clinical setting. Fam Pract. 2005;22 (6):617–23.
43. Weiss SJ, et al. Development of a screening for ongoing intimate partner violence. Violence Vict. 2003;18(2):131–41.

44. Campbell JC, Webster DW, Glass N. The danger assessment: validation of a lethality risk assessment instrument for intimate partner femicide. J Interpers Violence. 2009;24(4):653–74.

45. Snider C, et al. Intimate partner violence: development of a brief risk assessment for the emergency department. Acad Emerg Med. 2009;16(11):1208–16.

46. Stephenson R, et al. Towards the development of an intimate partner violence screening tool for gay and bisexual men. West J Emerg Med. 2013;14(4):390–400.

47. Ard KL, Makadon HJ. Addressing intimate partner violence in lesbian, gay, bisexual and transgender patients. J Gen Intern Med. 2011;26(8):930–3.

48. Sprague S, et al. Barriers to screening for intimate partner violence. Women Health. 2012;52(6):587–605.

49. Elliott DE, et al. Trauma-informed or trauma-denied: principles and implementation of trauma-informed services for women. J Community Psychol. 2005;33(4):461–77.

50. Miller E, Levenson R. Hanging out or hooking up: clinical guidelines on responding to adolescent relationship abuse. San Francisco: Futures Without Violence; 2012.

51. Miller E, et al. A school health center intervention for abusive adolescent relationships: a cluster RCT. Pediatrics. 2015;135(1):76–85.

52. Miller E, et al. A family planning clinic partner violence intervention to reduce risk associated with reproductive coercion. Contraception. 2011;83(3):274–80.

53. Awan A, Liang Q. Fenway Institute: TOD@S Collaborative, Boston; 2015.

54. Dutton MA, Goodman L, Schmidt RJ. Development and validation of a coercive control measure for intimate partner violence: final technical report. Bethesda: COSMOS Corportation; 2005.

55. Campbell JC, Webster DW, Glass N. The danger assessment: validation of a lethality risk assessment instrument for intimate partner femicide. J Interpers Violence. 2009;24(4):653–74.

56. Herman JL. Trauma and recovery. Rev. ed. New York: BasicBooks; 1997. xi, 290 p.

57. Morland LA, et al. Telemedicine versus in-person delivery of cognitive processing therapy for women with posttraumatic stress disorder: a randomized noninferiority trial. Depress Anxiety. 2015;32(11):811–20.

58. Egede LE, et al. Psychotherapy for depression in older veterans via telemedicine: a randomised, open-label, non-inferiority trial. Lancet Psychiatry. 2015;2(8):693–701.

59. Van der Kolk BA. The body keeps the score: brain, mind, and body in the healing of trauma. New York: Viking; 2014. xvi, 443 pages.

Community Responses to Trauma

19

R.J. Robles and E. Kale Edmiston

Purpose

The purpose of this chapter is to provide an overview of the existing community support structures commonly utilized by LGBT people, as well as to outline ways that providers can support and advocate for their LGBT patients.

Learning Objectives

1. Outline how systemic social marginalization contributes to the need for community support.
2. Discuss why intersectional identities can create varying needs for support when accessing healthcare and making healthcare decisions.
3. Describe ways that healthcare providers can advocate for their LGBT patients and connect them to community support resources.

Introduction: Linking Interpersonal and Structural Violence in LGBT Communities

In this chapter, we will use several theoretical frameworks to inform our discussion of LGBT community responses to trauma. The first is the distinction between interpersonal discrimination and systemic violence. Stokely Carmichael first made this distinction in reference to the experiences of Black people living in the USA, arguing that individuals with marginalized identities experience limited opportunities as a result of both forms of violence,

although systemic violence is less-often acknowledged [1]. Interpersonal rejection and discrimination, when coupled with structurally inscribed violence and trauma, create unique challenges for LGBT communities. For example, although some LGBT youth are now finding that their families of origin support their identities, parental rejection remains a significant challenge for many others. Parental rejection on the basis of LGB sexual orientation has been linked to increased internalized homophobia [2], a nearly six-fold increase in depression [3], and a three-fold greater likelihood of engaging in unprotected sex [3]. Many LGBT youth who experience familial rejection opt to leave home; national data suggest that more than 40% of homeless youth are LGBT [4]. Many of the disparities outlined above can also be explained by systemic violence. In the case of LGBT youth, examples of systemic violence include school policies or legislation, such as "bathroom bills," that restrict access to facilities for transgender people, or laws that codify discrimination in the provision of counseling services [5]. LGBT students who do not feel safe at school, or who do not have access to supportive adults in whom to confide, are more likely to drop out or run away from home [6–7]. Thus, interpersonal violence (i.e., familial rejection) and systemic or structural violence (i.e., policies that limit access to resources such as shelters, counseling, or restrooms) result in a "perfect storm" that causes healthcare disparities [8]. If clinicians focus solely on interpersonal violence, they miss opportunities to intervene in systemic inequality.

The minority stress model is another key theoretical construct we will use when discussing individual and community responses to trauma. In this model, discrimination or the fear of discrimination leads to increased isolation and stress, which in turn can cause higher rates of mental health problems such as anxiety and depression [9]. Experiencing bias can also create internalized negative feelings about one's identity. Such internalized self-hatred can perpetuate and amplify cycles of isolation and mental distress and also

R.J. Robles, BA • E.K. Edmiston, PhD (✉)
Vanderbilt University Medical Center,
Program for LGBTI Health, 319 Light Hall,
Nashville, TN 37232, USA
e-mail: ekale513@gmail.com

© Springer International Publishing AG 2017
K.L. Eckstrand, J. Potter (eds.), *Trauma, Resilience, and Health Promotion in LGBT Patients*,
DOI 10.1007/978-3-319-54509-7_19

result in less adaptive coping strategies [10]. The minority stress model helps to explain the context in which population-level health disparities occur and can help clinicians and researchers understand the ways in which systemic discrimination impacts the health of individual LGBT people.

Lastly, we will also employ an intersectional framework when discussing responses of LGBT individuals and communities to trauma. The concept of "intersectionality," a term first coined by Kimberlé Crenshaw, provides a basis for understanding the lives of people with multiple marginalized identities [11]. According to intersectionality theory, the impact of discrete social categorizations such as race, class, sexual orientation, and gender on a person's life experiences cannot be analyzed separately but, instead, must be considered in aggregate in order to understand how systemic social forces can foster both advantage and disadvantage. In the context of this chapter, we will frequently discuss how multiple identities intersect and frame the experiences of individuals within LGBT communities, and how these identities impact experiences of trauma and access to resources.

It is important to affirm diversity among LGBT people. However, one experience many LGBT people share is community memory of significant trauma [12–13]. In the absence of support from families of origin, many LGBT people form chosen families as a way to create support networks for accessing resources, and to provide emotional support [14–16]. Although such informal communities can be a source of resilience, chosen families can also intensify harm. For example, LGBT people may be less likely to access healthcare resources when the community norm is to mistrust healthcare institutions. This mistrust is caused by historical mistreatment of LGBT people by medical institutions, as well as individual reports of poor treatment from healthcare systems or providers [17]. Thus, historical trauma within LGBT communities creates a legacy burden that can be propagated among peers via word-of-mouth. Although there are many reasons to celebrate within-community responses to trauma, we must also emphasize the importance of institutional partnerships, support, and ally-ship in fostering the creation of sustainable change among communities experiencing trauma and discrimination.

Despite the potential for harm, we will argue, throughout this chapter, that the best strategies for healing from trauma in LGBT communities are local and led by LGBT people. This insistence on within-community responses to trauma acknowledges the resilience and the wisdom that already exist in the communities most impacted by systemic inequality. Community-led approaches allow for an increased sense of self-efficacy, which is an important aspect of trauma recovery [18]. We argue that community-led responses may be more effective than strategies that come from outside the community because they are created by those with the most intimate knowledge of the manner in which systemic inequality functions.

Trauma and Resilience in Vulnerable LGBT Populations

Adolescents and Youth

LGBT adolescents face particular challenges when accessing support resources, as their caregivers may not affirm their identities, thereby restricting access to community, and causing feelings of isolation and depression [14]. Providers working with youth should be able to talk about concerns that parents might have about their child's identity in a manner that is affirming of both the child and the parents. This approach helps support both parties, thus building rapport and trust, while at the same time modeling supportive language and behavior for the parents. Particularly in LGBT youth populations, support networks for parents can be as important as support networks for youth because they provide spaces for parents to model unconditional love for their LGBT children. PFLAG offers resources for the parents of LGBT teens [19]; for a list of LGBT community resources, see Table 19.1. Providers should be able to refer caregivers to local support groups where they will be able to discuss the coming out process, interfacing with school officials, and dealing with bullying in an understanding environment.

Youth frequently utilize technology resources to connect with support networks. A huge number of transgender youth and young adults also video blog, or "vlog," their experiences on YouTube. Such vlogs are presented as "how-to" guides for transition and provide a forum for transgender people to speak to an assumed transgender audience. Particularly with regard to the effects of cross-gender hormone therapy, such vlogs can allow other transgender people to witness the effects of hormones over time, creating a "visual account" of transition [20]. Importantly, these video archives link transgender people all over the world and can be particularly helpful to youth who would not otherwise be able to meet other transgender people. In-person resources also exist; Gay-Straight Alliances (GSAs) are now available at many schools, and recent research has shown that participation in a GSA provides LGBT youth with a greater sense of agency, independent of parental acceptance [16]. There are also many LGBT-led organizations that pair youth with supportive LGBT adults. These include, but are not limited to, local LGBT youth groups, LGBT youth homeless direct-care services [21], and the Point Foundation, which provides scholarships for

Table 19.1 Examples of LGBT community-led resources

Organization name	Description	Website
Black and Pink	Boston-based direct service and advocacy organization working to end the criminalization of LGBT people and the prison industrial complex. Maintains a database of LGBT prisoners looking for pen pals	http://www.blackandpink.org/
The LGBT Oral History Digital Collaboratory	An online archive with links to oral histories featuring diverse LGBT people from around the world	http://lgbtqdigitalcollaboratory.org
GLMA	National policy, advocacy, and healthcare provider professional organization working toward health equity for LGBT people	http://www.glma.org/
GSA Network	An organization that links GSAs throughout the country with the goal of supporting youth organizing for racial and gender justice	http://gsanetwork.org
Point Foundation	National LGBT scholarship fund and youth mentorship organization	http://www.pointfoundation.org/
RAD Remedy	Maintains a user-generated database of healthcare providers for transgender and queer people	https://www.radremedy.org/
Reconciling Ministries Network	Christian network of LGBT-affirming congregations	http://www.rmnetwork.org/
SAGE	Provides advocacy and resources for LGBT elders. There are SAGE chapters in most cities that also serve as social groups for LGBT elders	http://www.sageusa.org/
The Sylvia Rivera Law Project	New York City-based organization that provides legal services to low-income transgender people, with a focus on racial and immigration justice	http://srlp.org/
The Sisters of Perpetual Indulgence	An order of queer nuns that mix drag, community service, and performance art. Most major US cities have chapters	http://thesisters.org/
The Trans Buddy Program	Nashville-based program that provides trained peer advocates for transgender people seeking healthcare referrals or support at healthcare encounters	https://medschool.vanderbilt.edu/lgbti/trans-buddy-program
Trans Lifeline	A crisis hotline run by transgender people for transgender people	http://www.translifeline.org/

LGBT youth as well as mentorship [22]. Intergenerational support and mentorship can be helpful for youth, who may not otherwise have access to adult LGBT role models.

Elders

Like LGBT youth, LGBT elders face barriers when accessing resources. Similar to heterosexual and cisgender elders, aging in LGBT populations can be associated with increased social isolation [23–25]. Although many LGBT elders have children of their own, LGBT elders are less likely than heterosexual peers to have adult children to care for them [26]. A focus group study of gay or lesbian older adults found that concerns regarding aging included lack of familial or social support, lack of a long-term caregiver, and concerns about discrimination in healthcare settings or from home healthcare aides [25]. Another study of aging, lesbian-identified, transgender women found that most respondents were not prepared to have discussions with their providers about end of life care and were overall, "ill-prepared" for the medical and legal challenges associated with aging [27]. Many members of the current cohort of LGBT elders lived through the HIV/AIDS crisis of the 1980s and early 1990s and survived the death of their partners and friends [23, 28–30]. Thus, this generation has not only already endured significant community trauma [31], but is now faced with the prospect of aging in the absence of their social network. The limited research focusing on HIV+

elders suggests differing correlates of care adherence and psychosocial adjustment in HIV+ elders compared to HIV+ youth or young adults [28, 32] that may be due, in part, to social isolation. Social isolation associated with aging is compounded by the fact that many assisted-living facilities, retirement homes, and nursing facilities are not welcoming to LGBT people [33] because of bias among staff or fellow residents or institutional policies that assume that all residents are heterosexual (i.e., visiting policies that assume that caregivers must be spouses or children). As a result, some LGB elders find themselves back "in the closet" in old age due to the consequences of intersecting homophobia and ageism, after a lifetime spent fighting for recognition and survival [34].

Some cities have LGBT-specific retirement or assisted-living facilities, which provide avenues for social connection among LGBT elders. Due to the lack of availability in many regions and cost, such facilities are not options for most LGBT elders, and alternative solutions, such as inclusion of elders in LGBT social spaces and the creation of intergenerational LGBT organizations, benefit LGBT people of all ages. Elder-specific groups, such as SAGE [35], The LGBT Aging Project [36], and the National Resource Center on LGBT Aging [37], are important national advocacy organizations that promote the needs of LGBT elders. LGBT oral history projects record and archive the life stories of LGBT elders while simultaneously connecting LGBT people of all ages with shared history [38]. Such projects include the Trans Oral History Project [39], OutLoud [40],

ACT UP Oral History Project [41], the African American AIDS Activism Oral History Project [42], Untold Stories [43], the LGBT Religious Archives Network [44], Impact Stories [45], the LGBT Oral History Digital Collaboratory [46], and many more. These archives honor and preserve the wisdom and stories of LGBT people of diverse backgrounds, and can be an important source of connection and recognition for elders.

Members of Faith-Based Communities

Faith-based communities can provide a sense of belonging and are an important social outlet; however, many LGBT people have experienced rejection from faith-based communities [47]. Indeed, studies of the attitudes of heterosexual people suggest that religiosity, particularly when coupled with limited knowledge about other faith traditions [48], is the primary predictor of negative attitudes toward LGBT people [49–51]. LGBT people who have grown up in conservative faith traditions or religious communities can recount numerous examples of religious oppression and trauma [52–53]. Many LGBT people struggle to find a way to accept themselves due to internalized self-hatred on the basis of their home faith's view of LGBT people, while also struggling to figure out how to maintain their religious identity [54–55]. Studies that have examined the perceived conflicts between religion and sexual identity have found sources of conflict in denominational teachings, scriptural passages, and congregational prejudice [56–57]. Experiencing conflict between these identities is associated with reduced disclosure of sexual orientation identity [58] and internalized homophobia [57, 59–60]. Unsurprisingly, experiencing conflict between LGB and religious identity is also associated with higher rates of suicidal ideation in young adults [61], while a negative sexual identity mediates the relationship between religious rejection and poor mental health in LGB youth [62]. Taken together, this research suggests that religious conflicts significantly impact identity formation among LGBT people.

LGBT identities have become divisive in many religious communities [63–64]. Individuals need to negotiate the messages they hear from religious authority figures and family members about LGBT people with their own lived experiences. LGBT people may resolve these conflicts in various ways, including identifying as "spiritual" rather than "religious," reinterpreting religious teachings, changing religious affiliations, remaining religious but not attending worship services, or abandoning religion altogether [65–68]. Most studies do not discuss LGBT people and positive experiences with religion, even though there are many ways that religious traditions engage with LGBT identity both morally and spiritually [69]. Membership in a welcoming faith-based community is a positive determinant of reduction in risk behaviors among LGB youth. For example, LGB youth who are a part of a supportive religious community are less likely to abuse alcohol and have fewer sexual partners than LGB youth who are a part of an unsupportive religious community [70]. One recent study of sexual minority college students found that Christian and Jewish students had lower odds of suicidal ideation than students who identified themselves as Atheist [71]. No behavioral health studies to date have assessed the role of religious affiliation in the lives of transgender people, although one recent study found a positive association between transgender identity, religious engagement, and a larger and more diverse social network [72]. Thus, while it can be difficult for an LGBT person to integrate their sexual or gender and religious identities, faith-based communities can also be sources of strength, community support, and holistic care for LGBT people.

More and more communities of faith are LGBT-affirming [73]. Various communities identify as part of the Reconciling Ministries Network [74], the National LGBT Task Force Institute for Welcoming Resources [75], and other umbrella organizations that affirm LGBT identities. These faith communities are pivotal because they provide support and fellowship to LGBT individuals and their families. There are also a number of tools that can assist faith communities in becoming more welcoming [76], for example, using inclusive language in community gatherings/worship services; developing liturgy or rituals that support LGBT children and adults during gender transition, name changes or other life-cycle events; practicing and providing spaces for gender pronouns to be asked and shared on name tags and membership forms, affirming LGBT people from the pulpit; including sexual and gender identity in welcoming statements during days of worship; celebrating LGBT events and annual commemorations; and creating gender inclusive restrooms in all facilities [77–78]. Such practices can help break cycles of trauma that perpetuate internalized self-hatred.

Faith-based communities are an integral part of the LGBT community, and LGBT people are integral to faith communities. These stories must be noted and cannot be erased or co-opted by those who claim that LGBT people have no place in faith [79]. For example, Liberation Theology, a movement that began in the 1950s within the Catholic Church, has helped to create queer and transgender theologies [80–81]. Furthermore, there is a diverse group of people from all faith traditions that are out as LGBT and are ordained preachers, reverends, imams, ministers, and more. There are LGBT Christians, Jews, Muslims, Buddhists, Hindus, Sikhs, and beyond. There are LGBT spiritual healers, curanderos, espiritistas, indigenous people of color, elders and community healers, ancestral archivists, priests/priestesses, pagans, agnostics, and atheists who are creatively reinventing and adapting their spiritual practices to include LGBT identities [57, 60, 77, 82–85]. Faith is a way in which LGBT people can express and affirm their sacred selves, and can be an important source of community, healing, and strength for LGBT people with a history of trauma and rejection. Providers should be careful not to assume that their LGBT patients are not members of a faith-based community, and should be aware of affirming congregations as a source of support for their LGBT patients.

Geographically Marginalized Communities

LGBT people living in the US South and in rural areas are more likely to have lower educational attainment than both cisgender/heterosexual people and LGBT people living in urban areas in northern states. They are also more likely to live in poverty, use tobacco, and report low rates of health insurance coverage [86]. Transgender Southerners face astonishingly high rates of violence, with the risk particularly high among low-income transgender people of color [87]. Although Southerners of all genders and sexual orientations are more likely to live in poverty, experience higher rates of chronic illness, and have an overall shorter life expectancy [88], the intersection of LGBT identity and geographic location is particularly toxic. LGBT Southerners experience isolation due in part to conservative religious ideologies that are more prevalent in the South and in rural areas of the USA [89]. LGBT people living in rural areas also have difficulty accessing healthcare resources because of endemic poverty and geographic isolation [90]. Limited access to providers can mean that in order to see an affirming clinician, LGBT people must drive several hours, sometimes even out of state, to access healthcare. This is particularly true for transgender people seeking transition-related care. Likewise, areas with low population density are less likely to have large concentrations of LGBT people, making it challenging for LGBT individuals in rural areas to form communities of peers. Despite these challenges, many LGBT people living in geographically isolated areas are able to access resources via online forums, social media, in-person support groups, print subscriptions, telephone networks, and even the creation of rural LGBT communal living sites termed "homesteads" [91]. These practices challenge the common misconception that LGBT culture is centered in large coastal cities such as New York or San Francisco.

Historical Community-Based Responses to Trauma

Starting with the codification of LGBT as an identity in the twentieth century, LGBT people have created alternative resource networks in the absence of mainstream acceptance (Fig. 19.1). Early systems were often covert, such as mailing networks and private social clubs [92]. Throughout much of the latter half of the twentieth century, gay and lesbian bars became the primary mode of socializing with other LGBT people, as well as important sites of political organizing [92]. Two key moments in LGBT history linked to gay bar culture, the Stonewall Riots and the Compton Cafeteria Riots, were both responses to police brutality and harassment that were led by transgender people of color. Gay bars also became important for the development of LGBT culture and identity, particularly drag culture [93]. Although drag performance originated as a form of entertainment primarily aimed at heterosexual audiences, drag has become a foundational part of LGBT people's experience of social community as a part of gay bar culture in the latter half of the twentieth century [92].

Importantly, particularly (but not exclusively) in the pre-integration era US South, gay bars were not safe for Black LGBT people. As a result, Black LGBT people formed their own social organizations and house parties to meet other LGBT people and form friendships, romantic relationships, and familial bonds in response to trauma and rejection [92]. The most famous of these are the House Ball Communities that persist in the present day, most prominently in New York City. House Ball culture is set up around membership in specific houses, which have parental figures that nurture more junior members. Houses hold Balls, which involve performance and competition, and provide a social outlet in a supportive environment [94]. House Ball Communities are critical sites of culture, resistance, and resilience in response to discrimination and violence, both from the dominant heterosexual culture and from white LGBT spaces that perpetuate white supremacy and segregation [95–101].

As it became more possible for LGB people to be open about their sexual orientations, many lesbian- and gay-specific groups formed around common interests, including sports leagues, book clubs, and choral groups. These groups persist in the present day as important social outlets for LGBT people [102–103]. One such organization, the Sisters of Perpetual Indulgence, is a group of queer nuns that has chapters around the world [104]. The order merges parody, performance art, and political activism with the goal

Fig. 19.1 LGBT people have created alternative resource networks in the absence of mainstream acceptance

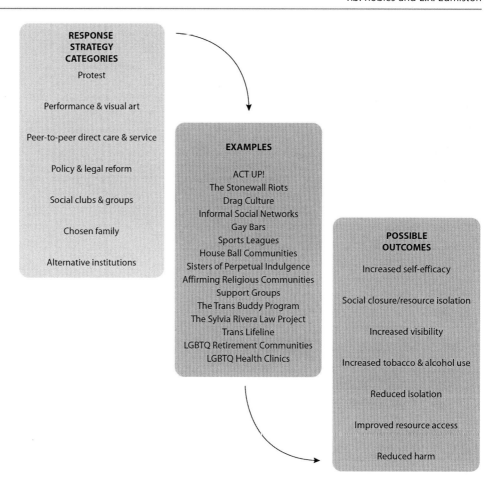

of "promoting human rights, respect for diversity, and spiritual enlightenment" [105]. Other groups formed beginning in the 1960s and 1970s around common political organizing goals, including Lesbian-feminist consciousness-raising, LGB anti-discrimination battles, and perhaps most famously, in response to the AIDS crisis of the 1980s and early 1990s.

The AIDS crisis is a benchmark for a generation of LGBT people. During the period from 1981 until 1996, numerous LGBT people and allies protested governmental obfuscation and inaction, worked to change federal policy, and took care of the sick and dying [106–107]. The minimal response from the federal government in the midst of the crisis [108] awakened a generation of activists and led to the formation of ACT UP!, or the AIDS Coalition To Unleash Power!, which successfully lobbied to change the allocation of federal funds for AIDS-related research, pressured the National Institutes of Health to streamline clinical trials and make them more transparent (a victory that has benefited not only AIDS patients, but countless patients awaiting clinical trial research for cancer and other illnesses), and provided support for people dying of AIDS [109]. These efforts resulted in reduced stigma surrounding HIV/AIDS, better education about transmission of the virus, and major medical advances

in HIV treatment. In addition to political organizing, the AIDS crisis inspired art and theater [110–111]. Most notably, the AIDS Memorial Quilt was first displayed on the National Mall in Washington, D.C. in 1987 to commemorate the lives of people who died of AIDS [112–113].

The experiences of people who survived the AIDS epidemic are quite different from those recently diagnosed [28]. Although many consider the AIDS crisis in the USA to be over, the rates of new HIV infections remain at epidemic proportions for the most marginalized members of the LGBT community: men of color, transgender women, and sex workers [114]. As of 2015, 50% of HIV+ people living in the USA were over the age of fifty, due in part to increasing life expectancies, as well as increasing rates of new infections in older adults [115]. Disparities in HIV prevalence are likely due to reduced access to healthcare that is caused by identity-based marginalization [116–117].

Limitations of Community-Led Responses

Although LGBT identity-based communities can be important sources of strength, they may also perpetuate cycles of violence. For example, when members of an LGBT community subgroup experience privilege in other aspects of their identities (i.e., white racial identity, cisgender identity, or middle-class socioeconomic status), they may deny resources to other LGBT people who experience multiple forms of marginalization or oppression. This practice is informed by prejudice, as well as fears about resource scarcity, and perpetuates systemic inequality. Furthermore, in the most marginalized LGBT communities, because the majority of people within a community have limited access to resources, the within-community social network often consists of people who are experiencing similar struggles and have limited access to long-term solutions. Resource dependence theory claims that access to resources creates power, and that organizations or groups are therefore contextually dependent on other groups in their environment [118–119]. Resource dependence theory mirrors the sociological phenomenon of social closure, first described by Parkin in 1979, and later expanded by others, which describes the ways in which social groups with access to resources limit their social networks to keep resources from outsiders [120–122]. When dominant members of society prevent access to resources, a small number of people within a marginalized community may be seen as hubs for support and resources, which can lead to fatigue and further trauma. In response to this phenomenon, several clinic- or hospital-based programs have been developed specifically to meet the needs of transgender people seeking healthcare, while other healthcare innovations have focused on using technology to combat social closure. These more recent approaches to within-community trauma are discussed in detail below.

Innovations in Community-Led Responses to Trauma

Because the challenges that LGBT people face are often specific to the communities in which they live, the most innovative and effective solutions to improving the lives of LGBT individuals are local. For example, LGBT information networks have developed lists of providers who have either self-identified themselves as LGBT or affirming of LGBT people, or providers who have been recommended by their LGBT patients as affirming. Such provider lists range from formal, publicly posted, and vetted directories to documents shared between members of a support group, to word-of-mouth knowledge that is shared in a specific social circle. Although these types of provider directories or lists can be a helpful starting point for LGBT people seeking healthcare, they are limited in that they do not adhere to any objective criteria, often lump lesbian, gay, bisexual, and transgender identities together, thus ignoring the significant differences that transgender and bisexual people experience compared to lesbian and gay cisgender individuals in terms

of stigma, health disparity, and health needs [123], and do not consider the impact of intersectional identities on the healthcare experience. More recently, a number of apps have been developed that rely on user report to recommend affirming providers. These apps, including RAD Remedy [124] and MyTransHealth [125], allow users to generate and review providers and staff, while also providing filters that allow users to select personal priorities for care (i.e., cost, location, etc.). These technologies are an exciting new development in LGBT healthcare and an important resource for LGBT people who have significant anxiety about clinical encounters.

Transgender people have created informal and formal support networks, often, though not exclusively, focused on the coming out process. Although such community support groups are in some ways similar to LGB-specific groups, they differ in responses to the types of interpersonal and structural challenges faced by transgender individuals. For example, community support groups discuss and problem-solve around challenges in accessing gender affirming care and/or insurance coverage to obtain necessary care. Furthermore, groups can provide support around the hardship of societal stigma and overt discrimination faced during gender transition. Because there is great diversity within transgender communities, many cities may have multiple transgender support groups based on individuals' needs and identities, including but not limited to religious practice, race/ethnicity, gender expression/identity, HIV status, and age. Providers should be aware of what support groups exist in their local area to be able to provide the most appropriate referral for their transgender patients.

In response to limited resources for transgender patients, as well as the immense difficulty many transgender people experience interfacing with cis-centric medical systems, several programs have begun offering transgender navigation or peer advocacy services. Most of these programs are based at LGBT-specific healthcare centers. In these programs, patient navigators are paid clinic staff, transgender or cisgender, who can consult with patients about how best to access healthcare resources. Programs of this kind exist at Fenway Health in Boston, Massachusetts [126], and as a part of the Center for Transgender Excellence at the University of California San Francisco [127]. These programs benefit from institutional funding, with paid staff members who have ties to institutional resources that can be shared with transgender clients, thereby reducing the burden of support for unpaid community members who may be struggling themselves.

Other programs combine direct-care services with advocacy, referral, and educational services. For example, the Sylvia Rivera Law Project in New York City offers legal services to low-income transgender people and incarcerated transgender people, many of whom who have been wrongfully incarcerated for defending themselves during violent hate crimes [8]. The Trans Buddy Program, founded in Nashville, Tennessee, by transgender people and cisgender allies, offers free direct-care services by pairing trained volunteer advocates with transgender people seeking healthcare [128]. Advocates can provide resources, referrals, and support, in collaboration with a wide spectrum of community organizations that serve transgender people. The Trans Buddy Program differs from other patient advocate programs in that it is staffed entirely by volunteer advocates who attend clinical visits with transgender patients. Volunteers also provide education and training for hospital staff on request, and have partnered extensively with inpatient nursing staff in the adolescent psychiatric hospital and other units to provide mandatory, all-staff trainings on the healthcare needs of transgender patients, particularly regarding how providers can best accommodate transgender patients in a biased healthcare system. Community-based peer advocacy programs, when coupled with healthcare institutions, are powerful intervention strategies to mitigate trauma and improve resource access.

Trans Lifeline is another peer-to-peer program that provides support to transgender people who are experiencing crisis and are in need of support, with the specific goal of preventing self-harm among transgender people. Founded in 2014 in response to gaps in existing crisis support services that were designed to serve cisgender people, Trans Lifeline is a free, national helpline staffed exclusively by transgender people to meet the needs of transgender clients [129]. Importantly, as a phone-based hotline, Trans Lifeline can offer services to transgender people who may not be able access crisis support due to location, economic or immigration status, or disability. The Trans Lifeline is an excellent example of how peer support can be an effective strategy for reducing trauma in marginalized communities.

It is important for providers to familiarize themselves with existing within-community support resources that are developed and led by LGBT people (see Fig. 19.1). Allied providers can play an important role in disrupting the cycles of trauma and resource isolation in LGBT social networks by connecting their patients with alternate modes of support. Strategies for provider engagement in community support networks are discussed in more detail below.

Provider Engagement in Existing Community Support Structures

Providers who have experience serving LGBT people may want to attend a support group meeting if it is open to the general public. Providers with knowledge regarding transgender health concerns, including but not limited to mental health, medical transition, and trauma-informed care, can be difficult to find, even for individuals embedded in transgender social networks. Community presence is an important part of building trust with populations that have experienced trauma in the healthcare setting.

Likewise, because of historical marginalization and shared community trauma, many LGBT people find health information and resources from alternate sources [130–131]. Examples of such trauma include the reluctance or refusal of many providers to care for gay men during the AIDS crisis [132–134], the abuse of LGBT people via reparative therapy [135], and restrictive requirements for medically necessary transition-related care that delay care and increase financial burden [136]. These are just a few examples of ways in which the medical establishment has caused mistrust within LGBT communities [17]. When coupled with readily available information online that is increasingly accessed by patients of all orientations [130], LGBT patients may enter a provider's office with misinformation and mistrust. Providers should be aware of how historical mistreatment may impact their interaction with LGBT patients even in situations where clinic staff has been affirming. Providers should also be aware of the most up-to-date and accurate online resources regarding LGBT health issued by their professional societies or LGBT health advocacy organizations and share these resources with their patients.

Advocacy Solutions: Ensuring Sustainable Models to Oppose Structural Violence

Providers can advocate for their LGBT patients in a number of ways, including writing letters of support for transgender patients attempting to access legal document changes, as access to accurate documents provides opportunity for employment and education, while reducing risk of arrest and transphobic violence [137]; educating parents or guardians about the needs of their LGBT child; or helping LGBT patients to identify supportive "chosen family" in the absence of an affirming biological family. Providers can also advocate for LGBT people by supporting healthcare and employment non-discrimination legislation and policies, although the efficacy of blanket non-discrimination legislation in improving the lives of the most marginalized LGBT people has been contested [138]. Providers can also speak out against discriminatory legislative measures, including legislation that is counter to the policies of their professional societies. Examples include the recent passage of "religious freedom" legislation that allows counselors or therapists to deny care to LGBT people on the basis of their identities, or so-called bathroom bills that require transgender people to use public restrooms counter to their gender identities. A recent study found that transgender people who have experienced discrimination in accessing public restrooms were more likely to attempt suicide than transgender people who have not experienced such discrimination [139], confirming that such discriminatory legislation poses a threat to the health of transgender people. In sum, engagement in patient advocacy is crucial in mitigating the structural violence that further traumatizes LGBT people.

Because the systems that restrict access to resources for LGBT people are so pervasive, it is critical for providers to work with their patients to ensure that community-led responses to trauma can be nurtured and sustained over time [140]. In addition to making connections with existing community organizations, providers should be aware of the local landscape for LGBT people. What are the major barriers to attaining optimal health? Where are the key sites in which community building takes place? Who are the leaders and potential early adopters of health-promotion strategies? With this knowledge, clinics and hospitals can better meet the needs of diverse LGBT patients, whether that means offering a specific clinic day reserved for pelvic exams for transgender people, integrating behavioral health into primary care and cross-gender hormone-therapy appointments, or making sure that HIV prevention is an integral aspect of primary care. Because of the powerful combined effects of interpersonal and systemic violence, if hospital administrators and clinic managers create policies that not only consider, but center on the needs of LGBT patients, there is significant hope for disrupting LGBT marginalization.

As an increasing number of LGBT providers are coming out and entering healthcare professions, it is important to acknowledge the ways in which LGBT patients' trauma can be transferred to LGBT-identified providers. To date, the literature has focused on the attitudes of providers toward LGBT patients [48, 141–146]; almost no research has examined the experiences of LGBT providers. One survey of presumed heterosexual and cisgender physician assistants found little stated bias against LGBT coworkers [147]. However, a recent study of LGB surgical residents found that over half (57%) of respondents reported hiding their identity from their attending physician, indicating significant problems with discrimination [148]. Another online survey study of LGB-identified physicians found that 65% of the sample reported hearing derogatory comments about LGBT people from their coworkers and 27% had witnessed discriminatory treatment of an LGBT coworker [149]. In addition to discrimination from colleagues, LGB providers may also experience discrimination from patients [150–151]. Importantly, all studies to date have used self-report measures in online convenience samples of LGB providers and there have been no studies of the experiences of transgender providers.

The discrepancy between the reported workplace experiences of heterosexual and LGB providers suggests that many well-intentioned individuals have implicit biases based on sexual orientation and gender identity, and that discrimination is underreported. When combined with the high rates of LGBT community trauma and the risk of over-identification with their patients, LGBT-identified providers are in particular need of peer and institutional support. There is growing recognition of the needs of LGBT providers and healthcare researchers; professional organizations such as GLMA serve an important role as social spaces for LGBT healthcare professionals, sources of professional support, and by providing political advocacy [152].

Conclusion

This chapter illustrates ways that LGBT communities respond to trauma. These strategies include creating art, sharing histories, forming social support networks, building alternatives to homophobic and transphobic institutions, and creating community-led organizations to support LGBT people. We have described some of the strategies employed by diverse LGBT people to manage trauma, but must acknowledge that there are likely many other ways that LGBT people cope, process, and heal. This acknowledgment is an act of cultural humility, a term that describes the limitations of approaches that emphasize mastery of knowledge about groups or cultures that one is not a member of, while simultaneously embracing the ongoing and personal nature of education [153]. In naming the limits of our own knowledge, we are best able to create room for all of the LGBT people in our lives to name their trauma and respond in the ways that best fit their needs.

References

1. Carmichael S. Black power, a critique of the system of international white supremacy and international capitalism. In: Cooper D, editor. The dialectics of liberations. New York: Penguin; 1968.
2. Bregman HR, Malik NM, Page MJ, Makynen E, Lindahl KM. Identity profiles in lesbian, gay, and bisexual youth: the role of family influences. J Youth Adolesc. 2013;42(3):417–30.
3. Ryan C, Huebner D, Diaz RM, Sanchez J. Family rejection as a predictor of negative health outcomes in white and Latino lesbian, gay, and bisexual youths. Pediatrics. 2009;123(1):346–52.
4. Grant JM, Mottet LA, Tanis J, Harrison J, Herman JL, Keisling M. Injustice at every turn: a report of the National Transgender Discrimination Survey. Washington, DC: National Center for Transgender Equality and National Gay and Lesbian Task Force; 2011.
5. Herman JL, Mallory C, Wilson BDM. Estimates of transgender populations in states with legislation impacting transgender people. The Williams Institute; 2016. Available from: http://

williamsinstitute.law.ucla.edu/wp-content/uploads/Estimates-of-Transgender-Populations.pdf

6. Bidell MP. Is there an emotional cost of completing high school? Ecological factors and psychological distress among LGBT homeless youth. J Homosex. 2014;61(3):366–81.

7. Castellanos HD. The role of institutional placement, family conflict, and homosexuality in homelessness pathways among Latino LGBT youth in New York City. J Homosex. 2016;63(5):601–32.

8. srlp.org [homepage on the Internet]. New York: Sylvia Rivera Law Project; 2016. [updated 2016 Apr 2; cited 2016 Apr 2]. Available from: http://srlp.org

9. Meyer IH. Minority stress and mental health in gay men. J Health Soc Behav. 1995;36(1):38–56.

10. Testa RJ, Sciacca LM, Wang F, et al. Effects of violence on transgender people. Prof Psych Res Prac. 2012;43(5):452–9.

11. Crenshaw K. Demarginalizing the intersection of race and sex: a black feminist critique of antidiscrimination doctrine, feminist theory and antiracist politics. University of Chicago Legal Forum. 1989;140:139–67.

12. Fowler RB. Community: reflections on definition. In: Etzioni A, editor. New communitarian thinking: persons, virtues, institutions, and communities. Charlottesville: University of Virginia Press; 1995.

13. Loue S. Community health advocacy. J Epidemiol Community Health. 2006;60(6):458–63.

14. McConnell EA, Birkett MA, Mustanski B. Typologies of social support and associations with mental health outcomes among LGBT youth. LGBT Health. 2015;2(1):55–61.

15. Tabaac AR, Perrin PB, Trujillo MA. Multiple meditational model of outness, social support, mental health, and wellness behavior in ethnically diverse lesbian, bisexual, and queer women. LGBT Health. 2015;2(3):243–9.

16. Poteat VP, Calzo JP, Yoshikawa H. Promoting youth agency through dimensions of gay-straight alliance involvement and conditions that maximize associations. J Youth Adolesc. 2016. Epub ahead of print.

17. Utamsingh PD, Richman LS, Martin JL, Lattanner MR, Chaikind JR. Heteronormativity and practitioner-patient interaction. Health Commun. 2016;31(5):566–74.

18. Cieslak R, Benight CC, Caden LV. Coping self-efficacy mediates the effects of negative cognitions on posttraumatic distress. Behav Res Ther. 2009;46(7):788–98.

19. www.pflag.org [homepage on the Internet]. PFLAG; 2016 [cited 2016 Apr 1]. Available from: http://community.pflag.org/

20. Ruan T. Archiving the wonders of testosterone via YouTube. TSQ. 2015;2(4):701–9.

21. www.nashvillelaunchpad.com [homepage on the Internet]. Launch Pad; 2016 [cited 2016 May 1]. Available from: http://www.nashvillelaunchpad.com/

22. www.pointfoundation.org [homepage on the Internet]. Point Foundation; 2016 [cited 2016 May 1]. Available from: https://www.pointfoundation.org/

23. Haber D. Gay aging. Gerontol Geriatr Educ. 2009;30(3):267–80.

24. Woody I. Aging out: a qualitative exploration of ageism and heterosexism among aging African American lesbians and gay men. J Homosex. 2014;61(1):145–65.

25. Czaja SJ, Sabbag S, Lee CC, Schulz R, Lang S, Vlahovic T, et al. Concerns about aging and caregiving among middle-aged and older lesbian and gay adults. Aging Ment Health. 2015;6:1–12.

26. Croghan CF, Moone RP, Olson AM. Friends, family, and caregiving among midlife and older lesbian, gay, bisexual, and transgender adults. J Homosex. 2014;61(1):79–102.

27. Witten TM. Elder transgender lesbians: exploring the intersection of age, lesbian sexual identity, and transgender identity. J Lesbian Stud. 2015;19(1):73–89.

28. Halkitis PN, Kupprat SA, Hampton MB, Perez-Figueroa R, Kingdon M, Eddy JA, et al. Evidence for a syndemic in aging HIV-positive gay, bisexual, and other MSM: implications for a holistic approach to prevention and healthcare. Nat Resour Model. 2012;36(2). Epub 2013 Nov 12.

29. Heckman TG, Halkitis PN. Biopsychosocial aspects of HIV and aging. Behav Med. 2014;40(3):81–4.

30. Hughes AK, Waters P, Herrick CD, Pelon S. Notes from the field: developing a support group for older lesbian and gay community members who have lost a partner. LGBT Health. 2014;1(4):323–6.

31. Fredriksen-Goldsen KI. Despite disparities, most LGBT elders are aging well. Aging Today. 2014;35(3). Epub 2014 Nov 25.

32. Siconolfi DE, Halkitis PN, Barton SC, Kingdon MJ, Perez-Figueroa RE, Arias-Martinez V, et al. Psychosocial and demographic correlates of drug use in a sample of HIV-positive adults ages 50 and older. Prev Sci. 2013;14(6):618–27.

33. Orel NA. Investigating the needs and concerns of lesbian, gay, bisexual and transgender older adults: the use of qualitative and quantitative methodology. J Homosex. 2014;61(1):53–78.

34. Gardner AT, de Vries B, Mockus DS. Aging out in the desert: disclosure, acceptance, and service use among midlife and older lesbians and gay men. J Homosex. 2014;61(1):129–44.

35. sageusa.org [homepage on the Internet]. SAGE USA; 2016 [cited 2016 Apr 1]. Available from: http://sageusa.org

36. fenwayhealth.org [homepage on the Internet]. The LGBT Aging Project; 2016 [cited 2016 May 1]. Available from: http://fenwayhealth.org/the-fenway-institute/lgbt-aging-project

37. www.lgbtagingcenter.org [homepage on the Internet]. The National Resource Center on LGBT Aging; 2016 [cited 2016 May 1]. Available from: http://www.lgbtagingcenter.org/index.cfm

38. Brown EH. Trans/feminist oral history. TSQ. 2015;2(4):666–72.

39. transoralhistory.com [homepage on the Internet]. The Transgender Oral History Project; 2016 [cited 2016 May 1]. Available from: http://transoralhistory.com

40. storycorps.org/outloud [homepage on the Internet]. OutLoud; 2016 [cited 2016 May 1]. Available from: https://storycorps.org/outloud

41. www.actuporalhistory.org [homepage on the Internet]. Act Up Oral History Project; 2016 [cited 2016 May 1]. Available from: http://www.actuporalhistory.org/index1.html

42. afamaidsoralhistory.wordpress.com [homepage on the Internet]. The African American Aids Activism Oral History Project; 2016 [cited 2016 May 1]. Available from: https://afamaidsoralhistory.wordpress.com

43. www.lgbt-stories.org [homepage on the Internet]. Untold Stories: The Leicester LGBT Centre Oral History Project; 2016 [cited 2016 May 1]. Available from http://www.lgbt-stories.org

44. lgbtran.org [homepage on the Internet]. The LGBT Religious Archives Network; 2016 [cited 2016 May 1]. Available from http://www.lgbtran.org/OralHistory.aspx

45. www.impactstories.org [homepage on the Internet]. Impact Stories: An Oral History Project from the California LGBT Community; 2016 [cited 2016 May 1]. Available from: http://www.impactstories.org/aboutus.htm

46. lgbtqdigitalcollaboratory.org [homepage on the Internet]. The LGBTQ Oral History Digital Collaboratory; 2016 [cited 2016 May 1]. Available from: http://lgbtqdigitalcollaboratory.org

47. Etengoff C, Daiute C. Clinicians' perspective of the relational processes for family and individual development during the mediation of religious and sexual identity disclosure. J Homosex. 2015;62(3):394–426.

48. Wilson CK, West L, Stepleman L, Villarosa M, Ange B, Decker M, et al. Attitudes toward LGBT patients among students in the professions: influence of demographics and discipline. LGBT Health. 2014;1(3):204–11.

49. Dinkel S, Patzel B, McGuire MJ, Rolfs E, Purcell K. Measures of homophobia among nursing students and faculty: a Midwestern perspective. Int J Nurs Educ Scholarsh. 2007;4(24). Epub 2007 Nov 30.

50. Hooghe M, Claes E, Harell A, Quintelier E, Dejaeghere Y. Anti-gay sentiment among adolescents in Belgium and Canada: a comparative investigation into the role of gender and religion. J Homosex. 2010;57(3):384–400.

51. McDermott RC, Schwartz JP, Lindley LD, Proietti JS. Exploring men's homophobia: associations with religious fundamentalism and gender role conflict domains. Psychol Men Masculinity. 2014;5(2):191–200.

52. Siraj A. "I don't want to taint the name of Islam": the influence of religion on the lives of Muslim lesbians. J Lesbian Stud. 2012;16 (4):449–67.

53. Morrow DF. Cast into the wilderness: the impact of institutionalized religion on lesbians. J Lesbian Stud. 2003;7 (4):109–23.

54. Walker JJ, Longmire-Avital B. The impact of religious faith and internalized homonegativity on resiliency for black lesbian, gay, and bisexual emerging adults. Dev Psychol. 2013;49(9):1723–31.

55. Sowe BJ, Brown J, Taylor AJ. Sex and the sinner: comparing religious and nonreligious same-sex attracted adults on internalized homonegativity and distress. Am J Orthopsychiatry. 2014;84(5):530–44.

56. Jackson PA. Thai Buddhist accounts of male homosexuality and AIDS in the 1980s. Aust J Anthropol. 1995;6(3):140–53.

57. Kubicek K, McDavitt B, Carpineto J, Weiss G, Iverson E, Kipke MD. "God made me gay for a reason": young men who have sex with men's resiliency in resolving internalized homophobia from religious sources. J Adolesc Res. 2009;24(5):601–33.

58. Ross MW, Rosser BR. Measurement and correlates of internalized homophobia: a factor analytic study. J Clin Psychol. 1996;52 (1):15–21.

59. Bowleg L, Burkholder G, Teti M, Craig ML. The complexities of outness: psychosocial predictors of coming out to others among black lesbian and bisexual women. J LGBT Health Res. 2008;4 (4):153–66.

60. Shilo G, Yossef I, Savaya R. Coping strategies and mental health among religious Jewish gay and bisexual men. Arch Sex Behav. 2015. Epub ahead of print.

61. Gibbs JJ, Goldbach J. Religious conflict, sexual identity, and suicidal behaviors among LGBT young adults. Arch Suicide Res. 2015;19(4):472–88.

62. Page MJ, Lindahl KM, Malik NM. The role of religion and stress in sexual identity and mental health among LGB youth. J Res Adolesc. 2013;23(4). Epub 2013 Feb 4.

63. Ross LD, Lelkes Y, Russell AG. How Christians reconcile their personal political views and the teachings of their faith: projection as a means of dissonance reduction. Proc Natl Acad Sci USA. 2012;109(10):3616–22.

64. Schnabel L. Gender and homosexuality attitudes across religious groups from the 1970s to 2014: similarity, distinction, and adaptation. Soc Sci Res. 2016;55(1):31–47.

65. Sullivan-Blum CR. Balancing acts: drag queens, gender and faith. J Homosex. 2004;46(3–4):195–209.

66. Minwalla O, Rosser BR, Feldman J, Varga C. Identity experience among progressive gay Muslims in North America: a qualitative study within Al-Fatiha. Cult Health Sex. 2005;7(2):113–28.

67. García DI, Gray-Stanley J, Ramirez-Valles J. "The priest obviously doesn't know that I'm gay": the religious and spiritual journeys of Latino gay men. J Homosex. 2008;55(3):411–36.

68. Lapinski J, McKirnan D. Forgive me Father for I have sinned: the role of a Christian upbringing on lesbian, gay, and bisexual identity development. J Homosex. 2013;60(6):853–72.

69. Mood D. Beyond the dichotomy: six religious views of homosexuality. J Homosex. 2014;61(9):1215–41.

70. Hatzenbuehler ML, Pachankis JE, Wolff J. Religious climate and health risk behaviors in sexual minority youths: a population-based study. Am J Public Health. 2012;102(4):657–63.

71. Lytle MC, De Luca SM, Blosnich JR, Brownson C. Associations of racial/ethnic identities and religious affiliation with suicidal ideation among lesbian, gay, bisexual, and questioning individuals. J Affect Disord. 2015;178:39–45.

72. Erosheva EA, Kim HJ, Emlet C, Fredriksen-Goldsen KI. Social networks of lesbian, gay, bisexual, and transgender older adults. Res Aging. 2016;38(1):98–123.

73. Scheitle CP, Merino SM, Moore A. On the varying meaning of "open and affirming". J Homosex. 2010;57(10):1223–36.

74. www.rmnetwork.org [homepage on the Internet]. Reconciling Ministries Network; 2016 [cited 2016 May 1]. Available from: http://www.rmnetwork.org/newrmn

75. www.welcomingresources.org [homepage on the Internet]. National LGBTQ Task Force Institute for Welcoming Resources; 2016 [cited 2016 May 1]. Available from: http://www.welcomingresources.org

76. Barbosa P, Torres H, Silva MA, Khan N. Agapé Christian reconciliation conversations: exploring the intersections of culture, religiousness, and homosexual identity in Latino and European Americans. J Homosex. 2010;57(1):98–116.

77. Vidal-Ortiz S. "Maricón," "pájaro," and "loca": Cuban and Puerto Rican linguistic practices, and sexual minority participation, in U.S. Santería. J Homosex. 2011;58(6–7):901–18.

78. Sanders S. Compassionately caring for LGBT persons in your faith community. J Christ Nurs. 2012;29(4):208–14.

79. Wilcox MM. Outlaws or in-laws? Queer theory, LGBT studies, and religious studies. J Homosex. 2006;52(1–2):73–100.

80. Gutierrez G. A theology of liberation. 1st ed. Maryknoll: Orbis Books; 1973.

81. Cheng PS. Radical love: an introduction to queer theology. 1st ed. New York: Seabury Books.

82. Jaspal R, Cinnirella M. Coping with potentially incompatible identities: accounts of religious, ethnic, and sexual identities from British Pakistani men who identify as Muslim and gay. Br J Soc Psychol. 2010;49(4):849–70.

83. Reese AM. "But of course he is led by God": pastoral influence on an HIV/AIDS ministry. J Homosex. 2011;58(6–7):919–31.

84. Liboro Jr RM. Community-level interventions for reconciling conflicting religious and sexual domains in identity incongruity. J Relig Health. 2015;54(4):1206–20.

85. Radojcic N. Building a 'dignified identity': an ethnographic case study of LGBT catholics. J Homosex. Epub 2016 Feb 8.

86. Hasenbush A, Flores AR, Kastanis A, Sears B, Gates GJ. The LGBT Divide: a data portrait of LGBT people in the midwestern, mountain, and southern states. The Williams Institute; 2014. Available from: http://williamsinstitute.law.ucla.edu/wp-content/uploads/LGBT-divide-Dec-2014.pdf

87. Bradford J, Reisner SL, Honnold JA, Xavier J. Experiences of transgender-related discrimination and implications for health: results from the Virginia Transgender Health Initiative Study. Am J Public Health. 2013;103(10):1820–9.

88. Centers for Disease Control and Prevention. MMWR 2013;62 (Suppl 3):9–104.

89. Barton B. "Abomination"—life as a Bible belt gay. J Homosex. 2010;57(4):465–84.

90. Kano M, Silva-Bañuelos AR, Sturm R, Willging CE. Stakeholders recommendations to improve patient-centered LGBTQ primary care in rural and multicultural practices. J Am Board Fam Med. 2016;29(1):156–60.

91. Maher MJ. A voice in the wilderness: gay and lesbian religious groups in the Western United States. J Homosex. 2006;51 (4):91–117.

92. Sears JT. Rebels, rubyfruits, and rhinestones : queering space in the Stonewall South. 1st ed. New Brunswick: Rutgers University Press; 2001.

93. Kaminski E, Taylor V. "We're not just lip-synching up here": music and collective identity in drag performances. In: Reger J, Meyers DJ, Einwohner RL, editors. Identity work in social movements. 1st ed. Minneapolis: University of Minnesota Press; 2008.

94. Kubicek K, Beyer WH, McNeeley M, Weiss G, Ultra Omni T, Kipke MD. Community-engaged research to identify house parent perspectives on support and risk within the house and ball scene. J Sex Res. 2013;50(2). Epub 2011 Dec 29.

95. McCready LT. Some challenges facing queer youth programs in urban high schools: racial segregations and de-normalizing whiteness. J Gay Lesb Issues Educ. 2004;1(3). Epub 2008 Nov 20.

96. Green AI. On the horns of a dilemma: institutional dimensions of the sexual career in a sample of middle-class, urban, black, gay men. Black Studies. Epub 2007 Apr 16.

97. Sanchez T, Finlayson T, Murrill C, Guilin V, Dean L. Risk behaviors and psychosocial stressors in the New York City house ball community: a comparison of men and transgender women who have sex with men. AIDS Behav. 2010;14(2):351–8.

98. Phillips G II, Peterson J, Binson D, Hidalgo J, Magnus M. YMSM of color SPNS Initiative Study Group. House/ball culture and adolescent African-American transgender persons and men who have sex with men: a synthesis of the literature. AIDS Care. 2011;23(4). Epub 2011 Jan 24.

99. Wong CF, Schrager SM, Holloway IW, Meyer IH, Kipke MD. Minority stress experiences and psychological well-being: the impact of support from the connection to social networks within the Los Angeles house and ball communities. Prev Sci. 2014;15(1):44–55.

100. Han C. They don't want to cruise your type: gay men of color and the racial politics of exclusion. Social Identities. 2007;13(1). Epub 2007 Jan 22.

101. McCready LT. Understanding the marginalization of gay and gender non-conforming black male students. Theory Pract. 2004;43(2):136–43.

102. Elling A, de Knop P, Knoppers A. Gay/lesbian sport clubs and events: places of homo-social bonding and cultural resistance? Int Rev Soc Sport. 2003;38(4):441–56.

103. Pruitt J. Gay men's book clubs versus Wisconsin's public libraries: political perceptions in the absence of dialogue. Libr Q. 2010;80 (2):121–41.

104. Glenn C. Queering the (sacred) body politic: considering the performative cultural politics of the sisters of perpetual indulgence. Theory Event. 2003;7(1):247–62.

105. thesisters.org [homepage on the Internet]. San Francisco: The Sisters of Perpetual Indulgence; 2016 [cited 2016 Apr 2]. Available from: http://thesisters.org/.

106. Cvetkovich A, Butler J. Legacies of trauma, legacies of activism: ACT UP's lesbians. In: Eng DL, Kazanjian D, editors. Loss: the politics of mourning. 1st ed. Berkeley: University of California Press; 2003.

107. Brier J. Infections ideas: U.S. political responses to the AIDS crisis. 1st ed. Chapel Hill: The University of North Carolina Press; 2011.

108. Poirier G. Neo-conservatism and social policy responses to the AIDS crisis. In: Johnson AF, McBride S, Smith PJ, editors. Continuities and discontinuities: the political economy of social welfare and labour market policy in Canada. 1st ed. Toronto: University of Toronto Press; 1994.

109. Elbaz G. Beyond anger: the activist construction of the AIDS crisis. Soc Justice. 1995;22(4):43–76.

110. Bader E. Coping and caring: films on the AIDS crisis. Cinéaste. 1989;17(1):18–9.

111. Della Luce K. ACTing UP against AIDS: the (very) graphic arts in a moment of crisis. In: Reed TV, editor. The art of protest: culture and activism from the civil rights movement to the streets of Seattle. 1st ed. Minneapolis: University of Minnesota Press; 2005.

112. Capozzola C. A very American epidemic: memory politics and identity politics in the AIDS memorial quilt, 1985–1993. In: Van Gosse R, Moser R, editors. The world the sixties made: politics and culture in recent America. 1st ed. Philadelphia: Temple University Press; 2003.

113. Morris CE, editor. Remembering the AIDS quilt. 1st ed. East Lansing: Michigan State University Press; 2011.

114. Baral S, Holland CE, Shannon K, Logie C, Semugoma P, Sithole B, Papworth E, Drame F, Beyrer C. Enhancing benefits or increasing harms: community responses for HIV among men who have sex with men, transgender women, female sex workers, and people who inject drugs. J Acquir Immune Defic Syndr. 2014;66(S3):S319–28.

115. Fredriksen-Goldsen KI, Espinoza RE. Time for transformation: public policy must change to achieve health equity for LGBT older adults. Generations. 2014;38(4):97–106.

116. Feldman MB. A critical literature review to identify possible causes of higher rates of HIV infection among young black and Latino men who have sex with men. J Natl Med Assoc. 2010;102 (12):1206–21.

117. Poteat T, Resiner SL, Radix A. HIV epidemics among transgender women. Curr Opin HIV AIDS. 2014;9(2):168–73.

118. Hillman AJ, Withers MC, Collins BJ. Resource dependence theory: a review. J Manag. 2009;35(1):1404–27.

119. Drees JM, Heugens PPMAR. Synthesizing and extending resource dependence theory: a meta-analysis. J Manag. 2013;39 (1):1666–98.

120. Parkin F. Marxism and class theory: a bourgeois critique. London: Tavistock; 1979.

121. Silver H. Social exclusion and social solidarity: three paradigms. Int Labour Rev. 1994;133(5–6):531–78.

122. Brown P. Cultural capital and social exclusion: some observations on recent trends in education, employment and the labour market. Work Employ Soc. 1995;9(1):29–51.

123. Institute of Medicine (US) Committee on Lesbian, Gay, Bisexual and Transgender Health. The health of lesbian, gay, bisexual, and transgender people: building a foundation for better understanding. Washington, DC: National Academies Press (US); 2011.

124. radremedy.org [homepage on the Internet]. Rad Remedy; 2016 [cited 2016 Apr 1]. Available from: http://www.radremedy.org.

125. mytranshealth.com [homepage on the Internet]. MyTransHealth; 2016 [cited 2016 Apr 1]. Available from: http://mytranshealth. com.

126. fenwayhealth.org [homepage on the Internet]. Fenway Health Center; 2016 [cited 2016 Apr 1]. Available from: http:// fenwayhealth.org/care/medical/transgender-health/.

127. transcare.ucsf.edu [homepage on the Internet]. Center of Excellence for Transgender Health; 2016 [cited 2016 Apr 1]. Available from: http://transcare.ucsf.edu/.

128. medschool.vanderbilt.edu/lgbti [homepage on the Internet]. The Trans Buddy Program; 2016 [cited 2016 Apr 1]. Available from: http://medschool.vanderbilt.edu/lgbti/trans-buddy.

129. translifeline.org [homepage on the Internet]. Trans Lifeline; 2015 [cited 2016 Apr 1]. Available from: http://www.translifeline.org.

130. Magee JC, Bigelow L, Dehaan S, Mustanksi BS. Sexual health information seeking online: a mixed-methods study among lesbian, gay, bisexual and transgender young people. Health Educ Behav. 2012;39(3):276–89.

131. Rawson KJ. Transgender worldmaking in cyberspace: historical activism on the internet. QED. 2014;1(2):38–60.

132. Daniels N. Duty to treat or right to refuse? Hast Cent Rep. 1991;21 (2):36–46.
133. Lang NG. Difficult decisions: ethics and AIDS. J Sex Res. 1991;28(2):249–62.
134. Schwartz AR. Doubtful duty: physicians' legal obligation to treat during an epidemic. Stanford Law Rev. 2007;60(2):657–94.
135. Flentje A, Heck NC, Cochran BN. Experiences of ex-ex-gay individuals in sexual reorientation therapy: reasons for seeking treatment, perceived helpfulness and harfulness of treatment, and post-treatment identification. J Homosex. 2014;61(9):1242–68.
136. Bouman WP, Richards C, Addinall RM, Arango de Montis I, Duisin D, Esteva I, et al. Yes and yes again: are the standards of care which require two referrals for genital reconstructive surgery ethical? Sex Relat Ther. 2014;29(4):377–89.
137. Smith N, Stanley EA, editors. Captive genders. 1st ed. Oakland: AK Press; 2011.
138. Spade D. Normal life: administrative violence, critical trans politics, and the limits of law. 1st ed. Durham: Duke University Press; 2011.
139. Seelman KL. Transgender adults' access to college bathrooms and housing and the relationship to suicidality. J Homosex. 2016. Epub ahead of print.
140. Mananzala R, Spade D. The nonprofit industrial complex and trans resistance. Sex Res Soc Policy. 2008;5(1):53–71.
141. Dinkel S, Patzel B, McGuire MJ, Rolfs E, Purcell K. Measures of homophobia among nursing students and faculty: a Midwestern perspective. Int J Nurs Educ Scholarsh. 2007;4(1). Epub 2007 Nov 30.
142. Klotzbaugh R, Spencer G. Magnet nurse administrator attitudes and opportunities: toward improving, lesbian, gay, bisexual, or transgender-specific healthcare. J Nurs Adm. 2014;44(9):481–6.
143. Porter KE, Krinsky L. Do LGBT trainings effectuate positive change in mainstream elder service providers? J Homosex. 2014;61(1):197–216.
144. Sherman MD, Kauth MR, Shipherd JC, Street Jr RL. Provider beliefs and practices about assessing sexual orientation in two veterans health affairs hospitals. LGBT Health. 2014;1(3):185–91.
145. Burke SE, Dovidio JF, Przedworski JM, Hardeman RR, Perry SP, Phelan SM, et al. Do contact and empathy mitigate bias against gay and lesbian people among heterosexual first-year medical students? A report from the Medical Student CHANGE Study. Acad Med. 2015;90(5):645–51.
146. Carabez R, Pellegrini M, Mankovitz A, Eliason M, Ciano M, Scott M. "Never in all my years… ": nurses' education about LGBT health. J Prof Nurs. 2015;31(4):323–9.
147. Ewton TA, Lingas EO. Pilot survey of physician assistants regarding lesbian, gay, bisexual, and transgender providers suggests role for workplace nondiscrimination policies. LGBT Health. 2015;2 (4):357–61.
148. Lee KP, Kelz RR, Dube B, Morris JB. Attitude and perceptions of the other underrepresented minority in surgery. J Surg Educ. 2014;71(6):e47–52.
149. Eliason MJ, Dibble SL, Robertson PA. Lesbian, gay, bisexual, and transgender (LGBT) physicians' experiences in the workplace. J Homosex. 2011;58(10):1355–71.
150. Druzin P, Shrier I, Yacowar M, Rossignol M. Discrimination against gay, lesbian and bisexual family physicians by patients. CMAJ. 1998;158(5):593–7.
151. Lee RS, Melhado TV, Chacko KM, White KJ, Huebschmann AG, Crane LA. The dilemma of disclosure: patient perspectives on gay and lesbian providers. J Gen Intern Med. 2008;23(2):142–7.
152. glma.org [homepage on the Internet]. GLMA: Health Professionals Advancing LGBT Equality; 2016 [cited 2016 Apr 1]. Available from: http://www.glma.org.
153. Tervalon M, Murray-Garcia J. Cultural humility versus cultural competence: a critical distinction in defining physician training outcomes in multicultural education. J Health Care Poor Underserved. 1998;9(2):117–25.

Resilience Development Among LGBT Health Practitioners

20

Carl G. Streed Jr. and Mickey Eliason

Objectives

- Identify three stressors experienced by LGBT health practitioners
- Describe how stress impacts LGBT health practitioners
- Identify three sources of resilience among LGBT health practitioners
- Discuss recommendations for fostering resilience among LGBT health practitioners in healthcare

Introduction

Most LGBT people who choose to pursue a career in the healthcare field have personally experienced stress related to coming out, bullying in school, or rejection. They may have grown into adulthood with few role models who are LGBT health practitioners, and unlike underserved racial/ethnic populations, there are no pipeline programs to recruit and support LGBT people in healthcare careers. Despite these challenges, or perhaps because of them, LGBT individuals can be drawn to careers in healthcare to improve the treatment and well-being of others because of their own lived experiences [1]. However, Sexual and gender minority stress may complicate their career paths, seeking employment, and ongoing clinical practice.

C.G. Streed Jr., MD (✉)
General Internal Medicine & Primary Care, Brigham & Women's Hospital, Boston, MA, USA
e-mail: cjstreed@gmail.com

M. Eliason, PhD
Faculty Development and Scholarship, College of Health and Social Sciences, 1600 Holloway Avenue HSS Building, Room 214, San Francisco, CA 94132, USA
e-mail: meliason@sfsu.edu

The inherent stress associated with working in a healthcare setting can be compounded by the stigma associated with a minority sexual or gender identity (e.g., LGBT identification); this "minority stress" is hypothesized to underlie the elevated rates of mental health concerns, substance use, and poorer physical health among LGBT individuals compared to the general population [2–4]. In healthcare work environments punctuated by high levels of such minority stress, fear of discrimination, harassment, or even job loss may adversely impact LGBT health practitioners' ability to achieve their full professional potential, and willingness to serve as needed mentors to LGBT individuals interested in pursuing careers in healthcare. Thankfully, research demonstrates a steady decline in discrimination and harassment of LGBT health practitioners and is beginning to address resilience among LGBT populations and health practitioners [5–7]. This chapter reviews literature on experiences of LGBT health practitioners, and proposes methods to reduce discrimination and foster resilience.

Case Scenario, Part 1

Laura is a 38-year-old female cisgender bisexual nurse at an urban academic medical center (Fig. 20.1). She has dated and been in long-term relationships with both men and women at various times in her life. Many of her work colleagues now know her to be bisexual and have been welcoming to her significant others, but she has experienced some negative comments from coworkers and one supervisor in the past. Laura participates in an Employee Resource Group (ERG) on LGBT issues that has successfully updated policies to protect against discrimination based on sexual orientation and gender identity, and has begun to address health insurance equity for transgender employees and training on LGBT issues for current employees as well as new hires.

© Springer International Publishing AG 2017
K.L. Eckstrand, J. Potter (eds.), *Trauma, Resilience, and Health Promotion in LGBT Patients,*
DOI 10.1007/978-3-319-54509-7_20

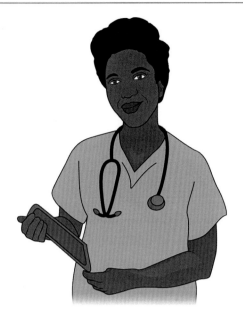

Fig. 20.1 Laura is a 38-year-old female cisgender bisexual nurse at an urban academic medical center

Trauma and Discrimination Experienced by LGBT Health Practitioners

Like racism and other structural inequities that create and maintain barriers between people, heterosexist, homophobic, transphobic, and gender normative attitudes affect individuals in the healthcare setting. These attitudes negatively influence the education of health practitioners, the quality of healthcare for patients/clients, and the healthcare environment [8]. Studies from the 1970s forward have demonstrated challenges coming out in the workplace along with experiences of harassment, discrimination, or differential treatment [8]. Most studies thus far have focused on physicians (or medical students) and nurses [9, 10]. The additional stress of being LGBT in the workplace combined with the experience of minority stress outside of work may underlie mental and physical health disparities [11–13]. In numerous healthcare practice and academic settings, LGBT staff and students/trainees may not feel safe being out as a consequence of a lack of institutional nondiscrimination policies and recognition or support of their identities (e.g., trans-inclusive health insurance policies) and/or relationships (e.g., domestic partner benefits). Sexual orientation and gender identity are rarely obtained when gathering demographic data [14], resulting in an inability to quantify how many faculty, staff, and/or students/trainees identify as LGB or T and to identify and address any disparities in their experiences. This institutional invisibility creates and maintains an environment of isolation and fear of being outed without permission, fired, or denied equal protection

and an inability to access needed healthcare *despite* being a member of the healthcare profession.

Case Scenario, Part 2

When Laura first came out as bisexual, an attending physician on her floor cornered her in the break room and asked her to join him and his girlfriend for a threesome. She politely said no, but he persisted in asking her out several times over the next few months and made her feel very uncomfortable. She also felt that her job might be threatened because of the greater power the physician had in the workplace.

Physicians, Medical Students, and Physician Trainees

Physicians tend to be seen as leaders within healthcare, and are thus in a unique position of authority and responsibility. Initial attempts to address LGBT health disparities have therefore focused on understanding physicians' knowledge, attitudes, and skills related to LGBT health, with competence associated with a more welcoming environment for both LGBT patients and employees. Studies of physician attitudes toward LGBT patients (i.e., homophobia/transphobia) have found a decline in overtly negative attitudes and biases toward working with LGB patients (19% in 1999 down from 58% in 1982) [15–17]; these negative attitudes have even been cited to limit referrals to LGBT physicians [18]. Negative and harmful attitudes and biases have also been found in students and trainees [19, 20]. More recent studies of bias, however, have found that while a majority of students still harbor some form of implicit bias against lesbian and gay patients, explicit bias against lesbian and gay patients is declining; similar attitudes toward gay and lesbian patients have been found among physicians [21–23]. These findings suggest that there is an understanding that LGBT patients are entitled to the same competent and compassionate care as their heterosexual, cisgender peers.

To understand the experiences of LGBT physicians, Schatz and O'Hanlan [24] conducted a survey in 1994 of the members of an LGBT medical organization. A quarter of respondents stated that most of their colleagues knew of their sexuality, and another quarter reported that less than 10% of their colleagues knew of their sexuality; half fell somewhere between these extremes. A follow-up to this study in 2011 [9] noted significant improvements in LGBT physician experiences. Table 20.1 compares some of the findings of these two studies across time.

Table 20.1 Comparison of experiences of LGB physicians in the early 1990s and late 2000s [9]

Finding	Shantz and O'Hanlon, data from 1993 [24] (%)	Eliason et al., data from 2008 [9] (%)
Refused privileges or denied promotion	17	
Denied referrals	16	10
Experienced verbal harassment	34	15
Experienced social ostracism	37	22
Heard disparaging remarks from colleagues	88	65
Witnessed poor care of LGBT patients	52	33

Arguably, an intolerant or unwelcoming climate in healthcare work settings partially stems from the lack of training in healthcare professional education. Obedin-Maliver and colleagues [25] found medical school curricula had only a median of 5 h dedicated to teaching LGBT-related content in the entire curriculum with nearly a third of schools reporting 0 h of LGBT-related content. Other research reported that fewer than half of medical students always asked their patients about same-sex behaviors, and the majority rarely or never discussed a patient's sexual orientation; 28% reported they were uncomfortable addressing an LGBT patient's health needs [26]. Further, whereas 58% of US internal medicine residency programs covered the health of racial/ethnic minorities in their curricula, only 30% addressed health of gay men and 11% health of lesbians [27].

In addition to the lack of formal curricula addressing LGBT issues, exclusionary and sometimes even anti-LGBT sentiment is often found in the hidden curriculum of clinical training. The hidden curriculum includes interactions with other students outside of the classroom, extracurricular activities and clubs, conversations and advising from faculty, and the wide diversity of experiences in clinical settings. Medical students, residents, and physician teachers report witnessing medical colleagues behave in a discriminatory fashion or make derogatory remarks about LGBT patients to about the same extent as they observe gender and racial discrimination [28, 29]. Unfortunately, homophobic attitudes can have profound effects on workforce development; nearly a quarter of family practice program directors would not match openly gay residents to their programs [30].

Therefore, it is not surprising that 95% of LGBT students applying for medical school did not disclose their sexual orientation for fear of discrimination, and 46% did not disclose when applying for a residency [31]. While some may judge this vigilant behavior to be overly cautious, several studies suggest that fears of disclosure are valid [32]. Patients may also discriminate against physicians they know to be LGB. A study of LGB internists in Canada revealed that 30% had been subjected to homophobic remarks by patients on three or more occasions [33]. In a related study, researchers found that 12% of randomly selected adults would refuse to see an LGB family physician [34].

A national random sample survey of individuals in the USA found that 30% said they would change their provider if they found out the provider was LGBT, and 35% would switch to a different clinic or practice if they found the practice employed openly LGB healthcare providers [35]. Some LGB physicians choose to "pass" as heterosexual to avoid these potential problems with patients [36]. Thus far, no studies have examined patient attitudes about transgender physicians.

With physician job dissatisfaction as one of the most powerful predictors of "departure" from medicine [37], discrimination and harassment from supervisors, colleagues, and patients are likely to be important factors influencing the decisions of LGBT physicians to continue careers in medicine, as well as specialty and geographical practice location selections.

Case Scenario, Part 3

When Laura first came out to colleagues, they seemed to have no idea what bisexuality was—several asked her if it meant she was gay, and others implied that it was a phase she was going through. One coworker put a pamphlet from a church-run ex-gay ministry in her mailbox.

Nurses and Nursing Students

In addition to a high degree of job stress in the nursing profession, the added stress of discrimination toward LGBT nurses is likely a significant contributor to high turnover [38–41]. Evaluation of nurses' attitudes toward LGB patients has found results similar to their physician colleagues. In one early survey of nurse educators [42], more than half believed lesbians to be "unnatural" or disgusting (34%), or immoral (23%). A review of the nursing literature addressing LGB patient care found evidence for negative attitudes toward LGB patients in all 17 papers reviewed [43], and interviews with practicing nurses revealed shockingly low levels of knowledge [44]. Moreover, Sabin and colleagues [22] found that nurses collectively had widespread implicit preferences for heterosexual people, and heterosexual male nurses had the greatest degree of implicit bias.

However, research documents increasing acceptance over time. Participants in the largest study of LGBT nurses [10] were drawn from a wide variety of nursing settings: 57% were out to all of their coworkers, 4% were not out to anyone at work, and 88% were out to no or few patients. Less than 30% of respondents reported overtly negative workplace climates, but those who did had been outed, lost jobs, saw patients being ridiculed or even physically abused, and had experienced harassment. More promisingly, a majority (73%) reported that their workplace was generally LGBT-friendly; factors that made these environments friendlier included LGBT-inclusive policies, open-minded coworkers, openly LGBT coworkers, urban as opposed to rural geographical location, type of institution (less friendly if a religious-based hospital, more friendly in educational settings), and an institutional commitment to diversity.

Nursing education is comparable to medical education in the absence of LGBT health topics in the formal curriculum. However, recent studies show that attitudes about the importance of teaching on LGBT health are changing [45, 46]. A survey of over 1000 US nurse educators [45] found that just over 2 h on average were devoted to LGBT topics in nursing education, while 17% of programs had no LGBT content at all. A majority of respondents (70%) indicated that they were willing and ready to teach these topics, and 75% indicated they would be comfortable teaching LGBT topics but lacked knowledge of the content they should be covering. Thus far, no studies have addressed the hidden curriculum in nursing education.

Other Healthcare Practitioners and Trainees

Two surveys of dental school administrators [47, 48] found that although many were aware that they had LGBT students, few had any content in the curriculum about sexual and gender minority people. A survey of dental students [49] including 16 LGBT and 100 heterosexual students found that 30% of students disagreed that their school had a supportive climate for LGBT students, and 33% and 20% had observed unequal treatment of LGBT patients and providers, respectively. Over half (53%) had heard insensitive or disparaging comments about LGBT people from faculty members in their school and 87% from fellow students. Overall, 88% of students disagreed or were neutral about the statement that their program had adequately prepared them to work with LGBT populations. LGBT students felt less safe, included, or encouraged than heterosexual students, and witnessed more episodes of unequal treatment of both patients and LGBT providers. Seaborne, Prince, and Kushner [50] surveyed physician-assistant schools and

found a similar lack of LGBT health curricular content as reported at medical schools. To date, no studies have addressed the work experiences of LGBT physician assistants. Although a greater amount of literature has focused on inclusion of LGBT issues in the training of psychologists and social workers, little of this has examined workplace climate specifically.

An interdisciplinary study of LGBT healthcare practitioners currently underway [51] will offer the opportunity to compare experiences across different disciplines. A preliminary analysis of the data for over 200 LGBT healthcare professionals shows that over 80% were satisfied or very satisfied with their jobs, and over 80% showed resilience (ability to bounce back quickly after anti-LGBT incidents or comments). Many of the settings where respondents worked did not have LGBT-inclusive policies, and 30% of the sample reported that their workplace climate was not welcoming. Moreover, 64% reported an absence of training on LGBT issues for employees where they worked or went to school. When asked who gave them support when they experienced stress related to being LGBT at work, they relied mostly on partners and close friends, while less than 20% received good support from coworkers, 15% from bosses/supervisors, and 13% from professional organizations. Nearly half reported that LGBT-related work stress affected relationships with coworkers and job satisfaction; 42% reported mental health problems, and 38% reported work burnout.

While research on the experiences of LGBT healthcare practitioners and trainees in the workplace is sparse, available data suggest that both school and practice settings are perceived to be discriminatory or overtly hostile. These adverse environments may impede learning and productivity for LGBT healthcare practitioners, and may lead to poor job satisfaction and burnout. However, emerging research has demonstrated a decrease in discrimination and an increase in acceptance of LGBT health issues and LGBT health practitioners.

Case Scenario, Part 4

Laura was in a relationship with a woman when she first came out to coworkers, and no matter how often she explained that she was still bisexual, many of them referred to her as a lesbian. When that relationship ended, she started dating a man and a coworker asked, "So that means you aren't gay anymore, right?" Laura was in an LGBT employee support group and was able to share this experience and laugh about it. Because of the support she had from other LGBT coworkers, she was able to calmly address this comment and educate her coworker.

Resilience Among LGBT Health Practitioners

While LGBT health practitioners face many forms of discrimination from colleagues, patients, and society at large, many manifest a resilience that has not yet been well characterized. Resilience describes the ability of individuals and communities to bounce back or to cope successfully despite adverse circumstances [52, 53]. Resilience has been referred to as an inborn personality trait [54, 55] and/or a dynamic learned process [56]. A common theme is that individuals who are described as resilient are able to overcome challenging obstacles encountered over time.

What follows is a brief exploration of factors that may influence the resilience of LGBT health practitioners, examined at individual, institutional, organizational, and societal/public policy levels. An ecosocial model (see Fig. 20.2) has been applied to other aspects of LGBT health [57, 58]. This model proposes that no individual factors alone can predict health and well-being, because each individual is impacted by others close to them, the communities in which they live, the institutions where they receive education and work, and dominant societal-level discourses, laws, and policies. Factors across this sociocultural trajectory may support or prevent resilience development. The societal level is particularly critical, because if there were no stigma in society created by dominant discourses of law, medicine, media, education, and religion, there would be no minority stress for LGBT people. Primary prevention of stigma is a priority.

Societal/Public Policy Level

Societal changes related to civil rights and stigma reduction for LGBT populations would reduce much of the stress in the workplace for LGBT health practitioners. Examples of

meaningful changes at the societal level include relationship equality/recognition, workplace nondiscrimination laws, comprehensive sexuality education in schools, anti-bullying programs that address sexual orientation and gender identity, and changes in religious doctrines and dogma regarding LGBT people. The upsurge of Religious Freedom bills promulgated by several state legislators threatens the safety and equality of LGBT individuals, as these bills allow businesses and institutions to actively discriminate against people with diverse sexual orientations and gender identities. Further, national policies and laws affect the health and well-being of LGBT individuals. Most notably, marriage equality has been linked to the health and well-being of LGBT individuals and families [59–62] by allowing access to healthcare by partners; increasing overall health and longevity; protecting hospital visitation and decision making rights; increasing investment in the relationship; increasing family and community support for the relationship; and improving care of children of LGBT parents when their families are respected and accorded legal protections.

Despite the benefits afforded by marriage equality, now a reality in many countries worldwide, LGBT individuals can still lose their jobs based on their sexual orientation or gender identity. In the USA, a federal employment nondiscrimination law will be necessary to protect LGBT people from job loss. In addition, pipeline programs that encourage students to enter the health professions could further increase professional opportunities for LGBT youth and young adults.

Organizational and Professional Factors of Resilience

Macro-level factors at organizational, professional practice, and policy levels can profoundly affect the work experiences of LGBT health practitioners. Practices and policies range from hostile or apathetic toward LGBT individuals to supportive, affirming, and inclusive [63]. Organizations affect LGBT persons in a variety of domains, including institution- and unit-level policies and procedures; public statements and philanthropy; strategic planning; recruitment, hiring, promotion, and termination; and employee/trainee/staff benefits, training, and other support resources. These factors do not need to be overtly apparent to affect the resilience of LGBT health practitioners; individuals may not be aware of discrimination when they are not hired for a job or do not receive patient referrals. In addition, LGBT health practitioners may not be aware of LGBT-affirming practices used by their institutions. Mohr and Fassinger [64] noted that "lesbian-, gay-, and bisexual-affirming" practices and policies of institutions may indirectly create a positive influence by "attracting socially progressive workers who are

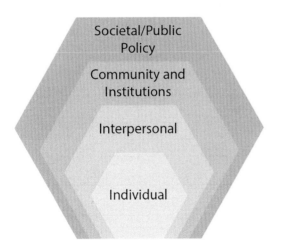

Fig. 20.2 An ecological model for understanding resilience in LGBT healthcare practitioners

more likely than others to contribute to a positive work environment for non-heterosexual colleagues." An example of LGBT-affirming practices includes recruiting and hiring openly LGBT health practitioners with the consequence that future LGBT hires may feel more welcomed and supported. Additional strategies to enhance climate and inclusion include nondiscrimination policies, same-sex partner benefits, training on LGBT-inclusive climate, and a commitment to diversity that includes sexual orientation and gender identity alongside all other categories of diversity.

Healthcare practitioners are also influenced by advocacy organizations. National healthcare professional organizations have begun to address LGBT employee issues via task forces, committees, or workgroups. Table 20.2 shows some of these resources. These groups play multiple roles in improving healthcare services for LGBT patients, improving the work and providing support and networking for LGBT healthcare practitioners.

Marriage equality notwithstanding, national policies do not yet provide protections against LGBT employment discrimination. Institutions can play a leadership role by incorporating robust nondiscrimination policies related to

employment (hiring, retention) and workplace conduct (sexual harassment); these "best business practices" focus on the importance of recruiting and retaining top talent [65, 66]. For example, employer-sponsored insurance plans with inclusive transgender heath care coverage may be beneficial in recruiting and retaining students, faculty, and staff. The oft-cited financial burden of providing such coverage has not been borne out in analyses of organizations and systems that have already instituted these benefits [67].

LGBT student groups are common on undergraduate campuses, but not as prevalent in graduate-level healthcare training programs, where they could be highly beneficial. Other aspects of climate include extracurricular activities, social events, and celebrations that often center on heterosexual students' experiences and are not sensitive to LGBT experiences or inclusive of same-sex partners. It is crucial to be attentive to the hidden curriculum – a composite of implicit and explicit biases, institutional climate, and ingrained behaviors of clinical personnel [68] – as trainees tend to retain and incorporate into their own practice what they observe and experience far more than what they are overtly taught. The challenges of the hidden curriculum for

Table 20.2 Resources for LGBT health practitioners

Resource	Link
GLMA: Health Professionals Advancing LGBT Equality	http://www.glma.org/
LGBT Caucus of Public Health Professionals	http://www.aphalgbt.org/
LGBT Committee of the American Medical Association	http://www.ama-assn.org/ama/pub/about-ama/our-people/member-groups-sections/glbt-advisory-committee/
LGBT Expert Panel of the American Academy of Nursing	http://www.aannet.org/ep-lgbtq-health
American Academy of Physician Assistants LGBT Physician Assistant Caucus	http://www.lbgtpa.org/
World Professional Organization for Transgender Health (WPATH)	http://www.wpath.org/
American Psychological Association, Division 44	http://www.apadivision44.org/
American Psychiatric Association, LGBT Caucus	http://www.psychiatry.org/psychiatrists/cultural-competency/minority-and-underrepresented-groups-caucuses
American Medical Student Association; Has an LGBT Handbook	http://www.amsa.org/advocacy/action-committees/gender-sexuality/lgbt-handbook/
Association of Gay and Lesbian Psychiatrists	http://www.aglp.org/
Lavender Health LGBT Resource Center	http://lavenderhealth.org
Human Rights Campaign (HRC) Corporate Equality Index and Healthcare Equality Index	http://www.hrc.org/resources/entry/corporate-equality-index http://www.hrc.org/campaigns/healthcare-equality-index
OutLists	Examples: George Mason University: http://lgbtq.gmu.edu/safezone/allylist.php Johns Hopkins University: http://studentaffairs.jhu.edu/lgbtq/outlist/ New York University School of Medicine: http://www.med.nyu.edu/school/student-resources/diversity-affairs/lgbtq-resources/outlist University of California, Berkley: http://lavendercal.berkeley.edu/out-list University of California, San Francisco: http://lgbt.ucsf.edu/out_outlist.html University of Maryland: http://www.umd.edu/lgbt/outlist.html University of Michigan: https://spectrumcenter.umich.edu/outlist/home University of Oregon: http://lgbt.uoregon.edu/GetInvolved/AnnualPrograms/Outlist.aspx University of Southern California: http://sait.usc.edu/lgbt/signature-programs/outlist.aspx

LGBT students and trainees are illustrated by continued consideration of Laura's training experience [69].

Case Scenario, Part 5

Laura relates that she was afraid to come out in nursing school because the curriculum never mentioned LGBT issues, faculty members never raised the topic, and other students made homophobic remarks that were never addressed by faculty. One staff member was rumored to be gay and was the source of much malicious gossip.

The hidden curriculum has been experienced by students/trainees as largely negative as a result of observing insensitive attitudes, derogatory statements, and even frankly discriminatory behaviors from faculty and staff about or toward LGBT patients [70, 71]. The power dynamic between students/trainees and professors and clinical supervisors often discourages speaking out against such bias. When sexual harassment and anti-discrimination policies explicitly cover LGBT employees, the training for these policies can create allies among heterosexual, cisgender students, faculty, and staff, who can share the burden of speaking up when they witness microaggressions or overt harassment. This method is especially critical as trainees absorb and mimic what they experience and perpetuate such behavior in the academic environments when they become teachers themselves. Establishment of reporting mechanisms and rapid response teams trained to promptly address instances of bias and inequity in the hidden curriculum are strongly recommended [71].

Examination of the formal curriculum for opportunities to integrate LGBT health content is also a valuable approach. A survey of third- and fourth-year medical students found that students with more clinical exposure to LGBT patients were more likely to take sexual histories on all their patients, had more positive attitudes about LGBT people, and had more accurate knowledge about LGBT health than did students with limited clinical exposure [25]. Knowing an LGBT person is a predictor of more positive attitudes, suggesting that the more LGBT students and faculty members disclose their identities, the more likely they will be to shift the attitudes of their peers. Healthcare providers also need to be made aware of the power of implicit bias, and how to mitigate one's biases.

Additional policies address LGBT healthcare competency by requiring demonstration of requisite knowledge, attitudes, and skills as part of health profession training or hospital accreditation [72, 73]. Implementation of these policies is slow, and inclusion of LGBT issues in health professions training programs remains unstandardized and not required by entities such as the American Association of Medical Colleges and the American Association of Colleges of Nursing. Examples of curricular integration include but are not limited to the following [72–74]:

- Courses or lectures on development across the life span that consider the coming-out process and how it changes across the life course;
- Lectures on discrimination, health disparities, and social justice that include the concepts of minority stress, heterosexism, and gender normativity;
- Units on family structure that discuss the myriad ways that LGBT individuals forge families, and consider expanded definitions of family;
- Units about specific diseases or disorders that include some case studies depicting specific issues an LGBT person with these conditions might experience;
- Gerontology modules that address health disparities and discuss how to treat LGBT elders with sensitivity and respect in institutional settings; and
- Sexual health units that consider a host of LGBT issues that extend beyond discussion of HIV and STIs.

In clinical clerkships, LGBT healthcare can be addressed via intersessions, departmental grand rounds, "lunch rounds," formal and informal faculty talks, online modules, and other venues; each educational opportunity emphasizes to students and trainees the importance and relevance of these issues to patient care.

Community Factors of Resilience

Mereish and Poteat [75] proposed that "growth-fostering" relationships provide the foundation for resilience. A growing professional network exists among LGBT health practitioners, with organizations centered in LGBT advocacy, such as GLMA: Health Professionals Advancing LGBT Equality (see Table 20.2 for other resources). Key characteristics of growth-promoting relationships include empathy, mutuality, and empowerment [75]. Community building can be promoted via LGBT clubs, organizations, mentoring programs, institutional celebrations of LGBT pride, and OUTLists. OUTLists are publicly accessible collections of faculty, staff, alumni, students, and trainees who identify as LGBT and are willing to serve as mentors and an informal support network for the LGBT community at their institutions. OUTLists can be useful tools for recruiting and retaining the most talented LGBT employees, in that the existence of these lists provides a visible example of the organization's commitment to diversity and inclusion (see Table 20.2 for examples).

Individual Factors of Resilience

Limited research has examined the development of resilience among health practitioners in general, and research specific to LGBT health practitioners is practically nonexistent. We know that challenging workplaces, psychological emptiness, diminishing inner balance, and a sense of dissonance in the workplace are factors that affect resilience in nurses and physicians , and that characteristics related to resilience include hope, self-efficacy, coping, control, competence, flexibility, adaptability, hardiness, sense of coherence, skill recognition, nondeficiency focusing, gratification from the patient-provider relationship, ensuring leisure time, self-reflection, and time for family and friends [76–82].

Although this research has not focused on LGBT health practitioners, data suggest that being out as an LGBT health practitioner can have positive consequences. For example, Eliason, Dibble, and Robertson [9] found that many respondents (46%) had received referrals of LGBT patients, over half (52%) had been sought out as experts on LGBT health, and some (34%) had been asked to do grand rounds on LGBT topics. This suggests a new level of support and valuing of the knowledge and experiences of LGBT healthcare practitioners, but on the other hand, these requests may also increase workload and add to stress as noted by two respondents [51]:

> Often called on to teach anything having to do with human sexuality. Expected to be expert on anything LGBT...There is no protected time for these responsibilities and as a result I feel that my research productivity is diminished. In addition, the LGBT teaching I do seems to be less valued than basic science teaching.

> Currently we are trying to improve the curriculum at our school and the climate. It's overwhelming because the administration is "supportive" in that they will let us do the work we're trying to do but it is 100% on us. I don't have time to do all my classwork, as well as re-write their curriculum as the one of a handful of our people on campus. It's more work than I did when I worked full time, and no one pays me to do this.

Conclusions

This chapter highlights the challenges LGBT healthcare practitioners face during training and in their day-to-day professional practice and workplace. A growing body of research on the experiences of healthcare practitioners has identified key factors associated with burnout; an accompanying body of research on resilience is now blossoming. Nevertheless, little research has addressed the unique stressors and challenges faced by LGBT healthcare practitioners with regard to experiences of stigma and discrimination. We have provided a series of recommendations based on available evidence that can be used to transform healthcare settings into more welcoming and inclusive environments for LGBT people, thereby reducing trauma and burnout and fostering resilience at individual, institutional, and national levels.

Case Conclusion

Laura was able to find supportive colleagues in the Employee Resource Group on LGBT issues and work for policy change at her institution. This support allowed her to become more resilient so that she could educate her coworkers and patients on LGBT issues without experiencing stress and anxiety herself.

Discussion Questions

1. What role do institutions have in supporting LGBT health practitioners?
2. How do federal policies and laws affect the development of resilience among individual healthcare practitioners? How can healthcare practitioners become better advocates for systems-level change? What strategies can health practitioner institutions (human resources departments, academic programs) use when trying to promote health among fellow LGBT health practitioners?
3. What community resources are available to support LGBT health practitioners and their families?

Summary Practice Points

- Currently, LGBT healthcare professionals lack support from federal, institutional, and interpersonal levels that would enhance individual resilience.
- Employee acceptance and connectedness support resilience development among LGBT health practitioners.
- Organizational commitment and support in the form of Employee Resource Groups (ERGs) and inclusive policies, procedures, and language are crucial in enhancing employee resilience.

References

1. Baumle AK, Compton D, Poston D. Same-sex partners: the social demography of sexual orientation. Albany: State University of New York Press; 2009.
2. Lewis R, Derlaga V, Griffin J, Krownski A. Stressors for gay men and lesbians: life stress, gay-related stress, stigma consciousness, and depressive symptoms. J Soc Clin Psychol. 2003;22(6):716–29.

3. IOM (Institute of Medicine). The health of lesbian, gay, bisexual, and transgender people: building a foundation for better understanding. Washington, DC: The National Academies Press; 2011.

4. Meyer IH. Prejudice, social stress, and mental health in lesbian, gay, and bisexual populations: conceptual issues and research evidence. Psychol Sex Orient Gend Divers. 2013;1(S):3–26.

5. Connelly CM. A qualitative exploration of resilience in long-term lesbian couples. Fam J. 2005;13(3):266–80.

6. Kwon P. Resilience in lesbian, gay, and bisexual individuals. Personal Soc Psychol Rev. 2013;17(4):371–83.

7. Meyer IH. Identity, stress, and resilience in lesbian, gay, and bisexual people of color. Couns Psychol. 2010;38(3):442–54.

8. Eliason MJ, Chinn PL. LGBTQ cultures: what health professionals need to know about sexual and gender diversity. 2nd ed. Philadelphia: Lippincott; 2015.

9. Eliason MJ, Dibble SD, Robertson P. Lesbian, gay, bisexual and transgender physician's experiences in the workplace. J Homosex. 2011;58(10):1355–71.

10. Eliason MJ, DeJoseph J, Dibble S, Deevey S, Chinn P. Lesbian, gay, bisexual, transgender and queer/questioning (LGBTQ) nurses' experiences in the workplace. J Prof Nurs. 2011;27(4):237–44.

11. Brogan DJ, Frank E, Elon L, Silvanesan S, O'Hanlan KA. Harassment of lesbians as medical students and physician. JAMA. 1999;282:1290–2.

12. Brogan DJ, O'Hanlan KA, Elon L, Frank E. Health and professional characteristics of lesbian and heterosexual women physicians. J Am Med Women Assoc. 2003;58:10–9.

13. Fidas D, Cooper L, Raspanti, J. The cost of the closet and the rewards of inclusion: why the workplace environment for LGBT people matters to employers. Human Rights Campaign. 2014. Retrieved 15 July 2015 from http://hrc-assets.s3-website-us-east-1.amazonaws.com//files/assets/resources/Cost_of_the_Closet_May2014.pdf.

14. Perkovich B, Veuthy T. Do ask, do tell: UCSF SOM asks applicants about sexual orientation and gender identity. Synapse UCSF student voices [internet]. 2014 [cited 2015 Nov 24]. Available from: http://synapse.ucsf.edu/articles/2014/07/31/do-ask-do-tell-ucsf-som-asks-applicants-about-sexual-orientation-and-gender.

15. Chaimowitz GA. Homophobia among psychiatric residents, family practice residents and psychiatric faculty. Canad J Psychiatry. 1991;36:206–9.

16. Mathews CW, Booth MW, Turner JD, Kessler L. Physicians' attitudes toward homosexuality: survey of a California County Medical Society. West J Med. 1986;144:106–10.

17. Smith D, Mathews WC. Physicians' attitudes toward homosexuality and HIV: survey of a California medical society-revisited (PATHH-II). J Homosex. 2007;52:1–9.

18. Ramos MM, Tellez CM, Palley TB, Umland BE, Skipper BJ. Attitudes of physicians practicing in New Mexico toward gay men and lesbians in the profession. Acad Med. 1998;73:436–8.

19. Klamen DL, Grossman LS, Kopacz DR. Medical student homophobia. J Homosex. 1999;37:53–63.

20. Kitts RL. Barriers to optimal care between physicians and lesbian, gay, bisexual, transgender and questioning adolescent patients. J Homosex. 2010;57:730–47.

21. Burke SE, Dovidio JF, Przedworski JM, Hardeman RR, Perry SP, Phelan SM, et al. Do contact and empathy mitigate bias against gay and lesbian people among heterosexual first-year medical students? A report from the Medical Student CHANGE Study. Acad Med. 2015 May;90(5):645–51.

22. Sabin JA, Riskind RG, Nosek BA. Health care providers' implicit and explicit attitudes toward lesbian women and gay men. Am J Public Health. 2015; e1–11. Retrieved from http://doi.org/10.2105/AJPH.2015.302631.

23. Phelan SM, Dovidio JF, Puhl RM, Burgess DJ, Nelson DB, et al. Implicit and explicit weight bias in a national sample of 4732 students: the medical student CHANGES study. Obesity. 2014;22(4):1201–8.

24. Schatz B, O'Hanlan K. Anti-gay discrimination in medicine: results of a national survey of lesbian, gay, and bisexual physicians. San Francisco: American Association of Physicians for Human Rights; 1994.

25. Obedin-Maliver J, Goldsmith ES, Stewart L, White W, Tran E, Brenman S, et al. Lesbian, gay, bisexual, and transgender-related content in undergraduate medical education. JAMA. 2011;306(9):971–7.

26. Sanchez NF, Rabatin J, Sanchez JP, Hubbard S, Kalet A. Medical students' ability to care for LGBT patients. Fam Med. 2006;38:21–7.

27. McGarry KA, Clark JG, Landau C, Cyr MG. Caring for vulnerable populations: curricula in U.S. internal medicine residencies. J Homosex. 2008;54(3):225–32.

28. Oancia T, Bohm C, Carr T, Cujec B, Johnson D. The influence of gender and specialty on reporting of abusive and discriminatory behavior by medical students, residents and physician teachers. Med Educ. 2000;34:250–6.

29. Dhalilwal JS, Craine LA, Valley MA, Lowestein SR. Student perspectives on the diversity climate at a U.S. medical school: the need for a broader definition of diversity. BMC Res Notes. 2013;6:154.

30. Oriel KA, Madlon-Kay DJ, Govaker D, Mersy DJ. Gay and lesbian physicians in training: family practice programs directors' attitudes and student perceptions of bias. Fam Med. 1996;28:720–5.

31. Merchant R, Jongco A, Woodward L. Disclosure of sexual orientation by medical students and residency applicants. Acad Med. 2005;80:786.

32. Risdon C, Cook D, Willms D. Gay and lesbian physicians in training: a qualitative study. CMAJ. 2000;162(3):331–4.

33. Cook DJ, Griffith LE, Cohen M, Guyatt CH, O'Brien B. Discrimination and abuse experienced by general internists in Canada. J Gen Intern Med. 1995;10:565–72.

34. Druzin P, Shrier I, Yacowar M, Rossignol M. Discrimination against gay, lesbian, and bisexual family physicians by patients. Canad Med Assoc J. 1998;158:593–7.

35. Lee RS, Melhado TV, Chacko KM, White KJ, Huebschmann AG, Crane LA. The dilemma of disclosure: patient perspectives on gay and lesbian providers. J Gen Intern Med. 2007;23:142–7.

36. Riordan D. Interaction strategies of lesbian, gay, and bisexual healthcare practitioners in the clinical examination of patients: qualitative study. BMJ. 2004;328(7450):1227–9.

37. Buchbinder SB, Wilson M, Melick CF, Powe NR. Primary care physician job satisfaction and turnover. Am J Manag Care. 2001;7:702–13.

38. Roberts SJ, DeMarco R, Griffin M. The effect of oppressed group behavior on the culture of the nursing workplace: a review of the evidence and interventions for change. J Nurs Manage. 2009;17(3):1–6.

39. Roche M, Diers D, Duffield C, Catling-Paull C. Violence toward nurses, the work environment, and patient outcomes. J Nurs Scholarsh. 2010;42:13–22.

40. Casey K, Fink R, Krugman M, Propst J. The graduate nurse experience. J Nurs Adm. 2004;34:303–11.

41. O'Brien-Pallas L, Griffin P, Shamian J, Buchan J, Duffield C, Hughes F, et al. The impact of nurse turnover on patient, nurse and system outcomes: a pilot study and focus for a multicenter international study. Pol Polit Nurs Pract. 2006;7:169–79.

42. Randall C. Lesbian phobia among BSN educators: a survey. Cassandra: Radical Nurses' J. 1989;6:23–6.

43. Dorsen C. An integrative review of nurse attitudes towards lesbian, gay, bisexual, and transgender patients. Can J Nurs Res. 2012;44(3):18–43.

44. Carabez R, Pellilgrini M, Mankovitz A, Eliason M, Ciano M, Scott M. "Never in all my years...": nurses' education about LGBT health. J Prof Nurs. 2015;31(4):323–9.

45. Lim F, Johnson M, Eliason M. A national survey of faculty knowledge, experience, and readiness for teaching lesbian, gay, bisexual and transgender (LGBT) health in baccalaureate nursing programs. Nurs Educ Perspect. 2015;36(3):144–52.

46. Sirota T. Attitudes among nurse educators toward homosexuality. J Nurs Educ. 2013;52(4):219.

47. More FG, Whitehead AW, Gonthier M. Strategies for student services for lesbian, gay, bisexual, and transgender students in dental schools. J Dent Educ. 2004;68(6):623–32.

48. Behar-Horenstein LS, Morris DR. Dental school Administrators' attitudes towards providing support services for LGBT-identified students. J Dent Educ. 2015;79(8):965–70.

49. Anderson JI, Patterson AN, Temple HJ, Inglehart MR. Lesbian, gay, bisexual, and transgender (LGBT) issues in dental school environments: dental student leaders' perceptions. J Dent Educ. 2009;73(1):105–18.

50. Seaborne LA, Prince RJ, Kushner DM. Sexual health education in U.S. physician assistant programs. J Sex Med. 2015;12(5):1158–64.

51. Eliason, MJ, Streed, C, Jr. Factors related to resilience in LGBT health care professionals. 2017.

52. Rutter M. Developing concepts in developmental psychopathology. In: Huziak JJ, editor. Developmental psychopathology and wellness: genetic and environmental influences. Washington, DC: American Psychiatric Publishing; 2008.

53. Zautra AJ, Hall JS, Murray KE. Resilience: a new definition of health for people and communities. In: Reich JW, Zautra AJ, Hall JS, editors. Handbook of adult resilience. New York: Guildord; 2010.

54. Fredrickson BL, Tugade MM, Waugh CE, Larkin GR. What good are positive emotions in crises? A prospective study of resilience and emotions following the terrorist attacks on the United States on September 11th, 2001. J Pers Soc Psychol. 2003;84:365–76.

55. Campbell-Sills L, Cohan SL, Stein MB. Relationship of resilience to personality, coping, and psychiatric symptoms in youth adults. Behav Res Ther. 2006;44:585–99.

56. Luthar SS. Resilience in development: a synthesis of research across five decades. In: Cicchetti D, Cohen DJ, editors. Developmental psychopathology: risk, disorder, and adaptation. New York: Wiley; 2006.

57. Eliason MJ, Fogel S. An ecological framework for understanding sexual minority women's health: factors related to higher body mass. J Homosex. 2015;62(7):845–82.

58. Choi KH, Yep GA, Kumekawa E. HIV prevention among Asian and Pacific islander American men who have sex with men: a critical review of theoretical models and directions for future research. AIDS Educ Prev. 1998 Jun;10(3 Suppl):19–30.

59. Wight RG, Leblanc AJ, Lee Badgett MV. Same-sex legal marriage and psychological well-being: findings from the California health interview survey. Am J Public Health. 2013 Feb;103(2):339–46.

60. Lehmiller JJ, Agnew CR. Marginalized relationships: the impact of social disapproval on romantic relationships commitment. Pers Soc Psychol Bull. 2006;32(1):40–51.

61. Herdt G, Kertzner RM. I do, but I can't: the impact of marriage denial on the mental health and sexual citizenship of lesbians and gay men in the United States. Sex Res Soc Policy. 2006;3(1):33–49.

62. Herdt G, Koff B. Something to tell you. New York: Columbia University Press; 2000.

63. Rocco TS, Landorf H, Delgado A. Framing the issue/framing the question: a proposed framework for organizational perspectives on sexual minorities. Adv Dev Hum Resour. 2009;11:7–23.

64. Mohr JJ, Fassinger RE. Work, career, and sexual orientation. In: Patterson CJ, D'Augelli AR, editors. Handbook of psychology and sexual orientation. New York: Oxford University Press; 2013.

65. Zwack J, Schweitzer J. If every fifth physician is affected by burnout, what about the other four? Resilience strategies of experienced physicians. Acad Med. 2013;88:382–9.

66. Snowdon S. Equal and respectful care for LGBT patients. The importance of providing an inclusive environment cannot be underestimated. Healthc Exec. 2013;28(6):52, 54–55.

67. Herman JL. Costs and benefits of providing transition-related health care coverage in employee health benefits plans: findings from a survey of employers. Williams Institute: Los Angeles; 2013.

68. Hafferty FW, Franks R. The hidden curriculum, ethics teaching, and the structure of medical education. Acad Med. 1994;69(11):861–71.

69. Hafferty FW. Beyond curriculum reform: confronting medicine's hidden curriculum. Acad Med. 1998;73:403–7.

70. Young S. What it means when 'the doctor is out.' Harvard Gazette [Internet]. 2015 [cited 2015 Nov 24]. Available from: http://news.harvard.edu/gazette/story/2015/10/what-it-means-when-the-doctor-is-out/.

71. Fallin-Bennett K. Implicit bias against sexual minorities in medicine: cycles of professional influence and the role of the hidden curriculum. Acad Med. 2015;90(5):549–52.

72. Hollenback AD, Eckstrand KL, Dreger A, editors. Implementing curricular and institutional climate changes to improve health care for individuals who are LGBT, gender nonconforming, or born with DSD. 1st ed. Washington, DC: Association of American Medical Colleges; 2014.

73. The Joint Commission. Advancing effective communication, cultural competences, and patient- and family-centered care for the lesbian, gay, bisexual, and transgender (LGBT) community. a field guide. Oak Brook: The Joint Commission; 2011.

74. Snowdon S. Recommendations for enhancing the climate for LGBT students and employees in health professional schools: a GLMA white paper. Washington, DC: GLMA; 2013.

75. Mereish EH, Poteat VP. The conditions under which growth-fostering relationships promote resilience and alleviate psychological distress among sexual minorities: applications of relational cultural theory. Psychol Sex Orientat Gend Divers. 2015;2(3):339–44.

76. Streed C. Attendees find support at the gay and lesbian medical association conference. Medscape Med Students. WebMD [internet]. 2010 [cited 2015 Nov 24]. Available from: http://www.medscape.com/viewarticle/731815.

77. Hodges HF, Keeley AC, Troyan PJ. Professional resilience in baccalaureate-prepared acute care nurses: first steps. Nurs Educ Perspect. 2008;29:80–9.

78. Glass N. An investigation of nurses' and midwives' academic/clinical workplaces. Holist Nurs Pract. 2009;23:158–70.

79. Kornhaber RA, Wilson A. Building resilience in burns nurses: a descriptive phenomenological inquiry. J Burn Care Res. 2011;32:481–8.

80. Simoni PS, Larrabee JH, Birkhimer TL, Mott CL, Gladden SD. Influence of interpretive styles of stress resiliency on registered nurse empowerment. Nurs Adm Q. 2004;28:221–4.

81. Ablett JR, Jones RSP. Resilience and well-being in palliative care staff: a qualitative study of hospice nurses' experience of work. Psycho-Oncology. 2007;16:733–40.

82. Gillespie BM, Chaboyer W, Wallis M, Grimbeck P. Resilience in the operating room: developing and testing of a resilience model. J Adv Nurs. 2007;59:427–38.

Index

© Springer International Publishing AG 2017
K.L. Eckstrand, J. Potter (eds.), *Trauma, Resilience, and Health Promotion in LGBT Patients*,
DOI 10.1007/978-3-319-54509-7

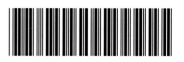